ADJUSTMENT OF SCHIZOPHRENICS IN THE COMMUNITY

ADJUSTMENT OF SCHIZOPHRENICS IN THE COMMUNITY

By **George Serban, M.D.**
Clinical Associate Professor of Psychiatry,
New York University Medical School
Principal Investigator,
New York University–Bellevue Medical Center

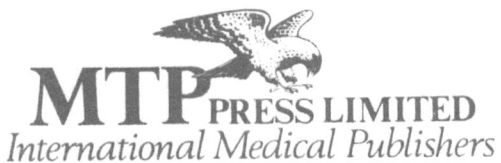

MTP **PRESS LIMITED**
International Medical Publishers

Published in the UK and Europe by
MTP Press Limited
Falcon House
Lancaster, England

Published in the US by
SPECTRUM PUBLICATIONS, INC.
175-20 Wexford Terrace
Jamaica, N.Y. 11432

ISBN-13: 978-94-011-5923-4   e-ISBN-13: 978-94-011-5921-0
DOI: 10.1007/978-94-011-5921-0

Contents

INTRODUCTION

The mental health movement of early release into the community of the chronic schizophrenic has been based on a set of old theoretical assumptions and expectations which, when tested on the community level, failed to meet the desired results. On the contrary, the first visible outcome of deinstitutionalization was the revolving door policy with the patients repeatedly in and out of the hospital, changing their previous status of inpatient to the new one of pseudoambulatory. Yet, this would not be a serious problem if the life of the patient in the community, in between rehospitalizations, was beneficial to him and to the community. However, the quality of life experienced by the patients in the community appears to be deplorable. Available statistics indicate that over 70% of chronic schizophrenics discharged into the community live a marginal, unproductive, aimless life in dilapidated hotels or private proprietary homes. Certainly, though there are various scattered community programs for the rehabilitation of the schizophrenic, the results are far from encouraging.

With these basic facts in mind, we have to ask ourselves: What went wrong with deinstitutionalization? Apparently in the process of hasty deinstitutionalization, too many issues were overlooked by the community mental health planners. The most critical factor neglected by the policy makers was the establishment of more realistic criteria for the patient who can or cannot function in the community. The indiscriminate selection of patients for discharge from hospitals was compounded by the lack of interest of community mental health centers in treating hard-core chronic schizophrenics. In fact, there were not any new modalities for the treatment of chronic schizophrenics which would have supported their community tenure or justified the rapid rate of discharge except for political or economical reasons. In addition to the indiscriminate discharge of patients into the community, another variable which has contributed to the high rate of return to the hospital is that of inadequate availability and coordination of existing services for offering the patient the variety of forms of support needed for his life in the community.

Naturally, in the community, the patient requires having at his disposal a well organized supportive system of services to assist him in solving his social needs. Yet, the expected loving care from the multidisciplinary team for the discharged mentally ill patient, promised by the community system, did not materialize. Even worse, when it was present, it was unprepared to rehabilitate the patient socially due to lack of adequate staffing or appropriate programs. At the root of all these difficulties is the philosophy of deinstitutionalization, evolved from incomplete research findings, which confused the medical issues with the social ones.

Full attention has not been paid to the fact that the post-hospital adjustment depends on many factors, such as regular attendance at an aftercare clinic, taking of medication, placement in a rehabilitative program, structured organization of daily activities, adequate family, relatives, or friends' support. Cursory evaluation was given to all of these elements of social interaction which require synchronization in order to enhance the schizophrenic's chance of integrating himself into the main stream of community life. At the same time, left out was the monitoring of the amount of stress experienced by the chronic schizophrenic in his daily activities. The patient's inability to sustain stress due to his psychological deficit appears to be the main cause contributing to his rehospitalization. His residual psychological deficit, persistent after his discharge, makes him appraise poorly the events of his daily life, thereby producing stress, which further impairs his ability to function adequately.

Though the difficulties in functioning of the chronic schizophrenic in the community are well known, no meaningful clinical method was developed for studying comprehensively the multivariate factors responsible for them. Until now, the low functioning was attributed, for justifiable reasons, mainly to the mental impairment of the discharged patient; the effect of stress as related to functioning and his mental status has been overlooked. It is wishful thinking to expect that a patient discharged into the community will manage, without any careful control of his tolerance to stress, in his interaction with family, relatives, and friends who represent the first line of his support in the community. In the same vein, it is important to know the expectations of the patient returning to his family and community, and their attitude toward and expectations of him. The more unrealistic the expectations on either side, the more difficult will be his integration into the community.

All these issues lead us to another major one, that of the quality of services and treatment available to the schizophrenic in the community. The literature which covers this area is highly controversial. This is primarily due to the lack of consensus as to what represents an effective and appropriate treatment for chronic schizophrenics in the community. There is almost general agreement that the range of existent modalities of treatment are inadequate due to incomplete data based on research in this area. In addition, even the existent forms of treatment are handicapped by the issue of voluntary approach to the "right to treatment" as decided by the courts and supported by legal activism. As a result, many discharged patients have refused any follow-up treatment.

All in all, it could be safely said that the enthusiasm for deinstitutionalization should have been supported by more conclusive research regarding what could or could not be done for chronic schizophrenics in the community.

Basically, the main question to be asked is whether the facilities offered by the community could service the same patient population as the mental hospital does. Those who feel that state hospitals should be phased out should remember that approximately one-third of chronic schizophrenics follow a deteriorating course and cannot stay in the community. Then it is only normal to attempt to determine, if possible, what type of schizophrenics have a poor prognosis as compared with ones who do not. More specifically, in what ways are they different from the other schizophrenics who recover? Are the ones who recover diagnosed incorrectly as schizophrenics? Is there any difference between these two groups in their response to medication and treatment? In other words, what could be the biological and psychosocial bases for the individual variations in the outcome of schizophrenia? To what extent do the criteria used for the division between reactive and process hold true with the advent of medication?

All these questions and others require more knowledge supported by scientific data than rhetoric or enthusiasm from the mental health activists—they require multidisciplinary research for the evaluation of the social and psychogenetic factors contributing to the schizophrenics' functioning and maintenance in the community. This has to start with a better definition of schizophrenia so as to differentiate clearly its outcome from other forms of psychosis. The importance of this knowledge for the outcome of schizophrenia cannot be minimized, particularly since the therapeutic approaches differ among various types of psychosis. In order to reach more effective solutions in organizing the community care network, all these issues require careful reevaluation by naturalistic and intervention studies.

An attempt to study all these interrelated dimensions of schizophrenia as affecting the patients' community integration was made at New York University-Bellevue Medical Center in a four year program from 1971 to 1975. Bellevue Psychiatric Division offered an ideal situation for the study, not only because at that time it received admissions from almost all New York City boroughs, but it also had the highest rate of admission of schizophrenics in the city (5,187), representing 16% of the schizophrenics admitted in all New York state hospitals at that time. Its association with three divisions of Manhattan State Hospital assured, in addition, the follow up of the patients transferred from Bellevue to those divisions. The decision made at that time to study intensively every fifth schizophrenic admission for a period of nine months and to follow them for a period of two years appeared to be a gargantuan task. Studying 900 admitted schizophrenics, each one with a battery of tests, is not an easy task, particularly when you depend on the good will of the patient and the fluctuation of his cooperative mood. In addition, the need for accurate social and personal data required a double verification of all the information provided by the patient, which made the assignment undertaken even more difficult. The schizophrenics were compared to 100 normals of similar social-demographic background.

As if this was not enough, the problem of assembling a highly qualified staff for meeting the specifications of this challenging project was an extremely difficult one. The difficulty was a double one; that of finding a dedicated, conscientious, professional team, one that was able to take the pressure of working with a group of patients who were not available when wanted because they were not supposed to be disturbed from their routine activities. Furthermore, they could have been transferred or discharged at a day's or sometimes at an hour's notice—which made it even harder for the staff in collecting the data. Under all these pressures, some of the members of the staff, unwilling to cope or function properly, required replacement in order to maintain the expected high quality standards for collection of scientific data. After overcoming all these obstacles, after elimination of patients who, due to their immediate transfer or release could not complete all the testing, the project was able to study fully 641 schizophrenics with five psychosocial and psychological instruments and to follow 419 schizophrenics for two years. At the same time, 228 informants of the patients were tested with psychosocial tests. Due to the lack of appropriate testing instruments for the aims of the study, two important research tests, one on the psychosocial measurement of functioning and stress and another on the measurement of motivation were developed and validated.

At this point, grateful acknowledgement should be given to the team of consultants: Ed Melnick, Ph.D., Associate Professor of Statistics, N.Y.U.; G. Raabe, Senior Research Scientist (Biometrics), Department of Epidemiology, Columbia University; P. Abrams, Research Dir., Calculogic Corporation, for their contribution to the statistical aspects of the Project, and to the team of research and clinical psychologists who participated actively in the preparation and write up of various articles resulting from the study. Among them, special mention is given to: C. Gidynski, Ph.D., Associate Research Project, N.Y.U.; G. Katz, Ph.D., Assistant Research Project, N.Y.U.; and G. Voloshin, Ph.D., Assistant Research Project, N.Y.U. Other researchers participated in the collection of data or in various phases of the computer processing and analysis. Mrs. A. Zimmermann was Administrative Coordinator of the Project. The project was supported in part by the Kittay Foundation. In addition, acknowledgement is given to C. Gidynski, Ph.D., who acted as manuscript consultant for this book.

The results of the Project permitted a comprehensive reevaluation of a series of issues related to prediction of outcome of schizophrenia—from those of social competence to that of family interaction, from that of psychosocial stress to that of motivational level. If this new information is integrated judiciously in the planning of discharge of the patient into the community and in his aftercare supportive program, we might be able to improve the quality of the treatment and the condition of life for the schizophrenic in the community.

CHAPTER 1

A Critical Appraisal of the Current State of Knowledge in Schizophrenia

Since a relationship between the cause and the outcome of schizophrenia has been always assumed, a summary review of the major theories of etiology of schizophrenia appears to be warranted as a starting point for our extensive study of factors involved in the prediction of this illness.

The elusiveness in identifying the etiology of schizophrenia for years resulted in a broad interpretation of its cause, with explanations ranging from psychosocial cultural factors to purely genetic ones. Regardless of a particular emphasis, the etiological hypothesis could be divided into three major conceptual formulations—two representing opposing points of view, the psychosocial one versus the organic one, while in the middle is the psycho-organic one, reflecting a more conciliatory position. Interestingly enough, each one of these approaches presents supporting arguments, based on empirical data which could justify, at least up to a point, their concept of schizophrenia. Yet, neither one is able to clarify the whole gamut of schizophrenic reactions. This will explain why, in the framework of psychosocial hypotheses (psychological, cultural, or psychodynamic concepts) several distinctive theories are vying for acceptance as major explanations for the development of the disease.

In this context, from an offshoot of the Sullivanian psychodynamic hypothesis of dysfunction in interpersonal relationships *(56)*, emerged the disturbed family interaction theory of Frieda Fromm-Reichman *(17)*, Wynne *(64,a)*, and Lidz *(37,a,b)*. The basic premise of this theory was that the child suffers from the negative influence of the so-called schizophrenogenic mother. According to this approach, the schizophrenogenic mother is highly neurotic, functions marginally in the family interaction, and acts negatively and destructively towards her child. Rosen *(47)* went even further to describe this mother as having a perverse sense of motherhood, that is, an individual who is unable to relate and to fulfill the role of mother. Yet, other authors within the same orientation disagree. Wynne and Lidz extended the interaction to the whole family relationship, which, as such, produces schizophrenia in the offspring. According to Arieti's *(3)* clinical observations, only 25% of mothers are indeed schizophrenogenic, that is unable to sustain normal interaction with their children because of their neuroses. But what about the other mothers who still have schizophrenic offspring?

They are relatively normal, but their image has been distorted by the fantasy of the schizophrenic who, in the process of years of poor interaction, changed the view of her, due to his illness. According to Arieti, this is mainly due to the schizophrenic process of thinking which made him respond differently to reality, which is possibly based on a genetic vulnerability. It is important to note that the distortions in the thinking of schizophrenics, particularly the misinterpretations of reality, are considered, by other proponents of the psychological school as well, as not stemming from a faulty interaction with their parents but, rather, from their constitutional predispositions.

In general, the proponents of the psychological school maintain the position that the distortion of perception, special sensitivity to anxiety, and fragmentation of reality bring about the schizophrenic response in an individual who, due to environmental circumstances, developed defective patterns of responding to reality. In this case, the genetic vulnerability is neither a necessary nor sufficient condition for the presence of schizophrenic syndromes. The etiology of thought disorders in schizophrenia was interpreted by the psychological school as stemming from either a reinforcement of a maladaptive learning process, due to negative intrafamilial stimuli (3) or to the formation of a deviant cognitive system resulting from conflicting intrapsychic interaction as formulated by psychoanalytic theories.

Another offshoot of the psychological environmental hypotheses is that schizophrenia is a disease of social adaptation. This concept is highly regarded by the sociological school, which emphasizes the social stresses as having a causal significance for schizophrenia. Yet, the cultural factor, as documented by social responses, is equivocal in its interpretation. It was felt that sociocultural factors are operating in two directions. The first one refers to predisposition to schizophrenia in some population groups more than in others. An example of this influence of the environmental factor is offered by the differences between the Irish and English populations, which have different rates of the illness (0.47% as compared to 0.33% in England) (42). The second cultural factor considered responsible for predisposition to schizophrenia is associated with social class (24). In contradistinction to the observation of the different prevalence of schizophrenia in various population groups, for which no comprehensive explanation exists except for sociological observations of possible stressful conditions related to conflicting sets of social values, sociologists were able to come up with a better formulation for the role of social class in the etiology of schizophrenia. From the observations of a higher rate of schizophrenia in the low social class group, some sociologists and researchers evolved the famous "drift" hypothesis (16, 14). Though social class has been implicated in the origin of schizophrenia, research findings in this area have been inconsistent. For instance, the findings of Goldberg and Morrison, in England, and those of Turner and Wagonfeld, referring to Monroe County, are at best contradictory *(20, 58)*. They indicate that there is evidence for another conceptualization of the drift theory: that of low social class being conducive to schizophrenia and that of schizophrenia drifting to the lower class.

Neither one of these positions is self-sustaining because, as concluded by other social studies, the latent development of schizophrenia interferes in some would-be schizophrenics with their ability to attain their potential occupational level before hospitalization. Thus, they become frozen into a lower occupational category, regardless of their original social class. In addition, it should be mentioned that since the lower class schizophrenics are more likely to be hospitalized in public facilities, as compared with those of higher occupational levels who might never end up in a hospital, or are treated under different diagnoses in private institutions, the impression is created that there are higher concentrations of schizophrenics in the lower class. The controversial issue of schizophrenia and social class is extensively discussed later in this book, in relationship to predictive value of sociodemographic variables.

Psychosocial theories based either on the psychodynamic models, intrafamilial relationships, or cultural hypothesis of social class failed to bring conclusive evidence to support any particular formulation for the causes of schizophrenia.

Basically all various hypotheses advanced by the Psychosocial School assume a maladaptive learning process, which viewed from another point of view presuppose a disturbance of neuropsychological adaptive mechanisms.

From all variations of the learning theory hypothesis, one of the most quoted in literature appears to be that of Mednick *(39)* who attempts to relate schizophrenia to a state of heightened drive. According to this approach, the personality of a preschizophrenic is characterized by a high drive level, a slow rate of recovery from anxiety, and a broad reactivity to anxiety situations. If such an individual is exposed to many anxiety arousing situations he is unable to control them because of reciprocal augmentation of anxiety due to the generalization of stimuli. Without any intention to discuss this theory in detail, it can be said that this hypothesis does not account for the reason why reciprocal augmentation leads to schizophrenia in some individuals and not in others. The premorbid personality, based on the three variables mentioned by Mednick does not justify in itself the precipitation of an acute schizophrenic attack when the individual is faced with antagonistic situations which are anxiety producing. His hypothesis is developed by Broen and Storms *(8)* who attempt to explain the disorganization of personality based on the limitation of the individual to respond to anxiety-provoking stimuli. As the anxiety mounts, the individual is assumed to reach his maximum response strength, at which point responses to different stimuli become the same, thereby disorganizing behavior. Obviously, Broen's analysis of disorganization is more complicated, presupposing such psychoschizogenic determinant factors of response as: (a) basic strength of dominant habits; (b) level of arousal, and (c) upper level of response strengths to various stimuli. Based on these neuropsychological determinants Broen and Storms attempt to explain various forms of schizophrenic psychopathology which are understood mainly as response disorganization. Without appraising the validity of the system of ceiling response, it can be said that this concept cannot be adequately supported by laboratory data. For instance, the hypothesis of response strength cannot explain obsessions, compulsions, or fixed delusions. In this respect, a more integrated theory is that of input dysfunction, as conceptualized by Venables (60), which tries to explain the cognitive disorganization of schizophrenia. Other learning theories, like that of the Russian school led by Pavlov (43), attempt to conceptualize schizophrenia in pure neuropsychological constructs defined in terms of excitation and inhibition, which within this theoretical framework determine all of human behavior. From the viewpoint of the learning orientation, Pavlovian theory of low threshold of transmarginal inhibition appears to offer the most integrated approach to the formulation of schizophrenia. All psychopathological process can be explained by them, due either to cortical inhibition or disinhibition of subcortical centers. In this view, schizophrenia is considered to be a disease of adaptation resulting from an over-stimulation of individual capacities for adaptation, particularly in persons with weak nervous systems who have a low threshold to transmarginal inhibition. Basically, all variants of learning theories are making two assumptions; one assumes an overload to the nervous system and the second one, spelled out better by the Russian school, contends an inborn proneness of the nervous system for inhibiting reactions under excessive stimulation.

The psychosocial theories or their neuropsychological correlates are unable to escape the basic assumption of either faulty neurometabolism or a constitutional vulnerability which ironically plays into the hands of supporters of the organic-genetic theory.

As it was previously mentioned, genetic and biochemical theories, at one end of the spectrum of theories, search out and attempt to explain the etiology of schizophrenia on a purely organic basis. The strength of the genetic factor appears to rely on the study of the concordance rates of identical twins who have an indisputably higher rate of schizophrenia than that found among nonidentical twins reared together (21, 52). The geneticists call attention, in support of genetic influence in the development of schizophrenia, to the rate of risk of schizophrenia in siblings of nonschizophrenics (9%) as compared with the incidence of schizophrenia when one parent (12%) or both parents (35%) are schizophrenic. In addition, the few cases of dual mating reported by Book and Hallgren indicated that the rate of schizophrenic offspring is about 45% (7, 23). Without dwelling on the value of the genetic position, it should be mentioned that the controversy between it and the environmental position is still unresolved.

One study which has attempted to resolve the problem is that of adoptive families of adopted schizophrenics (48). In this study the hereditary and environmental factors are separated to the extent to which the biological parents do not rear the infant who later becomes schizophrenic. The study had a few, almost unavoidable errors such as interviewer bias, lack of parental accuracy of self-reporting of their experiences, and finally, the evaluation of the difficulty of interaction between the child and parent brought about by the illness of the child, or by the preexisting problems of adoptive parents. The results of this study strongly support the notion of the genetic etiology of schizophrenia, indicating that the development of schizophrenia occurred independent of the psychopathology of the adoptive parents. Supporting data came from the study by Alanen comparing the psychopathology of adoptive parents *(48)* with that of biological parents (schizophrenic or neurotic), whose children showed schizophrenic or neurotic symtomatology depending on the respective category represented by the parents *(1)*.

Yet to the extent that genetic inheritance appears to account for only approximately 12% of the schizophrenic population—it does not explain the causes in the remainder of the schizophrenic population which has no clear-cut genetic heritage. This presupposes the operation of a contributing environmental factor responsible in the development of the disease, perhaps grafted onto a constitutional base.

It appears clear that neither the genetic hypothesis of schizophrenia, regardless of its powerful supporting documentation, nor the cultural-psychological formulations, were able to give a full account of the development of schizophrenia.

Other researchers have seen an interrelation between the environmental and genetic factors in schizophrenia. They believe it impossible to separate the genetic from the environmental factors because of the inextricable interaction between them. In the past the experimental argument has been formulated as follows: If the genetic constitution is similar (as in monozygotous twins) and the familial environment is similar, then the cause for the development of schizophrenia has to be of genetic origin. The weakness of this argument is self-evident. To start with, it is presumptuous to assume that the environment is always similar (even for monozygotous twins). The unacceptability of this argument is based on the logical deduction that the genetic factor, whether identical or not, may be associated with different environmental conditions, due to a variety of responses within the human environment and influenced by unknown variables which might lead to the development of schizophrenia. The difficulty of investigating the etiology of schizophrenia is always compounded by complications introduced by other psychological factors that intervene between the genetic and so-called controlled environmental variables such as birth order, maternal care, parental loss, ethnic and socioeconomic group membership, sex, or ''soft'' neurological signs in schizophrenia.

Documented by existing data, the psychobiogenetic approach assumes that it is more likely that the genetic factor is the predisposing one; a base on which types of environmental experience leave their imprint and lead to a spectrum of psychopathological reactions ranging from psychopathy to chronic schizophrenia.

Basically, to be able to explain the variety of factors responsible for or implied in the causation of schizophrenia, a multifactorial etiological concept has to be used'as a working hypothesis. This multifactorial position appears to be amply supported by the experimental work of Heston (25) in Oregon and Mednick (40) in Denmark. The elegant longitudinal studies of Mednick, Schlusinger (40) and their group attest to the multifactorial hypothesis; yet even the multifactorial approach appears incapable of identifying clearly the factors responsible for this illness. The mere collection of data and its classification into similar clusters of variables might produce findings of statistical significance but without any certain evidence of their validity in reproducing the disease under similar circumstances.

In general, the main failure of the commonly accepted etiological theories is that they succeed in explaining only some aspects from the totality of various conditions which predispose an individual to schizophrenia. Taking into account the genetic—environmental interaction, what appears to elude investigators are the conditions under which environmental factors produce the disease (in a preexisting disposition) and/or the effect of the genetic factor which progressively deteriorates one's psychosocial functioning, independent of the environmental conditions.

In an attempt to deal directly with this problem, a new psychophysiological concept—the individual biological capacity to respond to adverse life events, defined as "life stressors," was introduced into the study of schizophrenia.

The basic assumption was that the interaction between life stressors and the individual biological responses might lead to what is called biochemical abnormalities. Various biochemical mediators and neurotransmiters, such as catecholamine, indolamine precursors, and others, were believed responsible for producing the whole symptomatology of schizophrenia. The bioamine hypotheses were supported by the model psychosis created by some of the substances from the amphetamine group. Without discussing its merit, it appears that the dopamine hypothesis has gained the maximum support from all of these theories (30). The various brain metabolites considered responsible for hallucinogenic effects are linked to the catecholamine group. It is interesting to note that the catecholamine group together with the cortisol one were found to be responsible for producing stress in organisms as well. A circumstantial link between stress and schizophrenia was made when increasing amounts of epinephrine, hydrocortisole, and various products of degradation of dopamine were found in both conditions. This led to the biological explanation for the development of schizophrenia under conditions of psychosocial stress.

From all the theories attempting to explain schizophrenia, that of biogenic-amine combined with the social stress appears to be the most promising one for the understanding of the gamut of social conditions contributing to either the development of the disease or to the adjustment of schizophrenics in the community. In our attempt to predict the factors responsible for the community tenure of schizophrenia, we found this conceptualization the most valuable as a working hypothesis.

As if the problem of establishing more objective criteria for determining the factors contributing to the development of schizophrenia is not difficult enough, the investigators attempting to find new ways for understanding and controlling the illness face problems which appear to cloud their efforts even more: that is, the reliability of diagnosis. As long as psychiatrists are defining schizophrenia in different ways, then obviously it is very hard to arrive at any agreement as to what particular mental disturbance we are treating. American psychiatrists, until recently, disregarded the diagnostic categories believing that the treatment of the patient's symptoms was a more important issue. This led to a lack of general consensus regarding the criteria for the support of diagnosis which in turn affected the evaluation of the treatment outcome. For instance, the differences in diagnoses of schizophrenia in the U.S. and England illuminate so clearly this problem.

According to the study of Garland et al. (22), the ratio of schizophrenia to affective disorders as diagnosed by psychiatrists in U.S. hospitals was approximately nine to one (119 cases of schizophrenia to 13 affective disorders), while in London, the sample was approximately equal (59 cases of schizophrenia to 68 affective disorders). The study clearly indicated that New York psychiatrists have a tendency to give the diagnosis of schizophrenia to a greater proportion of patients with disturbance of thought and affect than do their London colleagues. This position helps to explain the high number of schizophrenics with good prognosis included in studies of schizophrenia who, in reality might be suffering from affective disorders.

This controversy brought into focus again the difficulty in classifying and defining schizophrenia as a syndrome. It is an old problem in psychiatry, going back to Kraepelin and Bleuler. When the concept of dementia-precox was redefined in terms of schizophrenias, which greatly broadened its scope, the problem of diagnosis was compounded by a lack of agreement in clarifying, operationally, the symptoms which distinguish this particular condition from other closely related ones. Aware of this situation, Langfeldt (35) and Schneider (56A) attempted to establish more exact criteria for clinically defining the disease; yet, their contribution went unnoticed in the U.S. until recently, though for research purposes this issue could not be minimized any longer.

For this reason investigators proceeded to solve the problem of classification of schizophrenia by developing standardized mental state inventories. These inventories were designed to capture symptomatology mainly in terms of thought disorder, delusions, disturbance of affect, and sometimes degree of social impairment. From the model of symptom categories proposed by Langfeldt (35), and particularly Schneider (56A), Kleist (32), and Leonhard (36), various mental status examinations have sprung up both here and abroad, such as that of Astrachan (1972) (4) of Yale or Spitzer and Endicott (1969) (54) of Columbia. Yet, none of these tests were evaluated on an international level. It became the task of an international pilot study of WHO to attempt to develop a system of classification of schizophrenia, based on an internationally tested structured mental status inventory. The research instrument developed by Wing, Cooper, and Sartorious (61), called "Present State Examination," with all its modifications, became, in its revised form, the only standardized test for psychiatric evaluation. One of the main difficulties of the inventory appears to be a short period of time covering the symptomatology and the length of the inventory. Its other limitation is that in its present form the test appears to be mainly a research instrument.

If the problems of etiology and diagnosis present serious obstacles to the understanding and classification of schizophrenia, in addition, they further compound the problem of predicting its course.

The predictions of outcome of schizophrenia have raised still another set of serious controversies. Obviously, the first difficulty with determining the course of the disease was created by the approach to the classification of schizophrenic illness. For instance, Langfeldt's (35) diagnostic system, which attempted to discriminate between "good" and "poor" outcome patients is questionable, since schizophreniform psychosis should not be considered with true schizophrenia, as we shall attempt to demonstrate in the course of the book.

According to Carpenter and Strauss (11), in a 2-year follow-up of symptoms, dividing the patients according to the Langfeldt criteria, significant differences between the groups were not found.

Apparently, the same fate is suffered by another classification of schizophrenia, that of the reactive-process, which has attempted to predict the course of the disease based on a combination of variables derived from Philipps' (44) or Elgin's (62) scales. The reactive-process division is practically based on the assessment of the critical level of functioning of the individual within the context of some psychosocial criteria identified by Langfeldt and modified by Vaillant (32). The validity of this approach appears to be highly questionable to start with, in view of its dependability on the age of onset of illness. Without discussing the merit of this approach, it appears that all the research generated by this classification has been basically fruitless for the advancement of new knowledge regarding the prediction of the course of schizophrenia despite the claims made by Higgins (26). For each set of findings supporting a set of claims for the "reactive-process distinction," there is another set of claims questioning or refuting it. This applies, for instance, to experiments linking arousal and responsiveness to the differentiation of reactive and process schizophrenics where the data on skin potentials of Crider, Greenspoon, and Maher (13) are contradicted by the work of Irwin and Renner (28), as well as others (31). This contradiction in findings is maintained with respect to general intellectual deficit or performance on the vocabulary subtests reported by Cancro *(10)* and Schwartz *(50)*. A study referring to the reinforcement effects found that "process" and "reactive" schizophrenics do not act differently to object-award reinforcers *(38)*.

If there is no question that process schizophrenics could be included in the classification of the chronic and the reactive ones in the acute category, where then should we place the acute episodic schizophrenics or the schizo-affectives who can move in either direction? The process-reactive approach is unable to clearly place these groups in terms of long term prediction and, thus, does not enhance our knowledge about either diagnosis or prediction.

In view of these contradictory or inconclusive data, the whole approach to the diagnosis of schizophrenia requires redefinition in more objective and precise terms in order to avoid the confrontation of extremist views supporting either the concept of it as a totally quantifiable disease in development and course or its existence as an identifiable clinical entity. The complication of the diagnosis of schizophrenia started when we attempted to integrate some forms of schizophrenic experiences within the realm of normal–borderline behavior in which mild delusions became considered overvalued ideas, while transient hallucinations were equated with sense memories *(29)*.

As a result of all this confusion in relation to etiology and diagnosis of schizophrenia, some radical psychiatrists [Szasz *(57)*, Goffman *(19)*, Laing *(33)*, Siirala *(51)*] disregarded whatever knowledge was accumulated about this illness and reached the conclusion that schizophrenia was not an illness at all. For example, one of the most popular of these theories is that of R.D. Laing who believes that schizophrenia is a form of alienation which occurs in human beings and is due to our intolerance of different fundamental structures of experience other than our own *(25)*. In this context, if the family is the one which "drives the child crazy," then the etiology of schizophrenia should be found in the social system itself, while the behavior of schizophrenics is explained as a special adaptive strategy invented by the person in order to cope with unliveable situations.

In this model of schizophrenia, the alleged patient is presented as a rebel who cannot accept social conformity with its sets of values and its oppressions and who is subsequently "jailed" in a mental institution and deprived of his legal rights and responsibilities. In this sense, the diagnosis is meaningless.

An even more momentous view of schizophrenia is presented by Siirala *(51)*, who envisioned the schizophrenic as a visionary, a prophet to whom nobody wants to listen. The message of schizophrenia is one of denouncing social injustice with its social and human crimes committed for centuries, which we try to forget and deny. In this context, the symptoms of schizophrenia are interpreted as a form of vision and rationality instead of a structured or unstructured delusionary system or faulty perception of reality. Whereas the true prophet attempts to denounce social insensitivity, intolerance, and corruption by preaching the coming of a new world, the schizophrenic, unable to adapt to his trivial life, becomes progressively more disorganized, incoherent, and irrational—his message, at best, is one of panic and despair at his inability to handle his own life.

Yet, with all these diversified views on the meaning of the concept of schizophrenia and its place in the continuum of human behavior, from normalcy to mental disease, schizophrenia still remains a clinical reality definable in terms of symptomatology, regardless of the degree of social acceptance of deviant behavior. A new, fresh look is required to reevaluate and redefine the vast amount of empirical data accumulated up to now in the classification of schizophrenia, the etiological significance of various contributory factors in the development of schizophrenia, and their predictive value for the courses of the disease if any conclusions are to be reached about its treatment.

In order to accomplish this, an innovative approach with a different methodology was required for testing the validity of these predictive assumptions about the adjustment of schizophrenics. In past research, investigators focused on observations about the patient and, using the collection of empirical data about him, claimed that this approach represented an objective and valid study of the patient. Yet, the patient's personal view of the factors leading to his acute psychotic episode were less understood. For instance, his style of life with its concomitant anxieties and stresses was reduced by researchers to precipitating events leading to hospitalization, as if only a particular life situation could induce serious emotional reactions to the point of mental disorganization in someone who previously had functioned more or less normally. Furthermore, assuming that this was correct, the question of why these life events played such a significant role in the life of some people and not in others was not answered. The experience of the patient, and the particular connotation it had for him, was somehow left out.

To rectify some of the errors of the past, one should attempt to take into account, to tap, and to measure the experiences of the patient within the context of his life patterns, to determine whether or not his experiences have any significance in the development of his illness. Such an approach is offered by the methodological concept of phenomenology. The phenomenological method, first introduced by Jaspers in the clinical study of schizophrenia, focuses only on the experiences of the subject and as such offers a unique possibility of quantifying the patient's inner and outer experience in relating to others and to himself, free of any scientific bias of the observer (27, 29).

For many years the main issue raised by many clinicians and investigators was that the observations made concerning the behavior of the patient were contaminated by the judgmental values of the investigator and particularly by his own views of what constitutes deviant behavior—the extent to which this type of behavior might violate the social norms and rules. Even the definition of symptomatology suffered from the same difficulty because of the vagueness with which the condition of the patient is described, particularly when he is not acutely hallucinatory or delusional. To trace such an inappropriateness of affect could be highly interpretative and would depend upon the ability of the investigator to tap the dysfunction between expressed ideas and their affective component. The same applies to behavior that, by standards of some subcultures, could be considered to be acceptable or not acceptable.

Against this background, the phenomenological approach offers a possibility of studying the adjustment of the patient to his environment within the framework of the patient's personal mode of viewing and reacting to situations. In order to capture the patient's evaluation of his level of functioning and stress in his daily living in the community, it was necessary that a new inventory be developed which could measure, test, and tease out these psychosocial variables. It is extremely interesting that, although there is a large body of literature describing the importance of psychological and environmental factors involved in the development of schizophrenia and emphasizing stress as a main causative agent—no quantitative or qualitative measurement of the stress itself has been conceptualized.

Stress has been primarily reduced to its clinical aspects of anxiety, or has been restricted to precipitating factors, as previously mentioned. It seems unrealistic to talk about the role of stress in schizophrenia and to reduce it to anxiety in a disease where anxiety cannot always be equated with stress. For instance, some schizophrenics, although experiencing intense anxiety due to their mental illnesses, do not have any stressful situations to cope with [Pichot (45)]. In schizophrenia, stress was measured only indirectly through biological tests related to the level of catecholamine and hydrocortisone output. Yet, the measure of functioning and the amount of clinical stress experienced by the individual before hospitalization will indicate the previous level of his adjustment to the community. Any disturbance in the fragile balance of ability to function due to internal or external stress could trigger an acute psychotic episode leading to rehospitalization. Only in this context are we able to discover the psychosocial predictors responsible for the patient's readmission.

Finally, but no less important in studying the predictive factors in schizophrenia, one has to take into consideration the fact that the classical features of chronic institutionalized schizophrenia (process) tend to disappear under the new prevailing policy of early discharge related to psychopharmacological treatment in the community. Therefore, the past division of schizophrenia into "reactive" and "process," as we have already discussed, does not present any predictive value. Under these circumstances it appears that only the traditional classification of patients into "acutes" and "chronics" is meaningful in comparing the causes of hospitalization in two groups. However, the definition of "acute" suffered various modifications according to the particular arbitrary classification of the investigator which led to confusion in the results. In general, the acute schizophrenic has been defined either in terms of the time variable of hospitalization or the type of onset and presence of precipitating events. The time variable as related to hospitalization was used for the classification of the "acutes" on a basis of three different and seemingly contradictory criteria: (a) length of hospitalization ranging from less than 1.9 months or less than 2 years (49) to 4 years or less (5); (b) the type of admission, first admission only (30), or new hospitalization for patients who had not been hospitalized 12 months previously (15); or (c) an "acute episode" with a duration of less than 3 months and a remission of at least 9 months before the present onset (53). The second set of criteria for defining "acute" schizophrenia was based on the type of onset, i.e., the presence of clear precipitating events (6), level of premorbid social functioning (9, 18), and mental status upon admission (59,55), particularly the presence of depression and confusion. Yet a close scrutiny of all of these classifications indicates that implied in the definition of "acute" schizophrenia is the concept of remission and favorable prognosis, which basically does not lead to chronicity (59).

Particularly, the validity of the second set of criteria for acutes appears even more questionable if we peruse the research literature evaluating their significance for outcome. For instance, some investigators have found a positive correlation between sudden onset and clear precipitating events in recovery from schizophrenia, while others reach the conclusion that these factors are weak indicators for the assessment of the course cf the illness. The same applies to confusion and depression. Vaillant (59) and Stephens (55) consider these mental symptoms as favorable, while Bleuler (6) and Casey et al. (12) found them of little value.

The debatable value of these allegedly predictive variables may be due to the possibility that not all patients used in these studies were schizophrenics. For instance, schizo-affectives, presenting the symptoms described above, could take any of these three directions: (1) a mixture of manic–depressive and schizophrenic symptoms; (2) relapse to full schizophrenia; or (3) change to manic–depressive in its course (2).

In order to eliminate these confusions which will affect the findings of any research on schizophrenia, acute patients should be identified, without any time variable bias, as first hospitalization cases. Chronic patients should be considered as those with multiple admissions over 2 years, representing a deteriorated phase in the spectrum of the same illness and, as such, with a higher impairment in psychosocial functioning. This approach attempts to take into account the effect of chemotherapy upon the acute–chronic distinction. Chemotherapy has totally changed the picture of formerly institutionalized chronic schizophrenics who, due to the treatment, can now maintain a peripheral community tenure between repeated hospitalizations, and as such represent a new type of schizophrenic—

the basically pseudoambulatory type. Yet, these patients could easily be confused in their episodes at admission with their acute counterparts because of their similar symptomatology.

Along with the study of the adjustment of schizophrenics in the community prior to hospitalization, one of the aims of this study was to prove that acutes and chronics do not differ substantially in terms of precipitating events, type of onset, or mental status at admission or discharge. The factors which make them different appear to be related to the level of their impairment of functioning that progressively affects their lives. Under stress, when they are unable to cope with these demands, they respond in a nonadaptive way by reacting with acute anxiety, exhibiting bizarre behavior and agitation, or withdrawing from reality, which leads to rehospitalization. The result is always a functional deficit and a consequent difficulty in maintaining community tenure (59, 60). The key to prediction of social adjustment is only in the study of their social performance, with its stress components.

The study undertaken at Bellevue with 125 acute schizophrenics and 516 chronics was specifically addressed to clarifying these problems, using the methodological approach of phenomenology, based on which new measurement instruments were developed.

With our unbiased clinical orientation, we attempted to approach the unsolved problem in prediction of outcome in the light of multifactorial elements such as acute–chronic distinction, influence of chemotherapy, and the stress of psychosocial interaction.

Since the previous empirically isolated set of predictors does not appear to determine, correctly, the outcome of the illness as already discussed, it was necessary to consider a multifactorial cluster of variables responsible for their nonfunctioning and rehospitalization. These could vary from social, familial or interpersonal relationships to lack of medication or inadequate programs for treatment in the community, not to mention the residual mental deficit which slants the reality of the patient's life in a peculiar and unique way leading to stress. In this context the level of motivation of the schizophrenic should also be mentioned. The distortions of motivation influence the duration and the ability of the patient to accept or not to accept the limitations of his functioning in the posthospital period.

These multifactorial variables appear to shift their forces, influencing individually or compounding the difficulties in the daily life of the patient according to the new situations he must face. If only one predictive variable is considered at a time, then it seems that it is a decisive factor for the patient's mental collapse. Yet, on closer scrutiny, other factors are also responsible for his deterioration, interacting with the first one, which naively was considered as the main precipitating factor.

Failure to pay attention to all of these elements discussed above has led to the present misrepresentation of the concept of schizophrenia, leading to sterile controversies, some of which end up questioning the existence of schizophrenia as an illness *per se*.

The Bellevue study has reevaluated all of these problems in an attempt to pin down available clinical evidence which has resulted in a new understanding of the course of schizophrenia as related to the latest developments in the treatment of patients in the community.

REFERENCES

1. Alanen, O.Y.: The families of schizophrenic patients. In "The Schizophrenic Syndrome." (R. Cancro, ed.). Vol. 1, pp. 235–239. Brunner/Mazel, New York, 1971.
2. Angst, J.: "Zur Atiologie und Nosologie Endogener Depressiven Psychosen." Springer Verlag, Berlin and Heidelberg, 1966.
3. Arieti, S.: An overview of schizophrenia from a predominantly psychological approach. *Am. J. Psychiat.* **113**: 3, 1974.
4. Astrachan, B.M., Harrow, M., Adler, D., Brauer, L., Schwartz, A., Schwartz, C. and Tucker, G.: A checklist for the diagnosis of schizophrenia. *Brit. J. Psychiat.* **121**: 529–539, 1972.
5. Bible, G.H., and Magaro, P.A.: Response hierarchy disorganization for chronic and acute schizophrenics. *Psychol. Rep.* **18**: 791–800, 1966.
6. Bleuler, E.: "Dementia Praecox." Int. Universities Press, New York, 1950.
7. Böök, J.A.: A genetic and neuropsychiatric investigation of a north Swedish population. *Acta. Genet. Basel.* **41**: 133–345, (1953).
8. Broen, W.E., and Storms, L.H.: Lawful disorganization. The process underlying a schizophrenic syndrome. *Psychol. Rev.* **73**: 265, 1966.
9. Bromet, E., Harrow, M., and Kasl, S.: Premorbid functioning and outcome in schizophrenics and non-schizophrenics. *Arch. Gen. Psychiat.* **30**: 203–207, 1973.
10. Cancro, R.: The relationship between premorbid adjustment, presenting picture and outcome in schizophrenia. *Proc. of the 76th Annual Convention of the Amer. Psychol. Ass.* **3**: 495–496, 1968.
11. Carpenter, T.W., Strauss, S.J., and Bartko, J.J. The diagnosis and understanding of schizophrenia. *Schizophrenia Bulletin.* **11**: 37–68, 1974.
12. Casey, J.F., Hallister, J.E., Klett, C.J., Lasky, J.J. and Caffey, E.N.: Combined drug therapy of chronic schizophrenics. *Am. J. Psychiat.* **117**: 997–1003, 1961.
13. Crider, A., Maher, B., and Grinspoon, L.: The effect of sensory input on the reaction time of schizophrenic patients of good and poor premorbid history. *Psycho. Sci.* **2**: 47–48, 1965.
14. Dunham, H.W.: "Community and Schizophrenia: an Epidemiological Analysis." Wayne State University Press, Detroit, 1965.
15. Evans, J.R., Goldstein, M.J., Rodnick, E.H.: Premorbid adjustment, paranoid diagnosis and remission. Acute schizophrenia in a community mental health center. *Arch. Gen. Psychiat.* **28**: 666–672, 1973.
16. Faris, R.E., and Dunham, H.W.: Mental Disorder in Urban Areas: an Ecological Study of Schizophrenia and Other Psychoses. University of Chicago Press, Chicago, 1939.
17. Fromm-Reichman, F.: Notes on the development of treatment of schizophrenics by psychoanalytical psychotherapy. *Psychiatry.* **11**: 263–273, 1948.
18. Garmezy, N., Rodnick, E.H.: Premorbid adjustment and performance in schizophrenia: implications for interpreting heterogeneity in schizophrenia. *J. Nerv. Ment. Dis.* **129**: 450–466, 1959.
19. Goffman, E. *Asylums. Essays on the social situation of mental patients and other inmates.* Garden City. N.Y. Doubleday. Anchor Books, 1961.

20. Goldberg, E.M., and Morrison, S.L.: Schizophrenia and social class. *Brit. J. Psychiatry* **109**: 785–802: 1963.

21. Gottesman, I.I.: Severity/concordance and diagnostic refinement in the Maudsly-Bethlem. Schizophrenic Twins Study. In "The Transmission of Schizophrenia." (D. Rosenthal and S. Kety, eds.) pp. 37–47, Pergammon Press, 1969.

22. Gurland, J.B., Fleiss, L.J., Cooper, J.E., Sharpe, L., and Kendell, R.E. Cross-National Study of Diagnosis of Mental Disorders: Hospital Diagnoses and Hospital Patients in New York and London. In "The Schizophrenic Syndrome." (R. Cancro, ed.). 1971. Vol. I, pp. 93–104. Brunner/Mazel, New York.

23. Hallgreen, B., and Sjogren, T.: A clinical and genetico-statistical study of schizophrenia and low grade mental deficiency in a large Swedish rural population. *Acta Psychiat. (Suppl.)* 140, 35, 1959.

24. Hare, E.H.: Mental illness and social conditions in Bristol. *J. Ment. Science* **102–349**: 57, 1956.

25. Heston, L.L.: "Psychiatric Disorders in Foster Home Reared Children of Schizophrenic Mothers in Contemporary Abnormal Psychology. (B. Maher, ed.), pp. 134–146. Penguin Books, Ltd., England, 1973.

26. Higgins, J.: Process-reactive schizophrenia. *J. Nerv. Ment. Dis.* **149**: 451–471, 1969.

27. Husserl, E.: "Ideas." Collier Books, New York, 1967.

28. Irwin, L., and Renner, R.L.: Effect of praise and censure on the performance of schizophrenics. *J. Abnormal Psychol.* **74**: 221–226, 1969.

29. Jasper, K.: "General Psychopathology." (Transl. J. Hoeinig and M.W. Hamilton) The University of Chicago Press, Chicago, 1963.

30. Kingsley, L., Struening, E.L.: Changes in intellectual performance of acute and chronic schizophrenics. *Psychol. Rep.* **18**: 791–800, 1966.

31. Klein, E.B., Cicchetti, D., Spohn, H.: A test of the censure deficit model and its relationship to premorbidity in the performance of schizophrenics. *J. Abnormal Psych.* **72**: 174–181, 1967.

32. Kleist, K.: Schizophrenic symptoms and cerebral pathology. *J. Mental Sci.* **106**: 246–255, 1960.

33. Laing, R.D.: "The Politics of Experience" Ballantine Books, New York, 1970.

34. Lamb, R.H., and Goertzel, V.: Discharged mental patients. Are they really in the community? *Arch. Gen. Psychiat.* **24**: 29–34, 1971.

35. Langfeldt, G.: The prognosis in schizophrenia. *Acta. Scandinavia (Suppl.* **110***)* 1956 (7–66).

36. Leonhard, K.: The question of prognosis in schizophrenia. *Inter. J. Psychiat.* **2**: 633–635, 1966.

37. Lidz, T., Fleck, S., and Cornelison, A.R.: The intra-familial environment of the schizophrenic patient. I. *The Father. Psychiatry* **20**: 329–342, 1957.

37a. Lidz, T., Fleck, S., and Cornelison, A.R.: IV. Parental personalities and family interaction. *Amer. J. Orthopsychiatry* **28**: 764–776, 1958.

37b. Lidz, T., Fleck, S., and Cornelison, A.R.: VI. The transmission of irrationality. *AMA Arch. Neurol. Psychiatry.* **79**: 305–316, 1958.

38. Little, I.K.: Effects of the interpersonal interaction on abstract thinking performance in schizophrenics. *J. Consult. Psychol.* **30**: 158–164, 1966.

39. Mednick, S.A.: A learning theory approach to research in schizophrenia. *Psychological Bull.* **55**: 316, 1958.

39a. Mednick, S.A.: Generalization as a function of manifest anxiety and adaptation to psychological experiments. *J. Consult. Psychol.* **21**: 491, 1957.

40. Mednick, S.A., and Schulsinger, F.: Studies of children at high risk for schizophrenia. *In* "Schizophrenia. The First Ten Dean Award Lectures" (S.R. Dean, ed.), pp. 247–293, M.S.S. Information Corp., New York, 1973.

40a. Mednick, S.A., and Schulsinger, F.: Factors related to breakdown in children at high risk for schizophrenia. *In* "Life History Research in Psychopathology." M. Roff and D.F. Rick, eds.), Vol. 1, pp. 51–93. University of Minnesota Press, Minneapolis, 1970.

41. Meyer, A.: Dynamic interpretation of dementia praecox. *Am. J. Psychol.* **21**: 385–403, 1910.

41a. Meyer, A.: The nature and conception of dementia praecox. *J. Abnormal Psycho.* **5**: 274–285, 1910.

42. Murphy, H.M.B.: Cultural factors in the genesis of schizophrenia. *In* "The Transmission of schizophrenia." (D. Rosenthal and S. Kety, eds.). pp. 144–145. Pergammon Press, Oxford, England, 1969.

43. Pavlov, I.P.: "Conditioned Reflexes and Psychiatry. (Translated by M.H. Gantt). International Univ. Press, New York, 1941.

44. Philips, L.: Case history data and prognosis in schizophrenia. *J. Nerv. Ment. Dis.* **117**: 515–525, 1953.

45. Pichot, P.: Quantification of psychological stress responses. *In* "Society, Stress and Disease." Vol. 1, pp. 49–53. Oxford Univ. Press, London, 1971.

46. Reich, R., and Siegel., L.: The chronically mentally ill: Shuffle to oblivion. *Psychiatric Annals* **3**: 35–55, 1974.

47. Rosen, J.: The concept of early maternal environment in direct psychoanalysis. Doylestown, Pa. Doylestown Foundation, 1963.

48. Rosenthal, D., Wender, H.P., Kety, S.S., Schulsinger, F. Welner, J. Ostergard, L. Schizophrenic offsprings reared in adaptive homes. *In* "The Transmission of Schizophrenia. (D. Rosenthal and S. Kety, eds.), pp. 239–377. Pergammon Press, Oxford, England, 1969.

49. Schooler, C., Silverman, J.: Differences between correlates of perceptual style and Petrie task performance in chronic and acute schizophrenics. *Percept. Mot. Skills.* **32**: 595–601, 1971.

50. Schwartz, M.I., Hunt, W.A., and Walker, R.E.: Clinical judgment of vocabulary responses in process and reactive schizophrenia. *J. Clin. Psychol.* **19**: 488–494, 1963.

51. Siirala, M.: Schizophrenia: A human situation. *American Journal of Psychoanalysis* **23**: 39–66: 1963.

52. Slater, E.: A review of earlier evidences of genetic factors in schizophrenia. *In* "Transmission of Schizophrenia." (D. Rosenthal and S. Kety, eds.). pp. 15–25. Pergammon Press, Oxford, England, 1969.

53. Spelman, M.S., Harrison, A.W., Graham, W.M.: Grid test for schizophrenic thought disorder in acute and chronic schizophrenics. *Psych. Med.* **1**: 234–238, 1971.

54. Spitzer, R.L., and Endicott, J.: DIAGNO II. Further developments in a computer program for psychotic diagnosis. *Am. J. Psychiat.* **125**: 12–21, 1969.

55. Stephens, J.H., Astrup, C., Magnum, J.C.: Prognostic factors in recovered and deteriorated schizophrenics. *Am. J. Psychiat.* **122**: 1116–1121, 1966.

56. Sullivan, H.S.: "Clinical Studies in Psychiatry." *In* "Schizophrenia, Paranoia, and Related Conditions." pp. 312–360. Norton & Co., New York, 1956.

56a. Schneider, K.: "Clinical Psychopathology." Grune & Stratton, New York, 1959.

57. Szasz, T.: "The Manufacture of Madness." Harper & Row, New York, 1970.

58. Turner, R.J., and Wagonfield, M.O.: Occupational mobility and schizophrenia, an assessment of the social causation and social selection hypothesis. *Am. Social Rev.* **32**: 104–13, 1967.

59. Vaillant, G.E.: Prediction of recovery in schizophrenia. *J. Nerv. Ment. Dis.* **135**: 534–543, 1962.

60. Venables, P.H.: In-put dysfunction in schizophrenia. *In* "Progress in Experimental Personality Research." (B.A. Maher, ed.). Vol. I, p. 1. Academic Press, New York, 1964.

61. Wing, J.R., Cooper, J.E., and Sartorious, N.: "The Measurement and Classification of Psychiatric Symptoms." Cambridge University Press, London, 1974.

62. Wittman, P., Steinberg, L.: Follow-up and objective evaluation of prognoses in dementia precox and manic–depressive psychoses. *Elgin State Hospital Papers* **5**: 216–227, 1944.

63. Wyatt, R.J., Schwartz, M.A.; Erdelyli, E. and Barchas, J.O. Dopamine 8 hydroxylase activity in brains of chronic schizophrenic patients. *Science.* **187**: 368–370, 1975.

64. Wynne, L.C., and Singer, M.T.: Thought disorder and family relations of schizophrenia. I. A research strategy. *Arch. Gen. Psychiatry* **9**: 191–198, 1963.

64a. Wynne, L.C., and Singer, M.T.: Thought disorder and family relations of schizophrenia. II. A classification of forms of thinking. *Arch. Gen. Psychiatry.* **9**: 199–206, 1963.

CHAPTER 2

Design and Procedures of the Schizophrenia Research Project: Subjects; Measures; and General Methods of Statisical Analysis

Part I - Subjects

This section describes in detail the sample used in this study. The subjects are described in terms of the selection criteria, social demographic characteristics, and diagnostic classification. In addition, comparisons of the present sample with New York State age and sex statistics for schizophrenics in psychiatric facilities are presented.

SELECTION OF SAMPLE

The subjects consisted of hospitalized schizophrenic patients and noninstitutionalized "normal" controls of both sexes. The patient sample was drawn from a population of schizophrenics admitted to Bellevue Hospital, New York City, between January and December, 1971. Bellevue Hospital is a municipal hospital located in Manhattan with a yearly admission of 8967 cases (1971) of which 5187 (56%) were designated as schizophrenia, 118 (1%) as affective psychoses, and 198 (2%) as other psychoses. The remainder were cases with primary diagnoses of mental retardation, chronic brain syndrome, drug addiction, alcoholism, and psychoneuroses.

From the list of all schizophrenic admissions to the hospital wards every fifth patient was selected for the study, provided that he or she met the following criteria:

1. Diagnosis. All patients with the admitting diagnosis of schizophrenia were considered eligible for selection to the project, except for cases whose diagnosis of schizophrenia was compounded with mental retardation, chronic alcoholism, long-term drug addiction, or organic brain syndrome. Patients exhibiting alcohol and drug abuse problems were admitted to the study only if these difficulties were secondary to the diagnosis of schizophrenia. Chronic alcoholics and heroin addicts over 35 years of age were excluded from the sample on the assumption that chronic problems in these areas are so intertwined with the diagnosis of schizophrenia as to contaminate the diagnostic criterion. Admission to the project

was based on the agreement between ward and project psychiatrists on the primary diagnosis of schizophrenia, irrespective of type, according to the nomenclature of the APA DSM II manual (1968).

2. Age. Only adult patients were selected as subjects. Their ages ranged from 17 to 52 years. The distribution of age is shown in Table 4.

3. Language. Adequate command of the English language was required. Strict adherence to this criterion was necessary to preclude invalidation of the measures by linguistic difficulties.

4. Sex. Although the sample was not specifically drawn to reflect the national distribution of male and female schizophrenics, an attempt was made to maintain an approximately equal ration of men and women in the sample.

5. Selection from the hospital wards. Patients were randomly selected from all adult wards in Bellevue Psychiatric Service, except the prison ward. Patients in transit were not eligible as subjects.

6. Selection of acute and chronic patients. Since the purpose of this study was to examine multiple factors underlying social functioning and associated stress in schizophrenics, the length of illness as well as effects of prolonged institutionalization were thought important. For these reasons, separate samples of first and multiple admissions were drawn. Acute patients have been classically defined as first hospitalization cases who either may have been first hospitalization cases or who may have been mildly ill and treated in the community for a maximum of 6 months prior to hospitalization. Chronic schizophrenics were defined as multiple hospitalization cases. The pool of eligible schizophrenic patients meeting all of the above criteria yielded a ratio of 1 acute to 4 chronic subjects.

Based on the six criteria, 904 schizophrenic patients were selected. Of these, 263 cases were subsequently eliminated as a result of incomplete testing due to rapid discharge or the discovery of a history of prolonged institutionalization, childhood schizophrenia, or mental retardation. The final schizophrenic sample consisted of 641 well defined and clearly diagnosed patients of whom 125 were acute (first hospitalization) and 516 chronic (multiple hospitalization) cases.

The "normal" control sample was drawn from a nonpsychiatric ambulatory population. None of the control subjects had been hospitalized for psychiatric illness or treated for mental disturbances. All control subjects volunteered for the study. They were selected from among New York University-Bellevue Medical Center employees, applicants at the New York State Employment Office, and clients in the Department of Social Services (welfare centers). Care was taken to select the controls from the same Catchment Area served by the Bellevue Psychiatric Hospital. From among the volunteers, a random sample of controls was selected based on the following criteria: The subjects had to be between 18 and 52 years of age with occupations and employment histories comparable to that of the schizophrenic sample. An attempt was made to obtain male and female controls in proportions similar to those in the schizophrenic sample.

CHARACTERISTICS OF THE SUBJECTS

Diagnostic Distribution of Patients

The distribution of subclassifications of schizophrenia in the patient sample is shown in Table 1. As can be seen in Table 1 among the 125 acute schizophrenics, the largest proportion of patients had the diagnosis of acute schizophrenic episode (40%, N = 50), closely followed by the paranoid subclassification (34.4%, N = 43); the schizoaffective subclassification ranked third (13.6%, N = 17); and Catatonic, simple, latent, and hebephrenic subclassifications ranked fourth (12%, N = 5).

Of the 516 chronic schizophrenics, the largest percent were diagnosed as the chronic undifferentiated type, (47.5%, N = 245), followed by paranoid (37.2%, N = 192), schizo-affective (12.2%, N = 63) types. Catatonic, simple, latent, and hebephrenic types accounted jointly for 3.1%, (N = 16).

Of the 125 acute patients studied, 97 (77.6%) had sudden onsets ranging from 1 week or less up to 3 months prior to their first hospitalization. Within this group, 57 (45.6%) reported that their psychiatric symptoms began within 1 week prior to Bellevue admission, 10 (8.0%) within 2 weeks, 17 (13.6%) between 2 weeks and 1 month, and 13 (10.4%) between 1 month and 3 months. For 9 acute patients (7.2%) the onset took place more than 3 months prior to hospitalization; for 5 (4.0%) it was over 1 year in duration. Of the 125 patients, 14 (11.2%) could not reliably determine the onset interval.

For the 516 chronic patients in the sample, the amount of previous hospitalization during the past 10 years ranged from 1 to 2 years; the average number of previous hospitalizations was 3.63. In the 5 years prior to the current hospitalization, 38 (7.4%) of the chronic patients did not require hospital treatment; 89 (17.2%) were hospitalized for a month or less; 167 (32.4%) were admitted for a

Table 1
Distribution of Diagnoses for Acute and Chronic Schizophrenics*

Diagnoses	Acute		Chronic		Total	
	N	%	N	%	N	%
Schizo-affective	17	13.6	63	12.2	80	12.5
Paranoid	43	34.4	192	37.2	235	36.7
Acute schizophrenic Episode	50	40.0	—	—	50	7.8
Chronic Undifferentiated Type	—	—	245	47.5	245	38.2
Catatonic	2	1.6	1	0.2	3	0.5
Others (simple, latent, hebephrenic)	13	10.4	15	2.9	28	4.4

*Diagnoses based on Diagnostic and Statistical Manual of Mental Disorders (DSM II) American Psychiatric Association, 1968.

period ranging from more than 1 month to up to 6 months; 82 (15.9%) were hospitalized for from more than 6 months to up to 1 year; 60 (11.6%) were in psychiatric hospitals for more than 1 year to up to 2 years; and 71 (13.8%) spent more than 2 years in psychiatric facilities. Of the 516 patients, 9 (2.0%) were unable to give reliable estimates. In the period 5–10 years before current rehospitalization, 282 (54.7%) did not require residential treatment; 29 (5.6%) were hospitalized for a month or less; 58 (11.2%) were admitted for from more than 1 month to up to 6 months; 40 (7.8%) for up to 1 year; 31 (6.0%) for up to 2 years; and 65 (12.6%) for more than 2 years. Of the 516 chronic patients, 11 (2.2%) could not provide information in this regard.

During the last 10 years, excluding the current hospitalization, 114 (22.1%) of the 516 chronic patients reported only one hospitalization; 91 (17.6%) two hospitalizations; 77 (14.9%) three hospitalizations; 62 (12.0%) four hospitalizations; 38 (7.4%) five hospitalizations; 30 (5.8%) six hospitalizations; 19 (3.7%) seven hospitalizations; and 63 (12.2%) eight hospitalizations. Of these, 8 (1.6%) could not determine the number of their hospitalizations, and 14 (2.7%) had none.

Inquiry into the psychiatric history revealed that of the 516 chronic patients, 2 (0.4%) had their first mental illness within 1 year of the current hospitalization and received no treatment; 2 cases (0.4%) reported their first illness within 5 years and no treatment, and 1 patient (1.2%) fell ill more than 5 years prior to current hospitalization and also had no treatment at that time. Of those who did receive treatment, 63 (12.2%) had their first symptoms within 1 year of current hospitalization, 183 (35.5%) within 5 years, and 258 (50.0%) more than 5 years before. Of the 516 chronics, 7 (1.4%) did not know or failed to disclose this information.

Table 2 shows types of first psychiatric treatment for the 516 chronic and 125 acute patients. As can be seen in Table 2, the largest percentage (50.4%,

Table 2
Distribution of Type of Previous Psychiatric Treatment
Received by Chronic and Acute Patients

Treatment of Type	Chronic		Acute	
	N	%	N	%
Private Psychiatrist	11	2.1	13	10.4
Outpatient Clinic	8	1.6	4	3.2
Psychiatric Hospitalization in General Hospital	260	50.4	11*	8.8
Voluntary Admission to State or VA Hospital	77	14.9	0	0.0
Commitment to State Hospital	151	29.3	0	0.0
Not Known	9	1.8	2	1.6
Never Treated	0	0	95	76.0

*Treated for 3–4 weeks or less.

Table 3
Distribution of Major Form of Past Psychiatric Treatment
for Chronic and Acute Patients

	Chronic		Acute	
Form of Treatment	N	%	N	%
Psychotherapy	345	66.9	24	19.2
Chemotherapy	115	22.3	2	1.6
Electroshock	10	1.9	0	0.0
Insulin shock	2	0.4	0	0.0
Lobotomy	0	0.0	0	0.0
Other	33	6.4	4	3.2
Unknown	11	2.1	0	0.0
Never treated	0	0.0	95	76.0

N = 260) of the chronic cases were previously treated in a general or private hospital, and the next largest (29.3%, N = 151) were committed to state hospitals. Of the 516 patients, 77 (14.9%) represent voluntary admission to State or VA hospitals, and 19 (3.7%) reported receiving first psychiatric treatment on an outpatient basis. Of these 11 (2.1%) were treated by private psychiatrists and 8 (1.6%) in outpatient clinics.

Table 3 shows the major form of treatment received by the chronic and acute patients. Of both types of patients who were treated, psychotherapy appears to be the most frequent form of past treatment [66.9% (N = 345) of the chronics and 19.2% (N = 24) of the acutes reported this form of intervention.] Chemotherapy ranked second, with 22.3% (N = 115) of the chronics and 1.6% (N = 2) of the acutes reporting this form of treatment. Other forms of therapeutic intervention were infrequent in both groups of subjects.

In terms of regularity of treatment received between hospitalizations by the chronic patients, it is of interest to note that, in the present sample, 221 (43.0%) received no treatment at all, 143 (27.7%) reported irregular treatment in outpatient clinics or with a private psychiatrist, and 146 (28.3%) attended regular treatment sessions either privately or on an outpatient basis.

Sociodemographic Characteristics of the Samples

Table 4 presents the distributions of age, sex, education, occupation, marital status, and race for the schizophrenic and normal samples.

The age of the subjects ranged from 17 to 52 years. Categorized into those 25 years or younger, 26–44 years of age, and 45 or older, the patient and normal sample distributions were as follows: 23.3% (N = 120) of the chronics, 45.6% (N = 57) of the acutes, and 28.4% (N = 27) of the normals were in the

Table 4

Sociodemographic Characteristics of the Schizophrenic and Normal Samples

Variable	Chronic N	Chronic %	Acute N	Acute %	Total Pts. N	Total Pts. %	Normal N	Normal %	χ^2
Age									
25 and under	120	23.3	57	45.6	176	27.5	27	28.4	
26–44	352	68.2	62	49.6	414	64.6	68	61.1	0.94
45+	44	8.5	6	4.8	50	7.8	10	10.5	
Sex									
Male	329	63.8	65	52.0	394	61.5	43	45.3	
Female	187	36.2	60	48.0	247	38.5	52	54.7	9.01*
Total	516		125						
Education (in grades)									
7–11	218	42.2	42	33.6	260	40.6	31	32.6	
12	186	36.1	48	38.4	234	36.5	32	33.7	5.44
13+	112	21.7	35	28.0	147	22.9	32	33.7	
Occupation									
Never employed	15	2.9	8	6.4	23	3.5	3	3.2	
Manual workers	281	54.5	55	44.0	335	52.3	43	45.3	
unskilled	230	44.6	41	32.8	271	42.3	16	16.8	
semiskilled	51	9.9	13	10.4	64	10.0	27	28.4	
skilled	28	5.4	6	4.8	34	5.3	5	5.2	
Occupation									
Intermediate level	161	31.2	45	36.0	206	32.1	34	35.8	
Owner, small business	2	0.3	1	0.8	3	0.5	1	1.0	
Technician	18	3.5	3	2.4	21	3.3	3	3.2	
Salesman	14	2.7	3	2.4	17	2.7	2	2.1	
Clerks	106	20.5	27	21.6	133	20.8	22	23.2	
Semiprofessional	21	4.1	11	8.8	32	5.0	6	6.3	2.01
Higher level	31	6.0	11	8.8	42	6.6	10	10.5	
Administration	13	2.5	5	4.0	18	2.8	1	1.0	
Lesser professional	16	3.2	4	3.2	20	3.1	9	9.5	
Owner, medium business	1	0.2	0	0.0	1	0.2	0	0.0	
Manager	0	0.0	1	0.8	2	0.3	0	0.0	
Marital status									
Single	306	59.3	80	64.0	386	60.2	25	86.3	
Married	67	13.0	20	16.0	87	13.6	34	35.8	45.94†
Separated	143	27.7	25	20.0	168	26.2	36	37.9	
Race									
White	292	56.6	60	48.0	352	54.9	42	44.2	
Black	192	37.2	57	45.6	249	38.9	33	31.7	
Puerto Rican	22	4.3	5	4.0	27	4.2	17	17.9	3.81
Oriental	1	0.2	2	1.6	3	0.5	1	1.1	
Other	9	1.7	1	0.8	10	1.5	2	2.1	

*$p < 0.01$.
†$p < 0.001$.

youngest age category; 68.2% (N = 352) of the chronic, 49.6% (N = 62) of the acutes, and 61.1% (N = 58) of the normals were in the intermediate age range, and 8.5% (N = 44) of the chronics, 4.8% (N = 6) of the acutes, and 10.5% (N = 10) of the normals were in the oldest group. Comparison of the total patient and normal controls in terms of age failed to yield significant differences ($X^2 = 0.94, df = 2; p > 0.05$).

In terms of sex distribution, 63.8% (N = 329) of the chronics, 52.0% (N = 65) of the acutes, and 45.3% (N = 43) of the normals were male; the percentages of female subjects were 36.2 (N = 187), 48.0% (N = 60), and 54.7% (N = 52) for chronics, acutes, and normals, respectively. There was a preponderance of males in the patient sample as compared to the normals ($X^2 = 9.01$; $df = 1$; $p < 0.01$), but a regression analysis failed to reveal significant sex effects on the dependent variables studied.

In terms of educational achievement, categorized into educational units of 7–11 grades completed, high school graduation, and 13 years of education or greater, there were no discernable differences between patient and control samples ($X^2 = 5.44$; $df = 2$; $p > 0.05$). Among the chronics 42.2% (N = 218) fell into the lowest educational category compared with 33.6% (N = 42) of the acutes and 32.6% (N = 31) of the normals. High school was completed by 36.1% (N = 186) of the chronics, 38.4% (N = 48) of the acutes, and 33.7% (N = 32) of the normals. In the highest education category there were 21.7% (N = 112) chronics, 28% (N = 35) acutes, and 33.7% (N = 32) normals.

Comparison of educational achievement of the patients to that of their family as a whole revealed that 6.4% (N = 33) of the chronics and 4.0% (N = 5) of the acutes had much less education than members of their family, 24.4% (N = 126) of the former and 19.2% (N = 24) of the latter reported less education than obtained by their family. For the majority of the 516 chronic patients (38.4%; N = 198), their educational levels as compared to those of their families were the same, and 27.7% (N = 143) reported having higher levels of education. Among the 125 acutes 36.0% (N = 45) acknowledged the same level of education as that of their family and 40.8% (N = 51) claimed having more education. Of the chronic group, 16 (3.1%) could not report these comparisons with any degree of accuracy.

Comparisons of educational achievements of the patients to that of their spouses and partners revealed that of the 516 chronics 15 (2.9%) had much less, 47 (9.1%) had less, 85 (16.5%) the same amount, and 75 (14.5%) more education. Of these, 293 (56.8%) had no spouses or partner available for comparison. For the same comparison, of the 125 acutes, 6 (4.8%) claimed to have much less, 17 (13.6%) less, 13 (10.4%) the same, and 16 (12.8%) more education than their spouses and partners. Of these, 73 (58.6%) were unable to make the comparison since they had no spouses or long term partners.

Inquiry into the history of on the job training and training school attendance revealed that of the 516 chronic patients, 361 (70.0%) never received any on the job training and 375 (72.6%) did not attend training school. Of the remaining 155 chronics, 45 (8.7%) started, but did not complete on the job training, 1 (0.2%) was receiving it currently, and 109 (21.1%) have completed such training at some point in the past. Of the 141 chronic patients who had training school experience, 56 (10.9%) started the training school programs but never completed these, 4 (0.8%) were currently enrolled, and 81 (15.7%) completed training school in the past. Among the 125 acutes studied, 100 (80.0%) never received any on the job training and 103 (82.4%) did not attend training school of any kind. Of the 25 patients who did receive job training, 2 (1.6%) started the program but failed to complete it, 1 (0.8%) was currently enrolled in it, and 22 (17.6%) successfully completed vocational training in the field. Among the 22 acutes who had some training school experience, 10 (8.0%) enrolled in training school but did not complete the training program, 1 (0.8%) was presently enrolled and 11 (8.8%) successfully completed it in the past.

Occupational classification of the subjects based on the Duncan classification system (1962) failed to reveal significant patient control differences ($X^2 = 2.01$; $df = 8$; $p>0.05$). The largest percentage of both patients (52.3%, N = 335) and normals (45.3%, N = 43) were unskilled and semiskilled manual workers, with 32.1% (N = 206) of the patients and 35.8% (N = 34) of the controls in intermediate levels of occupations such as technicians, salesmen, and clerks.

Perhaps more revealing than the occupational distribution of the samples is the information relating to employment history of the patients. Just before current hospitalization, of the 516 chronic patients (13 (2.5%) were never gainfully employed. A large percentage (68.0% N = 351) were unemployed prior to the Bellevue admission. Of those working prior to their hospitalization, 30 (5.8%) were employed on a part-time basis and 69 (13.4%) worked at full-time jobs; seven (1.4%) claimed to be employed but currently on sick leave. The remaining 46 chronic patients (10.4%) were either students or housewives, some of whom were employed. Among the 125 acute patients, 57 (45.6%) were unemployed just prior to their hospitalization, 9 (7.2%) were working on a part-time basis, and 25 (20.0%) were full-time employees. Of the remaining cases, 8 (6.4%) were never employed, 21 (16.8%) were students or housewives, some of whom were also employed. Four percent of the patients (N = 5) were employed but currently on sick leave.

Of those who reported to be unemployed, 234 (45.3%) of the chronic patients and 40 (32.0%) of the acute counterparts stated that their present unemployment was due to firing because of their mental condition, incompetence, irresponsibility, or friction with supervisors or co-workers. A small percentage of both types of patients attributed their unemployment to physical illness [9.1% (N = 47) of the chronics and 8.0% (N = 10) of the acutes]. Lack of gainful employment due to quitting or being laid off for noninvidious reasons was reported by 168 (32.6%) of the chronics and 34 (27.2%) of the acutes.

Inquiry into the length of unemployment in the past revealed that 13.2% (N = 68) of the chronics and 1.6% (N = 2) of the acutes have not worked for over 5 years prior to the key admission; 9.7% (N = 50) of the chronics and 4.0% (N = 5) of the acutes did not work for an interval of over 2 years; 10.5% (N = 54) of the former and 3.2% (N = 4) of the latter were unemployed for over 1 year. Of those whose unemployment period was under 1 year prior to admission to the project, 65 chronics (12.6%) and 14 acutes (11.2%) did not work from 6 months to up to 1 year; 50 of the former (9.7%) and 14 of the latter (11.2%) were unemployed for an interval of from over 3 months to up to 6 months, and 130 chronics (25.2%) and 43 of the acutes (34.4%) had no gainful employment for intervals ranging from 1 month to up to 3 months prior to key hospitalization. Present admission to Bellevue interrupted employment of 62 (12.0%) of the chronics and 16 (12.8%) of the acutes.

Inquiry into the length of time the patients worked continuously before present hospitalization revealed that 177 (34.3%) of the chronics and 32 (25.6%) of the acutes worked continuously for 3 months or less; 63 (12.2%) of the former and 10 (8.0%) of the latter were working for from more than 3 months to up to 6 months; 78 (15.1%) of the chronics and 17 (13.6%) of the acutes held jobs continuously for from over 6 months to up to 1 year; 56 (10.9%) of the chronics and 12 (9.6%) of the acutes were consistently employed for from more than 1 year to up to 2 years, and 108 (20.9%) of the former and 36 (28.8%) of the latter worked continuously for over 2 years prior to the current hospitalization. The remainder of the patients [6.6% (N = 34) of the chronics and 14.4% (N = 28) of the acutes] could not provide reliable information in this regard.

It is of particular interest to note that in the 5 years prior to their key admission, 66 (12.8%) of the chronics and 6 (4.8%) of the acutes did not work at all, and 179 (34.7%) of the former and 27 (21.6%) of the latter worked either irregularly or briefly during this time interval. Of the 516 chronics, 106 (20.5%) worked about half of the time in the past 5 years, as did 16 (12.8%) of the acutes in the study. One hundred twenty-seven (24.6%) of the chronics and 56 (44.8%) of the acutes worked most of the time for the past 5 years. The remainder [7.4% (N = 38) of the chronics and 16.0% (N = 20) of the acutes], although not employed, were students or housewives.

Of those who did work in the past 5 years (prior to the key admission) 364 (70.5%) of the chronics and 81 (64.8%) of the acutes were employed full time, 46 (8.9%) of the former and 16 (12.8%) of the latter worked at predominantly half-time and 4 (0.8%) of the chronics and 3 (2.4%) of the acutes worked at less than half-time in the 5 year interval period. One hundred and two (19.8%) of the chronic patients and 25 (20.0%) of their acute counterparts did not work at all due to either unemployment or their student or housewife status.

The intermittent employment history of the patients finds its reflection in the phenomenon of dependence on public assistance. At the point of key admission 40.7% (N = 210) of the chronic and 20% (N = 25) of the acute patients were receiving Welfare benefits and 10.1% (N = 52) of the former and 2.4% (N = 3) were on other agency assistance programs. Unemployment benefits were being collected by 2.7% (N = 14) of the chronics and 5.6% (N = 7) of the acutes. The remainder of the patients [46.5% (N = 240) of the chronics and 72% (N = 90) of the acutes) did not receive public assistance or other financial assistance from outside sources. Of the 276 chronic and 35 acute patients receiving welfare assistance, 156 (56.5%) of the former and 15 (42.8%) of the latter relied on these benefits for over 1 year. A considerably smaller percentage of both types of patients depended on welfare benefits for an interval of from over 6 months to 1 year [chronics 10.5% (N = 29); acutes 14.3% (N = 5)]. Similar distribution was obtained for the period of from 3 to 6 months with 12.0% (N = 33) of the chronics and 14.3% (N = 5) of the acutes reporting dependence on welfare for this time interval. Of those receiving welfare benefits for a period of from 1 to 3 months, 54 (19.6%) were chronic and 8 (22.9%) were acute patients. Four chronic (1.4%) and 2 acute (5.7%) cases could not reliably determine the length of time they were receiving public assistance.

Inquiry into the length of experience with Welfare revealed that although most of the patients [64.5% (N = 333) chronics and 81.6% (N = 102) of the acutes] reported no or very little experience with welfare, a sizeable proportion of the sample [21.9% (N = 113) of the chronics and 7.2% (N = 9) of the acutes] indicated receiving welfare benefits on and off as needed. Of the 183 chronics who reported varying amounts of experience with public assistance, 11 (2.1%) relied on welfare almost their entire life, 33 (6.4%) received welfare benefits for most of their adult life, 10 (1.9%) depended on welfare while growing up, and 16 (3.1%) reported having their parents on welfare while growing up. For the acute group, experience with welfare is less striking. Of the 23 patients who have had experience with public assistance, 3 (2.4%) relied on those benefits for almost their entire life, 9 (7.2%) were on welfare intermittently, and only one patient (0.8%) claimed to rely on welfare most of his adult life. Of the remainder, 4 (3.2%) grew up on welfare and 6 (4.8%) had parents who depended on public assistance while they were growing up.

The distribution of the parents' income just prior to hospitalization indicates that 189 (36.6%) of the chronic and 23 (18.4%) of the acute patients lived solely on public assistance income. Of the remaining 327 chronics, 84 (16.3%) reported incomes below $2000 a year, 72 (14.0%) in the $2001 to $4000 range, 42 (8.1%) from $4001 to $6000, 58 (11.2%) from $6001 to $8000 annually, and 36 (7.0%) were in the $8001 to $12,000 a year income bracket. Only 20 chronic patients (3.9%) reported having an income of above $12,000 a year. The remainder (2.9%; N = 15) refused to reveal this information. Of the 102 acutes who did not rely on public assistance, 27 (21.6%) reported an income of less than $2000 a year, 15 (12.0%) were in the $2001 to $4000 range, 17 (13.6%) from $4001 to $6000, 18 (14.4%) in the $6001 to $8000 range and 8 (6.4%) in the $8001 to $12,000 bracket. Only 8 (6.4%) of the acutes reported annual income of above $12,000. The remaining 9 cases (7.2%) refused to answer this question.

In terms of marital status a significantly higher proportion of controls were married as compared to the schizophrenics ($X^2 = 45.94$; $df = 2$; $p < 0.001$) which is consonant with the common clinical observation that more schizophrenics than normals remain single. Thus, 13% (N = 67) of the chronics, 16% (N = 20) of the acutes, and 35.8% (N = 34) of the normals were married.

No significant race differences were obtained for the patient and controls samples ($X^2 = 3.81$; $df = 8$; $p > 0.05$). The largest percentage of both patients (54.9%; N = 352) and controls (44.2%; N = 42) were White; 38.9% (N = 249) of patients and 31.7% (N = 33) of normals were Black.

CHARACTERISTICS OF THE FOLLOW-UP SAMPLE

Of the 516 chronic and 125 acute schizophrenic patients originally included in the study sample, 349 (67.6%) of the former and 70 (56.0%) of the latter were traced and made available for the follow-up observation period lasting 18 months.

In order to determine whether or not the follow-up sample was representative of the original population, the key admission and follow-up samples were compared in terms of social demographic characteristics as shown in Table 5. Inspection of Table 5 indicates that except for the occupation variable the two groups of patients were quite comparable. The follow-up sample did, however, contain a significantly larger proportion of unskilled and significantly smaller number of skilled and professional patients as compared to the key admission subjects.

Among the 349 followed-up chronic schizophrenics, 114 (32.7%) were readmitted to Bellevue Hospital while 144 (41.3%) were rehospitalized at other psychiatric facilities. Ninety-one of these patients (26.1%) did not require hospital care during the follow-up interval. Of the 70 acutes available for the follow-up observation, 11 (15.7%) were readmitted to Bellevue, 22 (31.4%) were rehospitalized at other institutions, while 37 (52.9%) were hospitalization free during the follow-up period.

In order to determine whether the readmitted and nonreadmitted patients differ in type of diagnosis and sociodemographic characteristics, the distributions of subclassifications of schizophrenia and the variables of age, sex, education, occupation, and marital status were compared for the two samples of acute and chronic patients by means of chi-square tests. The results of the first analysis, dealing with the diagnostic classifications are shown in Table 6. As can be seen from Table 6 no significant differences were found in terms of subtype of

Table 5

Comparison of Distributions of Social Demographic Characteristics for Key
Admission and the Follow-Up Schizophrenic Sample

Variable	Key admission (N = 641)		Follow-up (N = 419)		X^2
	N	%	N	%	
Age					
25	176	27.5	112	26.7	NS
25–44	414	64.6	276	65.9	
45–52	50	7.8	30	7.2	
Sex					
Male	394	61.5	244	58.2	NS*
Female	247	38.5	175	41.8	
Education (in grades)					
7–11	260	40.6	183	43.7	NS*
12	234	36.5	142	33.9	
13+	147	22.9	99	23.6	
Occupation					
Unskilled	358	55.8	336	80.2	66.39
Skilled and					$df=1$
Professional	283	44.2	83	19.8	$p < 0.001$
Martial status					
Single	386	60.2	245	58.5	
Separated	168	26.2	124	29.6	
Married	87	13.6	50	11.9	

*Not significant.

schizophrenia for either the acute ($X^2 = 1.24$; $df = 3$; $p > 0.05$) or the chronic schizophrenics ($X^2 = 4.28$; $df = 3$; $p > 0.05$). Comparisons of readmitted and nonreadmitted acute and chronic schizophrenics are shown in Tables 7 and 8, respectively. Examination of Table 7 reveals that none of the comparisons for the sociodemographic characteristics of age, sex, education, occupation, and marital status reached the acceptable levels of significance. By contrast, the distribution of these same characteristics for chronics present a different picture as shown in Table 8. It appears that the nonreadmitted chronics tend to be older than their readmitted counterparts ($X^2 = 10.93$; $df = 2$; $p < 0.01$) especially above 45 years of age. More males than females were rehospitalized ($X^2 = 13.63$; $df = 1$; $p < 0.001$), as were those of unskilled occupations ($X^2 = 5.01$; $df = 1$; $p < 0.05$). Readmissions were also more frequent in patients who were not currently married ($X^2 = 11.08$; $df = 1$; $p < 0.01$).

THE INFORMANTS

In addition to the schizophrenics and normal samples there were 228 informants who participated in the study. These were classified into close and secondary or distant informants. Close informants were defined as spouses and

Table 6
Distribution of Diagnoses for Readmitted and Nonreadmitted
Acute and Chronic Patients

Diagnosis	Readmitted acute (N = 33)		Nonreadmitted acute (N = 37)	
	N	%	N	%
Schizoaffective	3	9.1	7	18.9
Paranoid	10	30.3	12	32.4
Undifferentiated	8	24.2	5	13.5
Others (latent, simple, catatonic, hebephrenic)	12	36.4	13	35.2

$X^2 = 1.24; df = 3; p > 0.05.$

Diagnoses	Readmitted chronic (N = 258)		Nonreadmitted chronic (N = 91)	
	N	%	N	%
Schizoaffective	27	10.5	11	12.1
Paranoid	93	36.0	28	30.8
Undifferentiated	127	49.2	43	47.3
Others (latent, simple, catatonic, hebephrenic)	11	4.3	9	9.8

$X^2 = 4.28; df = 3; p > 0.05.$

such primary family members as parents and siblings. Secondary informants included aunts, uncles, cousins, friends, neighbors, clergy, and social workers who knew the patient for a minimum of 2 years prior to the current hospitalization.

Both types of informants were selected by the patients themselves, the choice being dictated primarily by availability. Of the 182 chronic patients who provided an informant, 148 selected a close informant and 34 a secondary informant. Among the 46 acute cases 34 chose close informants and 12 secondary informants.

The informants were accepted into the project only if they had close contact with the patient for 2 years preceding the latter's hospitalization and could be assumed to provide extensive information about the patient's behavior, attitudes, and past psychiatric history.

To maximize the reliability of data gathered from the informants, all participating respondents were questioned in depth about the extent of their familiarity with the patient before the actual interview. Those who met the criteria were then interviewed either at home or at Bellevue Psychiatric Hospital by a clinical psychologist or a specially trained social worker. The difficulties encountered in obtaining data from the informants were of two types: close informants (primary family members and spouses) tended to contaminate the information with feelings of guilt associated with their assumed contribution to the patient's hospitalization, and distant informants were often too eager to offer

Table 7

Distribution of Sociodemographic Characteristics for Readmitted and Nonreadmitted Acute Schizophrenics

Variable	Readmitted acutes (N = 33)		Nonreadmitted acutes (N = 37)		X^2
	N	%	N	%	
Age					
25 and under	14	42.4	19	51.4	0.5598*
26–44	17	51.5	17	45.9	
45+	2	6.1	1	2.7	
Sex					
Male	20	60.6	19	51.4	0.6024*
Female	12	39.4	18	48.6	
Education (in grades)					
7–11	12	36.4	14	37.8	0.7706*
12	11	33.3	15	40.6	
13+	10	30.3	8	21.6	
Occupation					
Unskilled	26	78.8	29	78.4	0.0812*
Skilled and Professional	7	21.2	8	21.6	
Marital status					
Single	20	60.6	25	67.6	0.7059*
Separated	8	24.2	6	16.2	
Married	5	15.2	6	16.2	

*Not significant.

information some of which appeared to be contrary to facts (contradictory evidence was obtained in different parts of interview). However, the first problem was often removed by a tactful approach which allowed free ventilation of guilt feelings and provided a genuine assurance that the information sought was not used to establish source of blame for either the patient's present illness or its recurrence.

The second source of bias (contradictory information) was significantly minimized by careful check of the data received against similar recurring questions as the interview progressed. To further verify the informant data, the parents and the spouse of the same patient were used whenever possible to obtain the same information from two independent sources.

To maximize the reliability of the information all informants were routinely requested to refrain from providing any data regarding the patient of which they were not absolutely sure. Areas of inquiry for which reliable information was not available were treated in the analyses as missing data.

Table 8

Distribution of Sociodemographic Characteristics for Readmitted and Nonreadmitted Chronic Schizophrenics

Variable	Readmitted chronics (N = 258)		Nonreadmitted chronics (N = 91)		X^2
	N	%	N	%	
Age					
25 and under	57	22.1	22	24.2	10.93
26–44	188	72.9	55	60.4	($p < 0.01$)
45+	13	5.0	14	15.4	
Sex					
Male	164	63.6	41	45.1	13.63
Female	94	26.4	50	54.9	($p < 0.001$)
Education (in grades)					
7–11	124	48.1	33	36.3	3.91
12	82	31.8	34	37.4	($p > 0.05$)
13+	52	20.1	24	26.3	
Occupation					
Unskilled	215	83.3	66	72.5	5.01
Skilled and					($p < 0.05$)
Professional	43	16.7	25	27.5	
Marital status					
Single	158	61.3	42	46.2	11.08
Separated	79	30.6	31	34.1	($p < 0.01$)
Married	21	8.1	18	19.7	

Part II—Measures

The selection of measures for the study was dictated by the overall plan, already detailed, to assess the degree of the schizophrenics' personality impairment, the severity of his or her illness, the quantity of his or her motivation, and the level of functioning in a wide range of interpersonal relationships. In addition, an important focus of the study was directed towards the measurement of distress associated with attempts to adapt to community and familial expectations.

The purpose of the extensive testing was twofold. First, it was deemed important to assess the multiple facets of functioning, stress, and motivation at different periods, prior to the current illness of the schizophrenics. In addition, the variables selected for the study were also tested in normal controls to provide a baseline for the comparisons. Second, the problem of identifying relevant factors for readmission in schizophrenia necessitated an extensive and detailed probe into a broad range of areas of behavior since it is well known that idiographic as well as more general factors may operate in readmissions.

THE CATTELL 16 PF TEST—FORM E

The Cattell 16 PF test was used for the general evaluation of personality structure. It was selected as a measure of choice because it claims to assess functionally, unitary source traits representing the main dimensions of personality. As such, it has shown promise for measuring individual differences in personality and describes the structure of the abnormal as well as normal personality, in terms of profiles, based on 16 bipolar dimensions. These dimensions, referred to as personality factors, tap such personality variables as introversion–extraversion tendencies, intelligence (in terms of concrete vs. abstract thinking), degree of ego and superego strength, dominance–submission, activity level, sensitivity and suspiciousness, social adequacy, conservatism–

radicalism, and levels of emotional integration and tensions. Form E of the test was employed since it was specially designed for use with educationally and culturally disadvantaged groups (less than a sixth grade reading ability), closely resembling the actual educational and cultural level of the Bellevue subject population. This particular test form was standardized on 1242 cases of both sexes, most of whom were rehabilitation clients, some psychiatric patients, and some persons with mental retardation, representing socioeducational characteristics of patients in state and general psychiatric hospitals.

The test was administered according to directions specified in the test manual and scored in terms of standard scores (stress) based on the combined male and female norms.

PSYCHIATRIC EXAMINATION

A modified version of the Problem Appraisal Scale (PAS) standardized by Spitzer and Endicott (29) was used to assess the signs and symptoms of psychiatric disorder, as well as the social functioning of the schizophrenics in the study. The Problem Appraisal Scale is basically a structured interview which covers traditional mental status categories and areas of impaired social and family functioning, generally included as supporting data in a comprehensive psychiatric examination. The areas covered by this psychiatric examination include physical function disturbance (sleeping and eating problems, enuresis and soiling, seizures and convulsions, and speech articulation problems); intellectual development (in terms of adequacy vs. mental deficiency); a set of social and family interaction (impairment in relationships with spouse, child, family members, others in the community); social performance disturbance in job, school, or housekeeping obligations; personality trends such as inferiority, hypochondriasis, and dependency; socially maladaptive behaviors (drug and alcohol abuse, sexual problems, and antisocial attitudes and acts); social manifestation of mental illness (anger and belligerence, assaultive tendencies, and impairments in daily routine and use of leisure time); and mental evaluation. In the last category classically considered as mental status proper, are assessed: anxiety symptoms (including fears and phobias); depression (suicidal thoughts, acts and gestures, depressed mood and feelings of inferiority); persecutory ideation (grandiosity, suspicion, persecution and homicidal tendencies); secondary thought disorder, i.e., delusions, hallucinations, obsessions; primary thought disorder, i.e., disorientation, incoherence, affect disorder, inappropriate behavior; and lack of insight into the illness. In addition, information was obtained regarding the duration and severity of illness and major and contributing stress.

The main modification of the PAS consisted of structuring the interview to provide clear specifications of information to be obtained by the interviewer, and the severity ratings to be applied to the data. Within each of the categories of the schedule, the disturbance was rated on a four point scale: absence of impairment was scored 0; low level of disturbance scored 1; mild disturbance scored 2; moderate disturbance scored 3; and severe disturbance scored 4.

For the purposes of the study, the items comprising the PAS were first scored according to the above mentioned instructions, and then categorized into 19 groups and 5 areas, to provide a comprehensive view of the mental and social condition of the patient upon admission (Table 9).

The first classification of the PAS items into 19 groups provided a more detailed delineation of functional impairment. Items relating to sleeping and eating problems, anxiety symptoms, fears, phobias, agitation, and hyperactivity were classified into the anxiety group (group 1). Intellectual functioning remained as an independent group (group 2) as did items relating to physical problems (group 3). Group 4 consisted of items dealing with disturbance with mate or spouse and general sexual problems. Social adjustment group (group 5) compiled items dealing with problems such as anger; belligerence; negativism; assaultiveness; and problems with children, family members, and other people. Absence of job, disruption of education, and impairment in ability to perform housekeeping chores were classified under activity maladjustment (group 6). Suicidal thoughts, acts, and gestures together with items relating to depressed mood and feelings of inferiority, made up the depression group (group 7). Somatic concern items were grouped under hypochondriasis (group 8). The paranoia group (group 9) consisted of items relating to grandiosity, suspicion, persecution, homicidal tendencies, as well as social withdrawal, isolation, dependency, and clinging. Obsessions, compulsions, delusions, and hallucinations were classified as general secondary aspects of schizophrenia (group 10). Abuse of alcohol, narcotics, and other drugs and antisocial acts formed group 11. Disorientation, impaired memory, speech disorganization, and incoherence made up the group of general primary schizophrenic symptoms (group 12); and lack of emotion, inappropriate affect, and slowing up were classified into a group of primary signs of schizophrenia (group 13). The objective signs group (group 14) comprised items dealing with inappropriate appearance and behavior. Groups 15, 16, 17, 18, and 19 consisted of information pertaining to duration of illness and severity, ratings of current psychiatric conductor, lack of insight, and major contributing stress, respectively.

The second grouping of the PAS items into 5 areas provided a broader classification of problem areas. Thus, items relating to disturbances with regard to children, family, other people, anger, belligerence, negativism, assaultiveness and impairments in functioning in job, school, and housekeeping comprised the social functioning area. Suicidal thought, acts, gestures, depressed mood, inferiority, guilt feelings, social withdrawal, and dependency made up an area labeled anxiety and depression symptomatology. This area consisted of items traditionally treated as mental status. Primary symptoms of schizophrenia (disorientation, impaired memory, speech disorganization, incoherence, slowing

Table 9

Problem Appraisal Scale—19 Groups of Mental Status and Their Item Content

Group	Item no.	Item content
1. Anxiety	15	Sleeping problems
	16	Eating problems
	17	Anxiety, fears, phobias
	45	Agitation, hyperactivity
2. Physical problems	18	Other physical problems
3. Intelligence	19	Inadequate intelligence
4. Sexual disturbance	21	Disturbance with mate or spouse
	42	Sexual problems
5. Social adjustment	20	Problems with children
	22	Problems with other family
	23	Problems with other people
	39	Anger, belligerence, negativism
	40a	Assaultiveness
6. Activity adjustment	24	Absence of job
	25	Absence of school
	26	Absence of housekeeping
7. Depression	27	Suicidal thoughts
	28	Suicidal acts and gestures
	31a	Depressed mood
	31b	Inferiority
	32	Somatic concerns, hypochondriasis
8. Depression (Masked) .	33	Social withdrawal, isolation
	34	Dependency, clinging
9. Paranoia	35	Grandiosity
	36	Suspicion, persecution
	40b	Homicidal
10. General secondary signs	30	Obsessions, compulsions
	37	Delusions
	38	Hallucinations
11. Antisocial activity	41	Alcohol abuse
	43	Narcotics, other drugs
	44	Antisocial acts
12. General symptoms	46a	Disorientation
	46b	Impaired memory
	47a	Speech disorganization
	47b	Incoherence (general thought disorders)
13. Disturbance of affect	48a	Slowed up
	48b	Lack of emotion
	49a	Inappropriate affect

Table 9 (continued)
Problem Appraisal Scale—19 Groups of Mental Status and Their Item Content

Group	Item no.	Item content
14. Observed behavior appraisal	49b	Inappropriate appearance and behavior
	52	Daily routine
15. Duration of Illness	56	
16. Severity of Illness	55	
17. Current psychiatric condition	57	
18. Insight level	50	(Lack of insight)
19. Major or contributing stress	51	

down, lack of emotion, and inappropriate affect) formed an independent area. The last dimension, antisocial activity, contained items dealing with alcohol and drug abuse, antisocial behavior, bizarre appearance, and daily routine.

On the basis of these two classification systems it was possible to compare subgroups of patients, in terms of various aspects of functioning impairments, as well as the overall level of disturbance, which represented the sum of the 50–odd items.

THE BELLEVUE MOTIVATION SCALE MAAIS. (MOTIVATIONAL, ACHIEVEMENT, ASPIRATION, INTEREST, SELF-APPRAISAL)

The construction of the MAAIS was based on the notion that motivation is an intentional state of readiness, which is actualized when an individual becomes committed to its execution. The working hypotheses underlying the test assumes that motivation consists of three components: (1) a mental construct of an act, which determines the direction and selectivity of motivation; (2) a driving force, leading to striving or accomplishments (the drive factor of motivation); and (3) these two activities take place within a framework of temporal perspective which links past experience with present decision as related to future aspirations. It is assumed that there is a meaningful interplay between past level of achievement, present self-appraisal of motivations and future actualization of one's aspirations, although the direction and strength of motivational components may vary with time. This notion is supported by the observation that all persons reevaluate themselves continuously, when presented with new situations, in which they have to project new and changing expectancies towards their achievements. In this sense, motivation may be thought of as an initiator and supporter of behavior, where one's potentialities, perceived in the context of one's socioeconomic environment, become the bases for one's choice of acts.

The MAAIS attempts to broaden the measure of motivation beyond that of general interest tendencies, or need of achievement, and directs its attention toward those intracomponents of motivation that may be impaired by psychotic disintegration.

The test itself consists of items pooled from universal motives similar to those used in such tests as Cattell's 16 PF (5), Hermans' Achievement Test (15), Barron's Ego Strength Scale, derived from the MMPI (2), Brainard's Occupational Inventory (3) and the Labor Department Statistics on Occupation (U.S. Labor Force Report, 1971; 30).

The test items represent two psychological dimensions. The first dimension deals with motivational self-appraisal and consists of five categories of items. Of the 50 items comprising the test, 10 items refer to goals (G), 10 to drives (D), 20 to vocation (V) divided equally into jobs (J) and professions (P), and 10 to status positions (S). The grouping of the items was dictated by the need to assess specific areas of human motivational behavior. Thus, items dealing with personal drives and goals attempt to tap the need for self-improvement. The status items measure needs for social recognition, a striving to compete and be successful, within the framework of the socioeconomic group to which the subject belongs. Vocational items, divided into jobs and career, represent lower and higher levels of work activities, and try to tap the individual's orientation toward his occupational fulfillment.

The second, and most important dimension of the test, encompasses the same areas of motivational behavior, but in terms of a time continuum. Thus, the same items are represented on four separate pages, first in terms of past activities, second as present self-appraisal, next as intentional learning and interests, and last, as future aspirations. Superimposed on the temporal dimension are the three basic components of motivation already described (achievement, self-appraisal, aspiration). In terms of the test structure, page one assesses patients' past achievements in terms of job (J), status (S), drive (D), profession (P), and goal (G), each containing 10 items. By asking the respondent to indicate whether he has ever engaged in these activities (see Table 10), the response is scored 1 or 2 depending on whether the answer is yes or no.

On the second page of the test, the same items are used to evaluate the subjects' present self-concept, in terms of the assessment of his ability to learn a particular skill or engage in a specific activity, independent of any commitment to actualize such behavior. The subjects' appraisals of their ability to learn, indicate self-rated competence in the five areas of motivation under study.

On the third page of the test, the subject is asked to reexamine the same items from the point of view of his present interest, that is the desire to achieve the stated potentials explored under intentional learning. The intentional learning and interests section of the test were designed to evaluate the subject's readiness for reaching goals in the near future. (The second and third pages introduce the items in terms of "could you learn? would you like?" terminology.)

The fourth page of the test asks the respondent to select from among the same items those activities which he would like to incorporate into his anticipated

Table 10
General Design of Test Items

Areas*	Motivational dimensions* (Self-appraisal)			
	Achievements	Ability to learn	Interests	Aspirations
Drives (D)	D1	D2	D3	D4
Goals (G)	G1	G2	G3	G4
Jobs (J)	J1	J2	J3	J4
Professions (P)	P1	P2	P3	P4
Status (S)	S1	S2	S3	S4

*Each of five areas consists of ten items.
†Each motivational dimension represents the five areas, consisting of ten items per area—50 items in total.

future. Thus, this section of the test is designed to measure the aspirations of the subject by selection of activities and tasks to which he is committed and which he is motivated to achieve. It is assumed that this section taps the highest level of the subject's achievement potential.

The general design of the test items is shown in Table 10a. The number accompanying the letters for each of the five areas of motivation indicates the test page number on which the specific items appear.

Table 10b shows an example of one item carried across all four motivational dimensions of past achievement, intentional learning, interest, and anticipated levels of performance.

SOCIAL STRESS AND FUNCTIONING INVENTORY FOR PSYCHOTIC DISORDERS (SSFIPD)*

Functioning Section

Adequate social functioning, broadly defined, is a constructive interplay between the individual and his social environment. On a behavioral level it is manifested as a satisfying performance of multiple social roles within the context of one's reference group. A more specific definition of social functioning in psychiatric populations and the delineation of its components is subject to the limitations of current understanding of mental health and arbitrary clinical

*The results can be found in: Serban, G.: Social stress and functioning inventory for psychotic disorders (SSFIPD): Measurement and prediction of schizophrenics' community adjustment. *Comp. Psych.*, **4, 19**: 337–346, 1978.

Table 10a

Example of one item of each category of MAAIS
across each temporal dimension

Page 1. Achievement: "Have you ever engaged"		
Cat.:* Job	(J_1)†	do office work
Status	(S_1)	lead a group
Drive	(D_1)	accept demanding tasks
Profession	(P_1)	instruct or tutor someone
Goal	(G_1)	drive a vehicle
Page 2. Intentional Learning: "Could you learn"		
	(J_2)	clerical work
	(S_2)	to direct organizations
	(D_2)	to cope with challenges
	(P_2)	how to teach
	(G_2)	how to drive (better)
Page 3. Interest: "Would you like"		
	(J_3)	typing, filing
	(S_3)	organizing people
	(D_3)	challenging situations
	(P_3)	teaching
	(G_3)	to drive vehicles
Page 4. Aspiration: "Intend to be"		
	(J_4)	an office worker
	(S_4)	a leader/manager
	(D_4)	resourceful/expedient
	(P_4)	teacher/instructor
	(G_4)	a (good) driver

*Ten items in each category per page = totaling 50 items.
†The number attached to the letter symbol shows the page designation.

standards. Despite the difficulties in establishing firm criteria for the measurement of social functioning stemming from as yet inadequately developed concepts of what is considered to be adequate social behavior and for whom, it is possible to identify areas of activity, which permit the clinician to make relatively reliable judgments about the individual's psychosocial performance. Attempts in this direction have been made by such investigators as Katz and Lyerly *(18)*, Clark *(7)*, Roen and Burnes *(27)*, and Linn *et al. (21)*.

The Katz and Lyerly scale tapped primarily clinical adjustment, that is, freedom from psychopathological symptoms as manifested in the patient's complaints and social behavior. Assessment of adequacy of social functioning was estimated on the basis of performance of occupational, social, and home responsibilities, personal adjustment and satisfaction in work, social and home areas, and general social behavior. Despite the apparent comprehensiveness of the KAS as a measure of community adjustment, the scale items sometimes

Table 10b
MAAIS
The Five Categories of Motivational Items
Presented in Their Temporal Dimensions

Past Achievement: factual self; "Have you ever engaged?"

---

    do office work (J)
    lead a group (S)
    accept demanding tasks (D)
    instruct or tutor someone (P)
    drive a vehicle (G)

Present Self-Concept: intentional learning; "Could you learn?"

---

    clerical work (J)
    to direct organizations (S)
    to cope with challenges (D)
    how to teach (P)
    how to drive (better) (G)

Present–Future Self-Concept: Interest; "Would you like?"

---

    typing, filing (J)
    organizing people (S)
    challenging situations (D)
    teaching (P)
    to drive vehicles (G)

Future-Aspiration: anticipated level of performance; "Intend to be"

---

    an office worker (J)
    a leader/manager (S)
    resourceful/expedient (D)
    a teacher/instructor (P)
    a (good) driver (G)

---

appear to suffer from vagueness which may affect the interpretation of the information sought from the patients. In seeking information from psychotic patients in general, and schizophrenics in particular, it seems crucial to address the test items to very concrete aspects of the patients' behavior, expectation, and self-attitudes. Another shortcoming of the KAS is the omission of inquiry into the extent and frequency of interpersonal relationships with important others such as family members, spouse or sexual partner, friends, and neighbors. Evaluations of employment seeking and dependence on public assistance are not made. Equally conspicuous by their absence are the quality and quantity of antisocial behavior, an important factor in community adjustment and a frequent precipitating factor in rehospitalization. In addition, the Katz scale appears to focus on current levels of community adjustment at the expense of premorbid instrumental and social performance which permits a more extensive evaluation of the patients' functioning.

The Personality and Social Network Adjustment Scale *(7)* is a self-report instrument with 17 globally defined items rated on a global 5 point scale. The items deal with adjustment in society, work, associational and family groups, and within the patient himself. As in the Katz scale, the period of assessment is restricted to the present. In addition, the scale provides limited coverage of social role performances, the most obvious omissions being represented by lack of assessment of marital and parental roles.

Roen and Burn's Community Adaptation Schedule *(27)* has the advantage of assessing both reliably and validly the behavior, affect, and cognition at work, within familial interactions (both marital and parental), and with social environment at large. It is extensive in scope (217 items) and is scored on a 6 point scale measuring intensity, attitude, and frequency. Its primary limitation is the global assessment of areas covered by the test, and its too detailed scaling of responses to be of practical use with schizophrenic patients who have difficulty dealing with too many response choices. Because it is a self-report measure and the items tend to be subject to wide range of interpretation by psychotics, this scale may have limited applicability for assessing adjustment among schizophrenics in the community, with additional difficulties emerging in its administration to hospitalized populations in acute stages of illness.

The Social Dysfunction Rating Scale (SDRS) *(21)* bypasses some of these problems by using a semistructured interview format to elicit information. The dangers inherent in a scale of this type, however, are the requirement of a skilled interviewer and the bias introduced by making clinical judgment regarding the patient's performance. Although this scale has been used with schizophrenics *(32),* it does not provide information regarding marital, parental, or extended family role functioning, and it assesses only a very brief period in the patient's life (today or last week).

One of the most glaring inadequacies in the construction of these measures is the restriction of their content to the evaluation of instrumental or affective functioning without any reference to the tensions and stresses which patients may experience in their community living. Although it cannot be denied that the level of role performance can provide a reliable indicator of the quality of the patient's interpersonal interactions and satisfactions in performance of roles, the amount of stress that may or may not be absorbed in the fulfillment of social expectation should be considered within the adjustment dimension.

This multivariate view of adjustment is even more important in the assessment of community adaptation among psychotic patients because of their inability to deal with stress.

The SSFIPD combines a comprehensive assessment of psychosocial functioning with a concomitant measure of subjectively experienced stress making it particularly relevant for the evaluation of readjustment difficulties in psychotics in general and schizophrenics in particular.

Rationale and Development of the SSFIPD

The content of the SSFIPD functioning and stress sections represent a wide sampling of daily interactions which make the instrument universally applicable to all populations. The multifactorial approach chosen for this measure also permits more detailed assessments of impairments which are useful in all outcome studies. At the same time, the item format, designed with psychotics in mind, is very concrete to compensate for the thought defect and short attention span of these patients. This type of format also minimizes misunderstanding by both the patient and the interviewer of the actual social performance level which the patient exhibits. Since psychotic patients rarely respond reliably to paper and pencil tests, the SSFIPD was designed as a structured interview with clearly delineated questions and precoded scoring guidelines.

The conceptualization of the functioning sections of the SSFIPD are partially modeled on previous adjustment scales particularly those of Roen and Burns (27) and Katz (18). The coverage of functioning extends to 21 dimensions covering not only social role performance but also antisocial behavior and detailed work history not covered in previous adjustment inventories.

It has been assumed that a meaningful assessment of psychosocial performance in psychotics has to be based on a comprehensive inventory of the individuals' activities in a variety of areas pertinent to their acceptance by the community after hospitalization. Since evaluation of the stress component is an integral part of any fruitful measurement of adjustment, the SSFIPD has a special section devoted to the assessment of stress. Unlike any other stress measures (18), the SSFIPD stress scale focuses on the experience of distress (upset) created by the patients' reaction to their life situations and the perceived nonfulfillment of their needs. It should be pointed out that the stress section of the SSFIPD, measuring subjectively experienced stress is scored and evaluated independently of the functioning section *per se*. The measure of experienced stress as designed in the SSFIPD rests on the assumption that the individual's perception of his life experience is highly personal and a systematic observation of the subjects's personal reaction to life events is required to indicate the degree of stress by the patients' inadequate coping with situations that to an outside observer may not appear stressful (22).

The SSFIPD stress scale was designed to verify both long-sustained stress and acute stress (events precipitating hospitalization). Stress stemming from impaired functioning is evaluated in terms of force (amount of experienced distress) and its effect (need for hospitalization, lowered functioning level, poor adjustment to community living).

The functioning and stress sections of the SSFIPD cover the same psychosocial behavior areas: instrumental performance, family interaction, social–interpersonal interaction and social maladaptive behavior.

Instrumental performance area, which basically evaluates the individual's ability for independent functioning and self sufficiency, has been further subdivided into the following sections: education; employment history; housekeeping ability; dependence on public assistance; management of finances; and general living circumstances. The area of family interaction attempts to measure relationship with parents, relatives, marital partner, and children. The category of social interpersonal interaction measures functioning and stress associated with relationships with opposite sex peers, dating sexual partners, close friends, neighbors, and the community at large. Within the category of antisocial activities and behavior, excessive drinking, drug abuse, and criminal behavior are measured and evaluated in terms of the stress they produce.

The basic concept underlying the measurement of functioning in the SSFIPD rests on the assumption that all individuals perceive their activities in relation to their own needs and the response of others, which gives their psychosocial behavior a particular meaning, and in the long run, predetermines their self acceptance or lack of it. Another aspect of individual functioning is based on the assumption that an individual will try to improve his performance, whether it be a result of his own need or desire for achievement and/or approval of others. It was the intention of the inventory to tap not only the patient's level of performance but also his acceptance of it.

In the preparation of the inventory, the construction of the specific items was guided by the awareness that self report of the psychiatric patient regarding specific aspects of his functioning is subject to distortion and, therefore, may represent an inadequate measure of his actual social performance, if the latter is based on commonly accepted norms. To minimize this danger each area of functioning was assessed in such a way as to provide information not only as to the presence or absence of a certain behavior, but also its frequency, duration, and the extent of interference in adequate social performance, due to the illness effects.

In addition, the items were designed to provide assessment of social functioning within specifically defined time periods, permitting the user to differentiate long standing patterns of behavior from short term effects.

The functioning section of the SSFIPD consists of 174 items used for direct assessment of the functioning level of patients. Other supportive items are also included in this section, but these serve as background for the functioning questions and help maintain the flow of the interview. The format of the 174 functioning items reflects five criteria thought to provide an indepth measurement of functioning, although their distribution may vary from one section of the inventory to another depending on the particular content of the dimension measured.

These five criteria are as follows: (1) factual evaluation of present activity and/or behavior; (2) comparison of the patients' performance with that of significant others (this type of item occurs only in the section covering instrumental performance); (3) attempt at self-improvement, occurring mainly in the evaluation of instrumental performance and socially maladaptive behavior; (4) functioning impairment due to uncontrollable events; and (5) personal appraisal of events. Examples of items reflecting each of these criteria are given in Table 11.

The specification of the different types of items for each of the 21 functioning dimensions are given below.

Table 11
Format of the Functioning and Stress Dimensions Assessed by the SSFIPD*

A.   Area—Instrument Performance: education, work, housekeeping, welfare dependence, management of finances, living circumstances

Information collected in each category	Example of the item as asked
Factual information	How far did you go in school?
Comparison with significant others	How much education do you have compared to your family as a whole?
Improvement	What have you done to improve your educational level?
Interfering situations	Why did you leave school and/or training program?
Personal appraisal of events	How well were you doing in school/job training program prior to hospitalization?
Subjective evaluation of stress	How much are you bothered (worried, distressed or upset) by the level of education you have achieved?

B.   Area—Social Interpersonal Interaction: dating, sex, relationship with close friends, neighbors, and community at large, use of leisure time, religion

Information collected in each category	Example of the item as asked
Factual information	Do you now have a girl/boy friend (steady relationship for at least 3 months)?
Interfering situations	Do you have difficulty in getting or holding a girl/boy friend?
Personal appraisal of events	How well do you get along with him/her?
Subjective evaluation of stress	How upset (bothered, worried, distressed) do you feel about that area of difficulty?

C.   Area—Family Interaction: relationship with parents, relatives, spouse, and children

Information collected in each category	Example of the item as asked
Factual information	How often are you in touch with your parents or people you consider parents?
Interfering situations	How dependent are you on your parents for emotional, social, or material support?

*Scoring: Answers to the items are scaled in terms of three possible levels of intensity, "very much" and "little or none" represent the two extremes; "somewhat" reflects the intermediate level.

Table 11 (continued)

Personal appraisal of events	How did you get along with your parents?
Subjective evaluation of stress	What kind of problems do you have with either or both of your parents that upset (bother, worry, distress) you very much?

D.   Area—Social Maladaptive Activities: excessive drinking, use of psychedelic drugs, use of addictive, drugs, and antisocial acts

Information collected in each category	Example of the item as asked
Factual information	How often do you drink?
Personal evaluation of events	What is your main reason for drinking?
Improvement	If you have tried to stop your heavy drinking, have you succeeded?
Subjective evaluation of stress	Does your drinking create serious problems with working, family life, social life, or sexual life?

In the education section, there were 16 functioning items. Of these, 4 dealt with factual information pertaining to the academic level achieved, 2 dealt with the comparison of one's education with that of close relatives, 4 provided information on the type of interferences which prevented achievement of expected educational goal, one question was directed at attempts to gain education as preparation for employment and 3 were evaluative items providing information on the level of acceptance of the respondent's educational level and achievement.

The job section of the questionnaire contains 19 functioning items, of which 7 dealt with past and present factual information regarding employment, 2 seek information on any attempts for improvement such as rehabilitation and job training, 6 inquire into the types of interference preventing adequate job performance and 4 are self-evaluative items of work performance.

The housekeeping section is a brief section, which although theoretically applicable to both sexes, is an area of functioning which does not generally affect the life of the patient to a great extent. The items in this category (5 in all) were primarily directed at the identification of interference in performance of housekeeping duties and selfevaluation of the level of performance of household tasks.

Although the section dealing with Welfare and other forms of public assistance is separated from that dealing with management of finances in the SSFIPD, both of these sections are interdependent, to some degree. The five items evaluating functioning in the section on Welfare are primarily focusing on factual information, attempting to obtain information on the extent, duration, and attitudes toward a life style based on public assistance. Improvement is not directly scored here, since forsaking Welfare dependence is considered to be a socially acceptable goal. Comparison with other close relatives regarding Welfare dependence is included in one item seeking factual information.

In the finances section, six questions deal primarily with facts on income level and source, comparison of one's financial status with that of his or her parents (specifically their attempts to save money), and evaluation of financial responsibility.

The Living circumstances section is also a brief one. Functioning is basically evaluated in terms of improvement of one's living condition.

The section dealing with parental relationships begins the evaluation of functioning along the dimension of family interaction. As in the subsequent sections of this general category, the items dealing with interference in attaining a goal become less objective as evaluation moves into the interpersonal dimension, and consequently, this item is scored under stress and is discussed later.

The functioning section concerning parents deals mainly with establishing facts regarding contact with mother and father (if living), the ability to get along with them, and with evaluation of the respondent's dependence, either financial or emotional, on the parents.

The section on relatives is similar. Functioning is basically evaluated on how well the patient gets along with his relatives, the frequency of contact maintained, and the extent of emotional and financial or social dependence.

Functioning in the marital relationship was estimated on the basis of three multiple choice questions providing information for the total of 19 items. The questions were directed toward the past and present problems leading to conflict, in past, as well as current marital relationships. These dealt with sexual difficulties, lack of support, unfaithfulness, inability to get along, interference from others, loss of love, and respondent's antisocial or irresponsible behavior. One question was used to tap the ability to discuss problems with spouse and the ability to explore feelings.

Functioning, in relationship to children, was measured by evaluation of extent of contact maintained, emotional involvement with offspring, support, and attempts at improving filial relationship.

The quality of interpersonal functioning with opposite sex peer (dating section) was measured by 5 items. These included factual information regarding attraction to opposite sex, ability to maintain the relationship, and exploration of emotional interferences in this regard.

The related section on sexual adjustment consisting of 3 items explored presence or absence of difficulties in developing a sexual relationship, type of sexual difficulties encountered, and any attempts at improvement.

Within the social life dimension of functioning, relationship with close friends was evaluated by 7 questions directed toward establishing difficulties in finding friends, the extent and duration of friendships and casual relationships, contacts with friends, and general evaluation of the quality of the relationship. Loss of friendship and reasons for it has also been determined.

Similar evaluation of functioning was obtained for relationship with neighbors. Amount and type of contact and the extent of friendliness are the basic measures.

Functioning in relationships with people in general was measured by 7 items ascertaining the degree of social isolation from others, enjoyment of participating in group activities, sharing activities with friends or acquaintances and evaluation of treatment by others.

A section on spare time interests consisting of 14 questions attempted to assess basically the extent of the patient's reading, movie attendance, involvement with TV, hobbies, and travel for pleasure. All of these items are basically factual. One evaluative item has been included dealing with assessment of travel difficulties.

A single item section on religion ascertained to frequency of church attendance and the degree of religious beliefs.

The last dimension of functioning in the SSFIPD deals with antisocial activities, subsumed under the categories of alcohol abuse, use of hard core and psychedelic drugs, and criminal behavior.

The section on drinking behavior consists of 6 functioning questions. Two of these deal with factual information such as frequency of alcohol use and the level of inebriation reached. One evaluative item deals with reasons for drinking, and one item is directed toward any efforts in ceasing alcohol abuse.

Similar distribution of items is found in the functioning sections inquiring into use of addictive and psychedelic drugs, the former consisting of 4 questions, the latter of 2. In both cases the inquiry is directed toward establishing the use of drugs, frequency of intake, reason for this behavior, and assessment of attempts to forsake the activity.

Antisocial behavior, defined primarily in terms of criminal activities, was assessed by means of 23 questions. The bulk of the items deal with arrest history, hospitalization, as a result of antisocial acts, various reasons for arrest, and evaluation of motivation underlying criminal activity.

Stress Section

The stress section of the SSFIPD, although independently scored, has been conceptualized as interrelating with the functioning level. Broadly envisioned, the stress measures of the SSFIPD evaluate the degree of imbalance between demands for psychosocial performance and the capacity for successful fulfillment of these demands. As in the case of the functioning measures, the assessment of associated stress is made in the four areas of social performance, family interaction, social interpersonal interaction, and social maladaptive behavior.

The stress items of the SSFIPD were designed to verify both long-sustained stress, primarily measured in terms of length of duration, and acute stress assessed by means of precipitating events. In addition to the aspect of duration, stress was also measured in terms of force, or quantity of distress (specific life situations evoking stress), and effect: need for hospitalization; lowered functioning level; and poor adjustment to community living.

Two additional aspects of stress were also investigated. Certain stress items were designed to identify internal stress, that is, a feeling of pressure placed by the individual on himself, due to his own projection of himself, in the psychosocial activity. The second aspect of stress, external stress, was tapped through items designed to show that the pressure experienced was due to psychosocial conditions in the life of the patient, to which he felt unable to respond constructively, and with which he was unable to cope successfully.

In order to avoid possible misinterpretation by patients of what was meant by stress, the items were worded using terms commonly associated with experience of stress. Such words as "worried," "upset," "distressed," "bothered," "feeling discomfort" were used to describe situations which created undue strain for the patient.

The evaluation of stress in each of the 21 areas subsumed under the 4 dimensions: social performance, family interaction, social interpersonal interaction, and social maladaptive behavior is discussed in more detail below.

In the area of education, the 15 stress items are addressed to worrisome preoccupation with the level of education achieved, its negative comparison to the educational achievement by the patient's family, spouse, or other significant persons, the worry associated with failing to complete school or vocational training, and by the level of one's intellectual capacity. Duration of stress associated with education and academic performance was tapped by inquiry into specific school situations which were upsetting to the patient, and the negative effect of academic achievement on the patient's self-esteem.

Stress associated with job performance was measured by 8 items focusing on being upset through current unemployment, worries and difficulties on last job and reasons for these, strain due to inability to find suitable work, and upset over the decline in working ability over the last 5 years.

Strain associated with housekeeping was measured by 2 items inquiring about upset, suffered as a result of housekeeping duties and the difficulties encountered in marketing.

Distress associated with Welfare dependence, management of finances, and living circumstances, measured by three items each focused on upset, brought about by reduced motivation to work, and lowered self esteem as result of dependence on public assistance, financial strain due to reduced income level, worries and subsequent upset precipitated by inability to handle money, discomfort experienced in dwelling place, and general strain due to having to deal with welfare authorities.

Stress associated with interaction with family members was tapped though items designed to discover which problems with parents were most upsetting to the patient (arguments regarding money, interference of parents in patient's marriage, his work, not meeting parental expectations, criticism and pressure to control by the parents, etc.). As regards stress stemming from relationship with close relatives, inquiry was made into degree of upset experienced in the relations with siblings, their refusal of help, and understanding of the patient.

Distress associated with marriage was measured in terms of past marital relationships (divorced or separated from spouse) and current marital problems (when remarried). Aside from an exhaustive list of marital problems, the patients were also asked to judge the degree of upset, due to the way the partners handled or solved their problems, and the disturbance due to the lack of the patient's spouse's concern with his problems.

For those patients who had children, the stress section evaluated the degree of upset experienced associated with the management of minor children away from home, worry about the relationship and the behavior of the children, and the feelings of guilt associated with the inability to care for the offspring.

Within the dimension of other social interpersonal relationships, stress experienced in relation to opposite sex peers, was evaluated in terms of degree of upset resulting from difficulties in obtaining and holding boy or girlfriends, uneasiness and guilt experienced in the presence of opposite sex, and lack of desire to get married.

Stress associated with sexual performance was estimated by three items focusing on worries associated with developing sexual relationships, degree of disturbance over sexual difficulties, and negative feeling about the spouse's affairs.

Stress experienced in relationship with close friends, neighbors, and others in the community, was measured in terms of upset over the degree of social alienation, the inability to obtain or hold friendships, uneasiness with others and general avoidance of participatory social activities.

Two items were directed at determining the extent of stress produced by lack of money to pursue interests and leisure activities and the strain due to difficulty in traveling.

Distress created by the religious beliefs and the race or ethnic origin of the patient was ascertained by 13 items. These basically focused on upset due to rejection or unfair treatment, precipitated either by religious affiliation or race, and spanning work, family situations, and social interactions in general.

Stress associated with antisocial activities was measured in the areas of alcohol abuse, use of drugs, and criminal activity.

Stress associated with drinking was measured in terms of problems created for the individual in the area of work, family interaction, social and sexual life; other items attempted to determine the extent to which drinking was precipitated by need to relieve anxiety as to relate socially.

Drug abuse and its accompanying stress was measured in terms of its interference with work, family, social and sexual life, and the main reason for the need for drugs.

Stress precipitated by antisocial "acting out" was measured in terms of degree of upset suffered upon arrest and conviction for criminal acts.

Psychiatric History Section

The history section of the SSFIPD contains 6 sections. The first section explores the reasons for and type of admission for the current illness. Length of onset of the illness prior to current admission and duration of onset and type of treatment received for the first mental illness episode are explored in section two. Section three is devoted to the examination of the duration of first mental illness and type of facility in which first psychiatric treatment took place. This section also explores type of treatment received. Section four inquires into length of hospitalization during the past 10 years, amount of hospitalization during the past 5 years, and during 5–10 years, prior to current hospitalization.

Section five explores the type of treatment received between hospitalizations and the extent of mental illness among family members. The last section determines the extent of upset experienced by the patient due to mental illness of his family members, delineates major life problems encountered prior to and subsequent to the age of 18, and requests an evaluation of general satisfaction with life prior to the first mental illness episode. Estimation of major stress contributing to first hospitalization is also included here.

Attitudes and Expectations (Appendix of SSFIPD)

The attitudes and expectations section of the SSFIPD has been designed to discover what the patients' attitudes toward Bellevue are, and what his or her plans may be, regarding readjustment to community living.

The section dealing with attitudes toward Bellevue focuses primarily on the perception of adequacy of treatment received, the degree of incentive for return to Bellevue in case of need of further hospitalization, and participation in outpatient treatment offered by the Hospital. Intentions regarding the following-through on discharge instructions and the extent of need for rehospitalization due to disregard of these instructions are also explored.

The major section of the Appendix is devoted to the exploration of patient's plans for extramural living. Attitudes toward and expectation of the benefits acruing from continuance of regular outpatient treatment are explored in detail. Reasons for nonattendance and beliefs in the beneficial effects of regular medication are also examined. A special section is included which explores the need for structured help in continuing medication and reasons which motivate the patient to withdraw from the prescribed medication programs.

One special section is devoted to employment plans. Here alternatives such as easing into the job market slowly, looking for a job, and remaining on public assistance are explored. Estimations of the patient's self-sufficiency, anticipation of living arrangements, preferences for social interactions, alcoholic abstinence, and drug use are also obtained.

The last section of the Appendix of SSFIPD is designed to provide a summary of attitudes and expectations and has been so phrased as to serve as a check on the consistency of the patient's answers. The accuracy check is accomplished primarily by asking for the same information in several different ways.

Scoring. The first set of scores for functioning and stress, labeled "D function" and "D stress" scores, was based only on responses which reflected the level of activity a behavior subsumed under each section of the Inventory. By contrast, the second set of scores, labled "E function" and "E stress," included both scorable responses and inapplicable items. Answers to the inapplicable items could not be coded in terms of either functioning or stress levels because the patient did not manifest a particular behavior or was not involved in a particular activity. For instance, if a patient never dates, the dating section of the SSFIPD was rated as inapplicable. The inclusion of inapplicable data in the E scoring system was based on the assumption that the absence of certain important relationships such as dating, unless the patient is already living with a mate, is indicative, however indirectly, of a poor level of social functioning of the patient.

In the derivation of D functioning and D stress scores, the precoded responses in the questionnaire were converted into scores representing three global anchor points—2 degrees of extremes and one intermediate one. Thus, for each item of the 21 dimensions of functioning and the 21 dimensions of stress a subject could earn one of three possible scores. For functioning the level of performance was scored as follows: nonfunctioning in a particular area depicted by a specific item was given a score of 1, low level of functioning a score of 2, and adequate functioning a score of 3. Level of stress was scored in the opposite direction, that is, presence of stress was assigned a score of 1, low level of stress a rating of 2, and absence of stress a score of 3. Under the scoring system in general, higher functioning scores indicated better level of functioning, whereas lower stress scores a higher level of experienced stress.

The sum of the raw scores obtained across all items within each of the 21 functioning and stress dimensions was then divided by the number of items that were rated. In this sense, the D function and D stress scores represent mean scores. The computation of these 21 mean scores for functioning (D function scores) and 21 mean scores for stress (D stress scores) was considered to be the best scoring solution to compensate for the unequal number of items within the 21 functioning and stress categories.

The E functioning and E stress scores were computed by assigning a score of 4 to each item of the SSFIPD (in whatever category of the 21 functioning and stress possibilities) whenever such item was deemed inappropriate for a patient. In this way, the E score computations are simply extensions of the D scoring system, the only modification being an addition of a score of 4 for each inappropriate item.

Inventory Versions

The inventory was prepared in two formats. One of these was designed for the interview with the patient, the other for an interview with an informant. Both versions contained identical questions, except for addition of several questions to the informant version, which sought information on the informant's view of the patient's attitudes and behaviors.

STANDARDIZATION AND RELIABILITY OF THE SSFIPD

The inventory was standardized on 130 schizophrenic patients at NYU–Bellevue Medical Center. The test–retest reliability (with a 6-month interval) of the measure, based on scores for seven dimensions of functioning computed for 78 cases ranged from 0.43 to 0.77. The correlations for the specific dimensions were: 0.48 for education; 0.43 for job; 0.51 for welfare dependence; 0.61 for alcohol abuse; 0.49 for use of psychedelic drugs; 0.77 for use of addictive drugs; and 0.68 for antisocial behavior. The items making up these seven subtests, used for establishing reliability, reflect 40% factual data and 60% attitudinal data, the latter subject to change within a 6-month interval, which may have correspondingly lowered the reliability coefficients. Interrater reliability in scoring of the individual items was measured by means of percent agreement between two independent raters and was found to range between 85% and 91%. Reliability of the obtained information was also ascertained by administering the SSFIPD to an informant (a member of the family such as parent, sibling, spouse, or an individual who has lived with the patient for at least 6 months prior to the subjects' hospitalization) and comparing the extent of agreement obtained for factual information. Computed on the basis of information gathered from 228 patients and their informants, the percent agreement ranged from 83% to 91%.

The validity of the Functioning Section of the Inventory was established based on the degree of concurrence between patients' reports and an independent source of information, in this case the close informant. This method of establishing preliminary validity is justified in light of the unavailability, at the time, of any other corresponding inventory against which the SSFIPD could be validated. This method of validation was later supported by the validation procedures used by Ellsworth et al. (10) and Gurland et al. (13) The independent source, represented by 148 close informants (parents, spouse, siblings, and other close relatives), was given the SSFIPD by a different interviewer than the one who administered the Inventory to the patient. The data from the informant and the patient were obtained on the same day in a majority of cases and, when not possible, at maximum within one week. The close informants were required to have full acquaintance with the patient to assure their intimate knowledge of the patients' behavior, attitudes, and feelings.

The correlation coefficients for the 21 functioning variables for the two sources are shown in Table 12.

There was significant agreement at minimum ($p < 0.05$) between the pairs of ratings obtained from patients and their informants on 17 out of the 21 functioning variables. The housekeeping and management of finances did not indicate a significant concurrence which can be best ascribed to the inapplicability of the items for a large proportion of the patients. The parents variable showed a low agreement indicating how little the informants know about the perception of this relationship by the schizophrenic patient. Living circumstances suggest the difficulty of informant to perceive the needs of the patient.

Validation of the Stress Section of the SSFIPD presented difficulty due to the nature of questions. Consensual validation against the informant source could not produce any significant correlation coefficients. For now the question of validity of the Stress section of the SSFIPD remains unanswered. It is possible only to assume at present that the lack of correspondence between patient and informant on stress items is due to the inability of the latter to appreciate and appraise the subjective stress experienced by the former.

Table 12
Correlation Between Patients' and Informants' Scores

Functioning variables	Correlation coefficient	p^*
Education	0.53	0.001
Job	0.38	0.001
Housekeeping	0.06	NS
Welfare dependence	0.59	0.001
Finances	0.21	NS
Living circumstances	0.25	NS
Parents	0.07	NS
Relatives	0.20	0.05
Marriage	0.27	0.05
Children	0.62	0.001
Dating	0.43	0.001
Sex	0.38	0.001
Close friends	0.26	0.01
Neighbors	0.34	0.001
Relations with others	0.17	0.05
Spare-time interests	0.33	0.001
Religion	0.30	0.001
Drinking	0.55	0.001
Addictive drugs	0.74	0.001
Psychedelic drugs	0.65	0.001
Antisocial acts	0.53	0.001

*NS, data not significant.

Part III—General Methods of Statistical Analysis

The purpose of this section is to describe basic principles and procedures of the statistical analyses used throughout this study. A number of tests, primarily The Problem Appraisal Scale, the SSFIPD, and the Test of Motivation, fully described in the last section, are complex in nature and purposely detailed to provide a maximum of information from the subject. Clinical experience indicates that evaluation of schizophrenics is not well served through the application of the statistical reductionistic model which restricts a number of variables under study. It is believed that only in investigating many areas of behavior and attitudes can one realistically appraise the realities of schizophrenic syndrome. The decision not to limit the study to a few "important" variables was further dictated by the belief that at this stage of our knowledge about schizophrenia such a preselection may preclude the investigation of those clinical aspects which may lead to the discovery of new and previously unconsidered factors in prognosis. Based on these considerations we have dealt with a wealth of data using various statistical approaches in an attempt to obtain the maximum amount of information which was in keeping with clinical realities.

Under ideal conditions all findings should be investigated by controlled experimentation; however, this in not possible because of the enormous time and resources required to conduct such studies. The findings reported in this book are based upon observed associations between specific psychosocial and emotional characteristics and schizophrenia. Randomized groups of schizophrenics (acutes and chronics) were compared to a matched socioeconomic group of normal individuals and the frequency with which personal factors were associated with the disease was recorded. Statistical methods were then employed to determine whether the observed differences were due to chance variations or to real differences between the various groups. Since the study represents a restricted population of schizophrenics at Bellevue Hospital, it was necessary to take a much higher sampling fraction of schizophrenics to controls than would be found in the general population. This manner of sampling is appropriate in our case since the classification of the disease is basically the presence or absence of schizophrenia and the objective of the research was to study etiological, psychological, and social factors as related to the course of disease. Although the computed summary statistics may vary from one hospital population to another, it is most unlikely that the magnitude and association of factors to the disease will differ greatly.

The overall aim of the study was to evaluate the predictive value of various factors considered determinant for the course of schizophrenics. In conjunction with it, it was necessary to demonstrate first that the acute chronic classification of schizophrenia is a valid one in terms of differentiating the outcome of illness. In this context the Chi-square tests have been used to test significance of differences when the data were expressed in terms of frequencies or in terms of percentages or proportions. This statistic is particularly useful when dealing with discrete data. In an attempt to differentiate acutes and chronics on various variables we set up contingency tables to test whether or not the arrays of variables were independent in the populations studied. Correlational analyses were employed whenever it was necessary to express the degree of correspondence between the values of two variables. Depending on the type of data available, three types of correlational procedures were used. The Pearson Product Moment Correlation Coefficient (r), which ranges in value from -1 to $+1$ provides two types of information. One of these is an indication of magnitude of the relationship, the other is the direction of the correspondence. When two variables are positively related, as one increases in value, so does the other. Some variables may be inversely related. Absence of a relationship is denoted by a correlation coefficient of .00 or thereabouts. The Pearsonian Correlation Coefficient is restricted to data where both variables are continuous. In some cases in the present study when one of the variables was a continuous one and the other could be conceived only as a dichotomy (yes–no, male–female) the point biserial correlation was used. This type of correlation represents a special case of the product moment correlation. Whenever the variables under study were basically continuous but were forced into a dichotomy, the tetrachoric correlation coefficient was employed. This method of obtaining information about the relationship between two variables was particularly useful when comparing responses of subjects to the most and the least important problem areas before and after the age of 18.

The second issue to be resolved was that of the extent to which functioning and stress levels of acute and chronic schizophrenics are different from each other and those of normals. To test the hypotheses regarding these differences both one-way and two-way analyses of variance were employed. Analysis of variance is a statistical technique designed to help the researcher (a) decide which of the several different kinds of variables operating simultaneously are important in differentiating the groups and (b) estimate their effects. The variations of the observations are separated into parts, each of which measures variation stemming from a specific source, included in the analysis. It can be a specific test measure, sex or age of the patient, subtype of diagnosis, etc. The intensity of the effect is measured by an F-ratio which compares variation between or among groups with that found within subject groups. In the comparisons of acute and chronic schizophrenics and normals, one-way analyses of variance were used to test significant differences between the mean values of the measures of functioning, stress, and sociodemographic determinants. Two-way analyses of variance were employed for the same three groups of subjects to determine the presence of any significant effect of functioning and stress, independent of the sex and the age of the patient, that arises from age–sex variables alone, and from a particular combination of age, sex of patient, and the functioning and stress variables. The two-way analysis of variance, thus, provides information regarding two independent factors and the effect of their interaction.

Whenever overall differences among the three groups of subjects were found to be statistically significant, as indicated by the high F-ratio, determinations of which of the pairs of comparisons has added a particular weight to the overall obtained difference were made by the Sheffe method. In such a case, acutes were compared only with chronics, chronics with normals, and acutes with normals. Whenever it was important to determine the differences in means between two groups of subjects, the t-ratio or the Student t-test was employed. In order to minimize the possibility of obtaining significant differences due to chance in computing a large number of comparisons, confidence limits were employed in evaluating data from these analyses, rather than accepting the conventional p levels of 0.05 or better.

The third related aim of the study was to determine that there are differences between schizophrenics and normals in motivational patterns. The measure specifically devised to test differences in the motivation of schizophrenics and normals required the use of factor analysis and quadratic discriminant function analysis. The principal components analysis was applied to the data obtained from the Motivation test and four factors each were extracted for the schizophrenic patients and normal controls. The orthogonal rotation (Varimax method) and the oblique rotation (Promax) yielded essentially identical structure. Factor scores derived on the basis of the principal component analysis were subsequently used in quadratic discriminant function analysis which was used to classify the population of respondents into patient and nonpatient groups on the basis of the factor scores.

Finally, the study attempted to prove that shortterm prediction of rehospitalization of acute and chronic schizophrenics is based on complex psychosocial patterns. The basic statistical approach in this context was through the use of multivariate and stepwise discriminant function techniques. The purpose of both of these techniques is to select, from a wide range of variables, a limited number of factors which best discriminate the groups under study. In a sense, the procedures provide a way of weighting the measures so as to provide a maximum separation of the groups. In the stepwise procedure the groups of subjects are compared on the most discriminating variable alone, and in an increasing combination with each of the next best discriminators until the addition of other variables fails to contribute significantly to the differentiation. In the multivariate analysis each of the variables under study is ranked in the order of importance in relation to the employed criterion, in this case short-term rehospitalization. The multivariate discriminant function analysis thus identifies the most discriminating linear combination of variables predicting this outcome. Irrespective of the type of the discriminant analysis used, the procedures were applied separately to acute and chronic populations.

In order to ascertain the effect of such extraneous variables as intelligence, years of schooling, and age and sex of the subjects on the social functioning and stress levels as well as motivational patterns regression analyses were employed. Determination of the absence of significant effects of these variables on the independent variables under study permitted a more concise evaluation of the significance of the findings derived from group comparisons on these factors.

The technique of factor analysis has been applied to the data on functioning derived from the SSFIPD in an attempt to determine the major clusters of functioning items for acute and chronic schizophrenics. The primary purpose in applying factor analysis to the data derived from the questionnaire was to reduce overlap and to determine whether or not the obtained factors could provide a set of scores which could be used in a clinically meaningful way in further group comparisons. It was believed, however, that such a reduction of items may not reflect the clinical reality regarding the social functioning of the patients and may mask some of the important variables which may operate in the phenomenon of readmission. For this reason group comparisons were made on the unreduced data derived from the SSFIPD.

REFERENCES

1. American Psychiatric Association: "Diagnostic and Statistical Manual of Mental Disorders" (2nd Ed.). Am. Psych. Assoc. Washington, D.C., 1968.
2. Barron, F.: An ego strength scale which predicts response to psychotherapy. *Journal of Consulting Psychology*, **17**: 327–340, 1953.
3. Brainard, P.P., and Brainard, T.R.: "Brainard Occupational Reference Inventory." The Psychological Corporation, New York, 1956.
4. Brown, G.W., and Birley, J.L.T.: Crises and life changes and the onset of schizophrenia. *Journal of Health and Social Behavior.* **9**: 203–214, 1968.
5. Cattell, R.B.: "The Sixteen Personality Factor Questionnaire (Form E)." Institute for Personality and Ability Testing, Champaign, Ill., 1968.
6. Cattell, R.B., Eber, N.W., and Tatsuoka, M.M.: "Handbook for the Sixteen Personality Factor Questionnaire (16 PF)." Institute for Personality and Ability Testing, Champaign, Ill., 1970.
7. Clark, A.W.: The personality and social network adjustment scale. *Human Relations*, **21**: 85–96, 1968.

8. Dixon, W.J. *et al.:* Program BMD02R, stepwise regression. *In* "Biomedical Computer Programs." pp. 233–257. Health Sciences Computing Facility, Department of Preventive Medicine and Public Health, School of Medicine, University of California, Los Angeles, 1964.

9. Duncan, O.D.: A Socioeconomic Index for All Occupations. *In* "Occupations and Social Status." (A.J. Reiss, Jr., ed.) pp. 109–138. Free Press of Glencoe, New York, 1962.

10. Ellsworth, R.B., Foster, L., Childers, B., Arthur, G., and Kroeker, D.: Hospital and community adjustment as perceived by psychiatric patients, their families and staff. *Journal of Consulting Psychology Supplement* 32 (No. 5, part 2), 1968.

11. Epstein, S., and Coleman, M.: Drive theories of schizophrenia. *Psychosomatic Medicine* 32: 114–141, 1970.

12. Ferguesan, T.: "Statistical Analysis in Psychology and Education." McGraw Hill, New York, 1966.

13. Gurland, B.J., Yorkston, N.J., Goldberg, K., Fleiss, J.L., Sloane, R.B., Cristol, A.H.: The structured and scaled interview to assess maladjustment (SSIAM). II. Factor analysis, reliability and validity. *Arch. Gen. Psychiat.* 27: 264–267, 1972b.

14. Harmon, J.J.: "Modern Factor Analysis." pp. 295–296. University of Chicago Press, Chicago, Ill., 1966.

15. Hermans, H.J.M.: A questionnaire measure of achievement motivation. *J. Appl. Psych.* 34: 353–361, 1970.

16. Holmes, T.S., and Rahe, R.H.: The social readjustment rating scale. *J. Psychosomatic Res.* 11: 213–217, 1967.

17. Institute for Personality and Ability Testing: Standardization Table for Form E of the 16 Personality Factor Test. Just for Personality and Ability Testing: Champaign, Ill.: August, 1971.

18. Katz, M.M., and Lyerly, S.B.: Methods for measuring adjustment and social behavior in the community. I. Rationale, description, discriminative validity and scale development. *Psychol. Rep.* 13: 503–535, 1963.

19. Korchin, S.J.: Stress. *In* "The Encyclopedia of Mental Health" (A. Deutch and H. Fishman, eds.), Franklin Watts, New York, 1963. Vol. 6, pp. 1975–1982.

20. Langfeldt, G.: The prognosis in schizophrenia. *Acta Psychiat. Scandinavica* (Supplement) 110, (1–66), 1956.

21. Linn, M.W., Sculthorpe, W.B., Evje, M., Slater, P.H., Goodman, S.P.: A social dysfunction rating scale. *J. Psychiat. Res.* 6: 299–306, 1969.

22. Mechanic, D.: Problems in Developing a Social Psychology of Adaptation to Stress. *In* "Social and Psychological Factors in Stress" (J.E. McGrath, ed.) pp. 104–123. Holt, Rinehart and Winston, Inc., New York, 1970.

23. Michaux, W.W., Gansereit, K.H., McCabe, O.L., and Kurland, A.A.: The psychopathology and measurement of environmental stress. *Community Mental Health Journal,* 3: 358–372, 1967.

24. Pasamanick, B., Scarpitti, F.R., and Dinitz, S.: "Schizophrenics in the Community. An Experimental Study in the Prevention of Hospitalization." Appleton-Century Crofts, New York, 1967.

25. Paull, A.E.: On a preliminary test for pooling mean squares in the analysis of variance. *Ann. Mathematical Statistics* 21: 539–556, 1950.

26. Press, S.J.: "Applied Multivariate Analysis." Holt, Rinehart and Winston, Inc., New York, 1972.

27. Roen, S.R., and Burnes, A.J.: "Community Adaptation Schedule Preliminary Manual." Behavioral Publications, Inc., New York, 1968.

28. Scheffe, H.: "The Analysis of Variance." pp. 362–363. John Wiley & Sons, Inc., New York, 1959.

29. Spitzer, R.L., and Endicott, J.: "Problem Appraisal Scales." Evaluation Section, Biometric Research, New York State Department of Mental Hygiene, New York, 1969.
30. U.S. Department of Labor, Bureau of Labor Statistics.: Work Experience of the Population, 1969. *Special Labor Force Report* **127,** pp. A–12, 1971.
31. Vaillant, J.: Prospective prediction of schizophrenic remission. *Arch General Psych.,* **11:** 509–517, 1964.
32. Weissman, M.: The assessment of social adjustment. A review of techniques. *Arch. General Psychiat.* **32:** 357–365, 1975.

CHAPTER 3

Value of Sociodemographic Data for Prediction of Outcome in Schizophrenia*

In the search for differentiating criteria for good and poor prognosis in schizophrenia, sociodemographic characteristics have received wide currency, particularly before the use of psychotropic drugs. However, age, education, occupation, work history, and marital status have continued to maintain a relevant and allegedly meaningful prognostic status. Let's see to what extent these assumptions are still valid.

AGE

One of the most frequently employed demographic characteristics has been age at the onset of illness, since schizophrenia itself, defined as dementia praecox attested to the early appearance of the disease. Although Bleuler *(4)* widened the concept of schizophrenia to include various groups of psychoses under the same title, age not only persisted as a significant variable in its prognosis, but also gained additional importance. Patients who developed schizophrenia at age 30 or later were assumed to have better prognosis than those who exhibited the illness under the age of 30. Empirically, it was known that the disease process was more damaging to a personality who still continues to grow and remold (until the third decade of life) than to the more firmly set and mature personality of an older individual. In the evolution of the concept of schizophrenic illness, a further distinction was made between adult and childhood schizophrenia, which has a direct bearing on prognosis *(3)*.

For adult schizophrenics, age still holds relevance inasmuch as the age at the onset appears to influence the course of the lifetime social adjustment of the

---

*The research results presented in this chapter have appeared in the following article: Serban, G., and Gidynski, C.B.: Significance of social-demographic data for rehospitalization of schizophrenic patients. *J. Health Social Behavior* **15**: 117–126, 1974 *(34)*.

patients. It was observed that schizophrenics developing symptoms at an early age, (20 years of age or younger), had a significantly poorer outcome than did those who became ill at a more advanced age (40 years or older) *(2)*. Ødegaard *(27)* also reported that low age at first admission correlated significantly with poor outcome.

On the basis of more documented research, Klein and Klein *(17)* determined that separation of onset of illness before or after the age of 23, permitted the authors to differentiate the readmitted and the nonreadmitted patients according to earlier and later onsets. Rosen *et al. (33),* in a related study, found further support for the relationship between early age of symptom onset and rehospitalization and demonstrated that a higher proportion of patients receiving treatment for schizophrenia, prior to age 23, tended to be rehospitalized, irrespective of other indicators of premorbid competence, than those receiving treatment after the age of 23. Stephens *et al. (38)* reported that onset of schizophrenia at age 20 or later serves as a good prognostic indicator. Perhaps some of the discrepancies in cut-off age scores stems from the fact that younger patients may be discharged earlier and more rapidly, since they are likely to have parents who assume care of them. This is particularly true when length of hospitalization is used as a criterion of outcome; in such a situation age may become an epiphenomenon of discharge policy, rather than a realistic measure of illness outcome.

The evidence regarding age and prognosis is by no means unequivocal. Other researchers tend to present evidence that low age at first hospitalization is not always related to poor outcome. Shofield *et al. (36),* for example, suggested that schizophrenics earning good posthospitalization adjustment ratings and who had no rehospitalization within 5 years of their original discharge, had lower mean age and a more restricted age range than did the patients who had poor outcomes (rehospitalization for 50% of the time since key admission, and difficulties requiring constant care). By the same token, Gabriel *(12),* in comparing the long-term course of schizophrenia arising late in life, with that of early onset, found that late onset schizophrenics tend to have poorer social adjustment and more chronicity than those whose onset appears at an earlier age. Gabriel interpreted his findings in light of old age complications present in his experimental group.

Reporting on the relationship of long-term hospitalization of schizophrenic patients in West Germany, Hartmann and Meyer *(15)* indicated that the average age at admission that leads to long-term hospitalization was 39.1 years. If risk of permanent hospitalization becomes an important factor in the prognostic evaluation of schizophrenia, this risk apparently increases with age.

However, in a recent study of a long term follow up of schizophrenics, Huber *et al. (21a)* found no direct relationship between the age at onset of the disease and the prognosis. A slight tendency for a more unfavorable prognosis was found when the onset of the disease took place in the patient's forth decade of life. Using still another criterion of outcome, the remission of schizophrenic symptoms in acute patients within 6 months of hospitalization, Walker and Kelley *(40)* found age to be a nonsignificant predictor variable.

It would appear that the relationship between age and prognosis in schizophrenia is especially confounded by the use of various outcome criteria, some of which may mask the particular effect of this variable.

EDUCATION

Educational level, per se, has received less attention as a specific prognostic indicator in schizophrenia. Traditionally, educational achievement has been combined with other demographic factors such as occupation under the rubric of social class. It is interesting to note, however, that when education was studied as one of the factors in prognosis, with the stringent criterion of outcome, i.e., social adjustment from 5 to 11 years of hospital discharge, no significant differentiation between good and poor outcome groups was obtained *(37)*. Using three separate criteria of outcome: discharge, within 6 months of admission; remission of schizophrenic symptoms (improved); and community tenure for 1 year after discharge (recovered), Walker and Kelley *(40)* found that the educational level in chronic schizophrenics was positively associated with the discharge criterion, but it did not predict readmission. For the acute patients, educational achievement was found to be a significant predictor of release within 6 months but, again, not significantly related to the remission of schizophrenic symptoms. It was suggested that the association between educational level and release may be an artifact of the intellectual level of the patient. Yet, Huber *et al.* *(21a)* in his 2-year follow-up study found that the individuals who received a higher education have a less severe schizophrenic psychological deficit, only 27.2%, while the noneducated have up to 50%. He assumes that there is a positive correlation between intelligence before disease and psychopathiological remission. Low intelligence with a corresponding poor school record handicaps the social adjustment of schizophrenics in the community *(15)*.

OCCUPATION

As with the educational variable, occupation as a demographic factor is traditionally subsumed under the determinant of social class. Consideration of occupational status spanning approximately 36 years of study suggests most consistently that the occupational variable reflects the incidence of schizophrenia to a greater extent than it does information regarding outcome *(8, 11, 22, 31)*. In this sense, it appears that unskilled laborers and the unemployed, or individuals in the lowest social class grouping, have the highest incidence of schizophrenia. Lowest rates for this disease have been found in managerial groups, and proprietors of small businesses or executives of large ones. Clark (8) suggests that the low prestige of the occupation increases the preschizophrenic's negative attitude toward themselves, accounting for the predominance of this illness in the lower classes. Occupation may also be viewed as reflecting general life style, values, and behavior, which may affect predispositions toward schizophrenia.

Occupational level as predictor of outcome has been considered by Astrup, Fossum, and Holmboe (2), who found that improved schizophrenic patients maintained their occupational level on a par with that of the affective psychotic patients, who have a more favorable prognosis. Astrup contended that the recovered schizophrenics were young people able to qualify, with increasing age, for better occupations. Perhaps his sample represented a group essentially less hampered by their illnesses than is generally true of most subjects in schizophrenic studies. Brown, Carstairs, and Topping (5) also demonstrated that in chronic patients, superior premorbid social achievement, in which occupational level is an important variable appears to be associated with posthospitalization success. Additional evidence of the prognostic value of occupational level comes from the research of Harris, Linker, Norris, and Sheppard (14) who found in their follow-up study that among the recovered schizophrenics, comparison of occupational status before admission and after discharge revealed little difference.

At the same time, there is some evidence that when the outcome criterion is more stringent, such as community tenure performance, occupation as a sole variable appears to be unable to differentiate good and poor outcome groups among schizophrenics (36).

WORK CAPACITY

A much more revealing prognostic indicator than occupational level is work or employment record. For the schizophrenic patient, finding and keeping a job can be considered an indication of achievement and a reflection of his social competence. This is particularly true since there is accumulating evidence that schizophrenics have difficulty in maintaining their jobs even before the florid symptoms of their illness become apparent (8a, 18). From the viewpoint of community adjustment, financial independence and self-support are perhaps the most accepted and expected aspects of adequate posthospitalization performance. It is not surprising that judgments of the patients' capacity to earn their own livings influence the clinical assessment of the patients' condition (14) and the prediction for posthospital success in the eyes of psychiatric raters. Good occupational history in the premorbid phase has been linked with good prognosis in schizophrenia (35) mainly because adequate working capacity helps keep the psychiatric patients out of the hospital (26) and bestows on them a status of a productive and active member of their community—a factor, which in the long run determines success or failure in the posthospitalization adjustment *(5)*. Corroboration of the importance of work record is further emphasized in the studies of Wirt and Simon *(41)* and Aldrich and Coffin *(1)*, who found a significant correlation between duration of productive employment and outcome. Astrup *et al. (2)*, for instance, reported that among recovered schizophrenics 82% had a good prepsychotic working capacity, whereas only 56% of the deteriorated patients manifested a similar level.

MARITAL STATUS

Marital status appears to be associated with both the incidence and outcome of schizophrenia. There is ample evidence that married persons have a lower first admission rate for schizophrenia than do the single, separated, divorced and widowed *(23, 24, 25)*. These differences are perceived as stemming from social factors associated with the availability of support and a home for married individuals as well as differential malignancy of the illness in the never married as compared with the married persons, which is often reflected in the age of onset. Such explanations appear to be all the more plausible in view of evidence that married schizophrenics tend to be discharged earlier and have comparatively shorter hospital stays *(27)*. As regards outcome, marital status has been demonstrated to be the best single demographic predictor in schizophrenic illness *(17)*.

This is not surprising when one considers that marriage reflects higher levels of premorbid adjustment, particularly on the interpersonal level. The investigation of Klein and Klein *(17)* provided ample evidence that the significance of marital status in prognosis reduces primarily to the better premorbid adjustment of the married patients, indicates only the presence of less severe asocial personality traits. Thus, presence of marriage as a prognostic sign appears to reflect the confluence of better premorbid functioning and personality traits rather than a demographic status, per se.

Presence of a marital partner also provides certain motivations and pressures for more adequate performance upon the return to the community. Sherman, Mosely, and Ging *(35)* have shown, for example, that the presence of a spouse in the community motivates the patient toward a more rapid recovery and is associated with lower rates of readmission *(27)*. The investigations of Farina, Garmezy, Zalusky, and Becker *(10)* and of Shofield, Hathaway, Hastings, and Bell *(36)* have shed further light on the role of marital status in prognosis. Farina *et al.* accounted for the prognostic significance of marital status in terms of social aspects of recent sexual life and the history of personal relationships in marriage among the recovered and unrecovered schizophrenics. These investigators demonstrated that it may not be the marital status which becomes the differentiating variable but rather the level of psychosocial premorbid adjustment which determines, in part, the patient's outcome. Corroborating evidence comes from the study of Shofield *et al.* *(36)* who found superior marital adjustment in the good outcome group, particularly affection for the spouse. It is interesting to note, however, that in their study, no differentiation between the good and poor group was obtained when the variable of marital status was considered, independent of the factor of marital adjustment. This may explain why some investigators have failed to obtain significant association between marital status and outcome of schizophrenic illness *(40)*.

It is reasonable to assume that sociodemographic characteristics may not only reflect underlying premorbid functioning levels of the patients but also tend to interact with one another, producing differential predictive effects. Age of the patient at the onset of illness has a particular influence on all other demographic factors in the final prediction equation. Early onset of schizophrenic symptoms certainly affects the acquisition of social and instrumental skills, comprising such demographic factors as education, level of occupational achievement, and working ability.

The awareness of this interactive effect has led Phillips and Zigler *(30)* to devise a theoretical framework that would meaningfully encompass biographical and sociodemographic data and provide a unifying explanatory principle for the alleged significance of case history items for prognosis. The central guiding principle in this endeavor has been the developmental approach to psychopathology, with personal and social maturity as the central pivot of this approach.

In the Phillips and Zigler view, a person progresses through successive levels of maturity, and individuals differ in the final maturation levels attained. At each phase, the individual must cope with complex tasks presented by society; some cope successfully and others deal with them inappropriately. Psychopathology represents, according to Phillips and Zigler, the inappropriate solutions to societal demands. The major emphasis of their approach focuses on the adaptive potential of the individual and the appropriate resolution of adaptive difficulties at any given level. Ideally, this represents maturity. Since a comprehensive index of maturity is difficult to construct, Phillips and Zigler unified the pertinent sociodemographic characteristic which showed prognostic promise under a concept of social competence. It was their contention that the variables of age, intelligence, education, occupation, employment history, and marital status provide an approximation of personal and social maturity, in that these variables reflect socioeconomic potential and likelihood of fulfillment of age and sex role expectations *(42)*. In a series of articles, Zigler and Phillips were able to show that premorbid social competence was associated with gross symptomatic pictures presented by process and reactive schizophrenics *(44)*, prognosis *(42)*, type of diagnosis received in a variety of psychiatric disorders, and outcome *(42)*. Using a broad and representative sample of schizophrenics, Turner and Zabo *(39)* found support for the relationship between time spent in hospital and social competence index, suggesting that the competence index may be of value as a practical tool in predicting hospital outcome.

In a cross-validation study of schizophrenic and other psychiatric patients, Rosen *et al.* *(33)* demonstrated that although social competence index predicted incidence of rehospitalization and, therefore, appeared useful as a predictor of outcome, its predictive value seemed to be confounded by the factor of age at first psychiatric treatment contact. Those whose illness appeared before age 23 had significantly poorer outcomes than those whose onset occurred after age 24. The authors suggested that although they found a positive relationship between social competence, as measured by the Zigler and Phillips index *(42)* and post-hospital outcome of schizophrenic patients, this association appeared to be entirely attributed to the age of the patient at his first psychiatric treatment.

It is quite plausible that the onset of illness at a later age would permit the patient to further his adult social attainment, increase his level of maturity, and develop more social skills which influence the outcome of schizophrenic illness by contributing significantly to readjustment after hospitalization. At the same time, the Rosen *(32, 33)* study of social competence in relation to both course and outcome of psychiatric illness has suffered from inclusions of broad psychiatric diagnoses, some of which have generally better prognoses than others; a fact which may have seriously affected the findings. In this particular study, the measure of social competence appears to be predictive of posthospital outcome of schizophrenics but not those with affective and character disorders.

From the clinical point of view, schizophrenia, affective disorders, and character disorders have a different course and outcome and, therefore, should not be used conjointly except as control groups. The confounding of the experimental group with a gamut of psychiatric disorders appears to be inherited from the original studies of Zigler and Phillips *(42)*, who viewed mental illness as a continuous process in which initial, middle, and final stages are meaningfully related *(44)*, and the psychopathologies are seen as variations of inappropriate solutions along the maturity dimension *(28, 39)*. In addition, another complicating factor in their studies is the unknown effect of medication on the outcome as related to sociodemographic variables.

It is our contention that some of the confusion regarding the prognostic validity of sociodemographic characteristics, whether considered singly or in an index of competence, as suggested by Phillips and Zigler *(30)*, may be clarified when these are studied in relation to well-defined diagnostic entities with predictable trends for community integration. We basically consider the Phillips and Zigler social competence construct to be of prognostic significance for schizophrenia, but not for other psychiatric syndromes, such as schizo-affective and affective disorders which appear more resilient in the course of illness. To the extent to which schizophrenics tend to remain with the chronic thinking disorder, even in a period of remission, the ability of these patients to readjust socially at a new level of functioning after hospitalization is minimal; the social competence gained in the premorbid phase becomes highly significant for their future adjustment to the community. Of course, the more extensive the period of hospitalization, and the greater the impairment suffered by the schizophrenic patient, the more difficult it is for him to function at his premorbid level upon release.

In view of the above considerations, we conducted a study relating social competence to outcome in two groups of schizophrenic patients, acute (first admission) and chronic (multiple hospitalization). The selection of acute and chronic schizophrenics was dictated by the following considerations: acute schizophrenics represent a clinical group consisting of some patients who will progressively deteriorate and in time become chronic schizophrenics. The acute group of patients also harbor those individuals who have less certain outcomes, particularly patients diagnosed schizo-affective (13.6% in our sample) and acute schizophrenic episode (40% in the study). The chronic schizophrenic group (in our case patients with the average of 3.63 hospitalizations) can be considered to have generally poor prognosis.

The sociodemographic variables employed in the study: age, education, occupation, and marital status were comparable to those used by Zigler and Phillips *(42)* in the construction of their social competence scale. Whereas their index contained six variables: age, intelligence, education, occupation, employment, and marital status, the present index was restricted to four variables: education, employment, occupation, and marital status. While intelligence was omitted because such data was unavailable for the samples studied, age was excluded on the basis of a regression analysis that showed that it was linearly unrelated to education, employment history, marital status, or dependence on welfare assistance in our population. The distribution of age in terms of the categories among the chronics (under 25, 25–44, and 45 or older), suggested by Zigler, was such that most of the sample (68.2%) fell into the middle range leaving few patients in the other extreme of the distribution (23.3% under 25 years of age; 8.5% 45 years or older), which would not provide an adequate test of the effect of age. Age for acutes showed a skewed distribution with the majority of cases (45.6% and 49.6%) falling in the first 2 age categories. In addition, age was eliminated from the index, since it was impossible to obtain the age at onset of illness for the chronic group, and present age is not a variable in the Zigler Phillips Scale. Deletion of age also permitted the determination of the weight of other variables in the social competence index and indirectly tested the Rosen *et al. (32)* hypothesis that social competence dimension reduces basically to age.

The possible effect of sex of the patient on his level of social competence was determined by means of two-way analysis of variance with sex and the variables of education, marital status, occupation, and employment comprising the two factors. The results disclosed no significant effect of sex on the social demographic factors considered.

Having determined that age and sex do not appear to influence the instrumental functioning of the patients, the variables of education, unemployment, occupation, and marital status obtained from the case histories of the patients at the time of admission to the project were used to construct a sociodemographic index along the lines suggested by Zigler and Phillips *(43)* for their social competence scale. Categorization of each of the four variables and their scoring values are given in Table 1.

Table 1

Description and Scoring Values of Sociodemographic Index Variables

Variable		Category	Score
Education	1.	7–11 years of school completed	0
	2.	Completed High School	1
	3.	13–15 years of school completed	1.5
	4.	15 + years of school completed	2
Employment	1.	Unemployed, receiving Welfare	0
	2.	Unemployed, no Welfare	0.5
	3.	Employed, part-time	1
	4.	Employed full-time (included housewives and students)	2
Occupation*	1.	Unskilled	0
	2.	Semi-skilled, manual	0.5
	3.	Skilled, manual	1
	4.	Semi-professional	1.5
	5.	Professional, administrative managerial	2
Marital Status	1.	Divorced (includes separated and widowed)	0
	2.	Single and homosexual	1
	3.	Married (includes common-law)	2

*Individual occupations were classified into these categories on the basis of the Dictionary of Occupational Titles (United States Government Printing Office, 1960).

The sociodemographic index provided two sets of scores. Each patient was first assigned four scores based on the ratings earned for each of the categories: education, employment, occupation, and marital status. The four scores representing each of the four areas of competence were subsequently averaged, producing for each individual, his total index score. The averaging procedure was necessitated by the fact, that for some patients, no score could be assigned in some of the four categories comprising the index. Once the individual total index scores were computed, they were grouped into three categories assumed to reflect three levels of social attainment defined as follows: Category 1 (low social attainment based on the average score of 0); Category 2 (medium social attainment based on the average score of 1); and Category 3 (high attainment, based on the average score of 2).

Since the sample of schizophrenics used in the study was composed of acute and chronic cases representing varying length and duration of illness, it was deemed important to compare sociodemographic data of these two groups, independent of outcome. The distributions of the variables of education, marital status, occupation, and employment status were compared for the 125 acutes and the 516 chronic schizophrenics by means of chi-square tests of independence. The comparisons revealed no significant differences between acute and chronic cases in terms of educational achievement ($X^2 = 3.74; df\ 2; p > 0.05$) or marital status ($X^2 = 3.32; df\ 2; p > 0.05$). As regards occupational attainment, a higher proportion of acute patients were classified in the skilled and professional category than their chronic counterparts, who predominated within the unskilled occupational brackets ($X^2 = 8.77; df\ 3; p < 0.05$). Comparisons of employment history for acute and chronic cases revealed that a higher number of acute patients had a housewife or student status or were employed and did not depend on public assistance than the chronic group ($X^2 = 22.56; df\ 3; p < 0.001$). It is of interest to note that, at least in this sample of schizophrenics, acutes and chronics show significant differences in two important facets of instrumental functioning that appear to be independent of outcome.

Table 2

Distribution of Social Competence Scores for Chronic and Acute Schizophrenics and Normal Controls for Key Admission and Follow-up Samples

Sample	N	Score 1		Score 2		Score 3	
		N	%	N	%	N	%
Chronics							
Key admission	516	267	51.7	189	36.6	60	11.6
Follow-up	349	184	52.7	127	36.4	39	11.2
Acutes							
Key admission	125	40	32.0	61	48.8	24	19.2
Follow-up	70	20	28.6	34	48.6	14	20.0
Normals	95	15	12.0	29	23.2	51	40.1

Before the relationship between social competence scores and outcome could be determined, it was necessary to establish whether or not the follow-up sample was comparable with the original schizophrenic cohort in terms of the variables studied. This was particularly so since 32.4% of the chronics and 44.0% of the acutes were lost to the follow-up, primarily due to change in residence. As can be seen in Table 2, the distributions of acute and chronic subjects within the three index categories were very similar for the original and follow-up sample. Among the chronics, 51.7% of the original and 52.7% of the follow-up samples were in the low social attainment category (Category 1); 36.6% of the original chronics and 36.4% of the follow-up chronics were classified into Category 2 (medium attainment); and 11.6% and 11.2% were represented in the high attainment category (Category 3), for original and follow-up chronic cases, respectively. Of the 125 acutes in the original study sample, 32.0% were classified in Category 1 of the index, 48.8% in Category 2, and 19.2% in Category 3. For the group of 70 acutes available to the follow-up, the percentages were 28.6%, 48.6%, and 20.0%, respectively. These results strongly suggest that the follow-up samples were indeed representative of the larger population from which they were drawn.

For the purposes of determining the relationship between case history data and outcome, the 70 acute and 349 chronic patients in the follow-up sample were divided into readmitted and nonreadmitted groups and compared by means of 2×3 contingency tables, in terms of the three categories reflecting the levels of social attainment. Results of these analyses were shown in Table 3.

Table 3

Distribution of the Combined Sociodemographic Scores for
Readmitted and Nonreadmitted Chronic and Acute Schizophrenics

Samples	N	Category 1		Category 2		Category 3	
		N	%	N	%	N	%
Chronics (total)	349						
Readmitted	258	147	57.0	87	33.7	25	9.3
Nonreadmitted	91	37	40.7	40	44.0	14	15.3
		$X^2 = 7.44; p < 0.05$					
Acutes (total)	70						
Readmitted	31	10	32.3	15	48.5	6	19.3
Nonreadmitted	39	12	30.8	19	48.7	8	20.5
		$X^2 = 0.033; p > 0.05$					

Examination of Table 3 reveals that a significantly higher proportion of the chronics who are readmitted (57%) were classified in Category 1 of the sociodemographic index (low social attainment) than were the nonreadmitted counterparts (40.7%). The nonreadmitted chronic patients had proportionally more individuals who were categorized in the medium and high social attainment categories (44.0% vs. 33.7% for Category 2 and 14.3% vs. 9.3% for Category 3). These differences appear to be significant as confirmed by a X^2 of 7.44 ($p < 0.05$).

Among the acute patients, sociodemographic categorization into the three levels of social achievement appears to be unrelated to outcome status ($X^2 = 0.03; p < 0.05$). The data suggests that for the acute group of patients in this study, outcome, as measured in terms of readmission within 2 years, cannot be reliably predicted from the level of premorbid social attainment, as measured by the sociodemographic categories.

To ascertain whether or not the obtained results with chronics reported in Table 3 may be affected by the fact that this group of readmitted patients consisted of individuals readmitted only after the first 6 months of observation

($N = 114$), as well as persons who were very frequently readmitted during the same interval (some as many as 15 times; $N = 144$), and thus representing a clinically different subsample of schizophrenics, the analysis was repeated limiting the readmitted group to those rehospitalized only after the first 6 months of observation.

Comparison of the 114 readmitted chronic patients and their 91 nonrehospitalized counterparts is shown in Table 4.

Table 4

Distribution of Combined Sociodemographic Scores for Readmitted and Nonreadmitted Chronic Schizophrenics*

Groups	N	Score 1 N	Score 1 %	Score 2 N	Score 2 %	Score 3 N	Score 3 %
Readmitted Schizophrenics	114	69	60.5	36	31.6	9	7.9
Nonreadmitted Schizophrenics	91	37	40.6	40	44.0	14	15.4

*$X^2 = 24.50; p < 0.001$.

As in the analysis using all the readmitted chronic schizophrenics, persons classified in Category 1 (low social attainment) were significantly more prone to readmission (60.5% vs. 40.6%) than were those in Category 2 (medium attainment 31.6% vs. 44.0%) or in Category 3 (high social attainment 7.9% vs. 15.4%). These differences appear to be quite reliable ($X^2 = 24.50$; df 2; $p < 0.001$). Elimination of the frequently readmitted group of chronics appears not to have changed the direction of the results, although it made the differentiation considerably more pronounced.

In order to delineate more precisely the individual contribution of each of the factors contributing to the overall value of the social demographic index, the variables of education, marital status, occupation, and employment were considered in relation to outcome status of both chronic and acute patients. For each of the studied variables, the proportion of subjects falling into the readmitted and nonreadmitted groups reflect the same categorization of the demographic factors as were used in establishing the individual scores on the index.

The educational level of chronic schizophrenics categorized into three levels, 7–11 grades completed, high school completed, and 13 years of schooling or higher, was found to be unrelated to readmission status ($X^2 = 3.90$; df 2; $p > 0.05$) and apparently does not have much value as an outcome predictor within the present sample of chronic schizophrenics.

The relationship between marital status and outcome for chronic schizophrenics is shown in Table 5.

Table 5

Marital Status by Readmission Status for Chronic Schizophrenics*

	N	Single		Separated		Married	
		N	%	N	%	N	%
Readmitted	258	158	61.3	79	30.6	21	8.1
Nonreadmitted	91	42	46.2	31	34.1	18	19.7

*$X^2 = 11.09; 2\, df; p < 0.01.$

Results of the 3 × 2 comparisons revealed a definite relationship between readmission and marital status ($X^2 = 11.09; df\, 2; p < 0.01$). Single patients tend to be most prone to readmission (61.3% readmitted, 46.2% nonreadmitted), whereas the married ones appear to be least rehospitalized (8.1% readmitted vs. 19.7% nonreadmitted). The status of being separated does not appear to contribute significantly to readmission in the present chronic sample.

Analysis of the relationship between occupation categorized into unskilled (including the never employed), semi-skilled manual (including housewives and students), and the skilled, managerial, and professional; and rehospitalization of chronic patients is shown in Table 6.

Table 6

Occupation by Readmission Status for Chronic Schizophrenics*

Group	N	Never Employed and Unskilled		Semi-skilled manual, and students–housewives		Skilled and professional	
		N	%	N	%	N	%
Readmitted	258	196	76.0	19	7.4	43	16.6
Nonreadmitted	91	57	62.7	9	9.9	25	27.4

*$X^2 = 6.68; 2\, df; p < 0.05.$

The 2 × 3 contingency table comparisons revealed that a significantly greater proportion of the readmitted chronics, 76.0% were either in unskilled occupations or were never employed, as compared with those not rehospitalized (62.7%). Similarly, 27.4% of the nonreadmitted, as compared with 16.6% of the readmitted, had skilled or professional occupations. The obtained differences may be considered quite reliable ($X^2 = 6.68; df\, 2; p < 0.05$) for this sample.

The last comparison, that of readmitted and nonreadmitted chronic patients with their employment records, revealed that when this variable was classified into dependence on welfare, unemployed status, part-time employment, and full-time employment (including housewives and students), work record did not contribute significantly to prediction of readmission ($X^2 = 6.18$; $df\ 3$; $p > 0.05$). In order to determine whether or not the attenuation of the work history variable led to the nondifferentiation of the groups, two additional chi-square tests of independence were performed comparing readmitted and nonreadmitted chronic patients in terms of three categories of work record. First the analysis considered employment history in terms of: welfare dependence, unemployment, and full-time employment. Part-time employment status was included in the full-time employment category. The results shown in Table 7, indicate that dependence on welfare appears to contribute most significantly to readmission in chronic schizophrenics and employment appears to be associated with nonrehospitalization ($X^2 = 8.25$; $df\ 2$; $p < 0.02$). In the second comparison, part-time employment was included in the unemployment category; similar results were obtained ($X^2 = 8.49$; $df\ 2$; $p < 0.02$). Both analyses suggest that of all the work history categories considered, it is the dependence on welfare which appears to contribute the greatest weight to the differentiation between readmitted and nonreadmitted chronics.

Table 7

Employment History by Readmission Status for Chronic Schizophrenics*

Group	N	Welfare		Unemployed		Employed	
		N	%	N	%	N	%
Readmitted	258	130	51.6	68	24.6	60	23.8
Nonreadmitted	91	30	37.5	33	20.0	28	42.5

*$X^2 = 8.25$; $2\ df$; $p < 0.02$.

Comparisons for the acute schizophrenics also based on 2×3 contingency tables for the 4 demographic variables failed to yield significant association with readmission status. The results unequivocally indicate that none of the sociodemographic variables single, or in combination, appear to be associated with outcome in acute schizophrenics.

The results strongly suggest that of the four variables comprising the sociodemographic index used in this study, education and employment record did not contribute significantly to prediction of readmission. It is interesting to note, however, that in connection with work record, it is the status of being on welfare that bears an important relationship to need for rehospitalization. In line with previous evidence, marital status appeared to differentiate readmitted and nonreadmitted chronic schizophrenics at the higher level of significance, with the remaining variable of occupation adding significantly to the overall prediction.

DISCUSSION

Although in the past, sociodemographic characteristics were assumed to form a meaningful cluster of social functioning variables predicting community tenure of schizophrenics, our study indicates that this is not necessarily the case. The results of the present study clearly show the inapplicability of the social competence dimension, as defined by the four factors of education, marital status, occupation, and work history, to prediction of outcome in acute or first hospitalized schizophrenics. Several factors may account for this. First, the acute group of patients, although diagnosed schizophrenic upon admission, may well include a conglomerate of schizophrenic-like forms (episodic) and true schizophrenia, either one of these groups presupposes a different prognosis. It is only with time that some of these patients will show the chronic course, while others, particularly if they are diagnosed schizo-affective, may not do so *(9)*. Futher discussion of the issue of diagnosis as it bears on outcome can be found in Chapter 8. Second, the social competence data may reflect the degree of social functioning impairment at a particular point in the continuum of the psychotic process. The acute group, younger and less exposed to the detrimental effects of multiple hospitalizations is still able to maintain its occupational category upon returning to the community. The acute patient, at the end of the first hospitalization, is more likely to retain the skills and thus be given an opportunity to resume his various social roles. The psychotic episode of the acute patient, responsible for his hospitalization, is usually short in duration and thus it is not likely to affect his general social functioning at this point in time. At the same time, the acute patients have closer ties with their families and receive greater financial support from this source than do the chronic schizophrenics.

Even with respect to chronic schizophrenics the prediction of community tenure on the basis of the cluster of sociodemographic variables appears somewhat tenuous. Although the index based on the four variables of education, occupation, work history, and marital status statistically differentiates the readmitted and the nonreadmitted chronic patients, the results show that educational level carries no significant predictive weight. Only marital status (being single), unskilled occupation (no employment history), and dependence on welfare appear to be the salient factors in readmission. A consideration of the underlying nature of these variables used in the index of social competence provides important clues as to why they have gained prominence in prediction of community adjustment of schizophrenics and other psychiatric patients.

Education, for instance, and marital status may be thought of as static factors of social competence, since they are often established before the schizophrenic process begins to unfold and appear to be subject to minimal variation afterwards. Since both of these factors precede the onset of the illness in most cases, they are not likely to be upgraded by the process of the illness itself. In fact, marital status has a good chance to be negatively affected by the illness process. Although education, in this review, cannot be expected to serve as a meaningful predictor of outcome, marital status is a complex variable which may operate in prediction in subtle ways. As Hammer *(13)* has shown, a married schizophrenic patient is more likely to be reaccepted by the family unit after hospitalization and may be more motivated to resume his family role and responsibilities than his single counterpart, for whom such expectations are nonexistent. The notion that the married schizophrenic patient's better outcome is a reflection of his response to external supports, as well as pressures and expectations of his mate, has also been suggested by the research of Garfield and Sundland *(12a)*. Another factor affecting the often obtained relationship between marital status and outcome may be the tendency, on the part of psychiatrists, to discharge a schizophrenic patient more readily and at an earlier time in care of a marital partner, than into his own care. This limits the married schizophrenic's length of hospital stay. Chapman *et al.* *(7)*, for instance, in studying 106 male schizophrenics, found that marital status predicted rapid discharge from the hospital. Obviously, marital status may cease to be a positive outcome variable in case of divorce, which in itself indicates the inability of the spouse to deal with the patient's aberrant behavior.

Some recent research has addressed itself to the question of whether or not marital status is a meaningful predictor, independent of the level of premorbid functioning which it may reflect. In keeping with previous studies, Klein and Klein *(17)* reported that, although marital status is empirically related to outcome, this relationship may be entirely explained by the more asocial premorbid adjustment of the single than of the married schizophrenics. The emphasis on the effect of premorbid adjustment patterns, particularly interpersonal relationships, on the predictor variable of marital status corroborates the findings of the earlier research of Farina *et al.* *(10)*. They suggested that when social aspects of recent sexual life and the quality of other close and recent social relationships are known, marital status, per se, adds very little to the prediction of outcome.

By contrast, occupation and employment are dynamic variables subject to change as a function of mental symptoms of illness. For instance, frequent hospitalizations disrupt working capacity, which, in our societal structure where competition tends to eliminate the less occupationally prepared and experienced, leads those unable to adjust to the demands of working conditions to be progressively eliminated. In this light, it is, therefore, not surprising that reliance on Welfare and level of occupation serve as meaningful predictors of outcome for the chronic patient. It is obvious that the chronic patient, who starts with a low social competence and who deteriorates in his social and vocational skills by numerous hospitalizations, becomes gradually rejected by the community at large and, thus, finds resumption of his social roles increasingly difficult. The chronic patient's deterioration, due to both the length of illness and the effect of custodial care, is furthered by the decreased tolerance of his deviant social behavior which accelerates the inevitable downward trend in his social functioning. In addition, the widespread practice of providing these patients with public assistance only exacerbates their lack of motivation to reenter the community as productive members. In our study, for example, 51.6% of the readmitted chronic schizophrenics received Welfare benefits as compared with 37.5% of their nonreadmitted counterparts. Contrary to the expectations of various government agencies who envisioned Welfare benefits as a solution to the social problems of the discharged schizophrenic patients, the life style engendered by reliance on public assistance appears to be a significant negative factor affecting outcome. The public assistance dependence which has become a way of life, particularly for the schizophrenics, does not increase these patients' social acceptance by the community; on the contrary, it isolates them in half-way houses in conditions of semi-isolated reclusiveness with other schizophrenics. These conditions lead to further impairment of the schizophrenics' self-image, loss of his or her social prestige, and, in the long run, to rehospitalization, which is one of the few places where he or she can take refuge.

Whatever the contribution of the concept of social competence to prediction of schizophrenics' tenure in the community, the dimensions of education, occupation, marital status, and employment history, which comprise the index, do not do justice to the area of the schizophrenic's social maladjustment. Other factors should prove to be more precise indicators of the patients' social dysfunction in the community than those reflected by the sociodemographic cluster. It seems that, in order to tap the true level of functioning of the schizophrenics in the community, one must provide a comprehensive evaluation of their social competence, encompassing, in addition to the above crude instrumental functioning, such areas as interpersonal relationships and other social behaviors that reflect the quality of their daily interactions in their own community settings. Such an assessment would serve as a more realistic indicator of the patients' social competence as judged by accepted community standards to which these individuals must conform if they are to be productive and fully integrated members.

Let's assume for the purposes of discussion that an acute schizophrenic, unmarried due to his relatively young age, on discharge from a hospital, retains his former job, and as such is considered to be fully reintegrated into his community and to be operating at his premorbid level, according to the Zigler and Phillips (42, 43, 44) and Turner and Zabo (39) criteria. Yet, a closer look at his total social functioning might well disclose that he has stopped dating, feels rejected by his friends, and quarrels continuously with his parents. Can we truly say that there is no change in his level of social functioning even though he is self-supporting? A follow-up of this case might well indicate that his rehospitalization has been precipitated by difficulties in interpersonal relationships that certainly would not be picked up by the crude criteria of social competence derived from sociodemographic data.

By contrast, let us consider two chronic schizophrenic patients who, at their first hospitalization were unmarried, performed unskilled work, were supported primarily by social Welfare, and graduated from junior high school. By the Zigler and Phillips and the Turner and Zabo criteria, both of these individuals would earn low scores on their premorbid social competence index. Let's assume further that one of the hypothetical chronics drinks heavily and, since his last hospital discharge, does not participate in an aftercare program. As a result of his excessive drinking and failure to take medication, he gets into difficulties with the authorities (due to his boisterous and disorderly conduct) and is soon rehospitalized. Our second case, however, follows through on aftercare treatment and requires crisis intervention occasionally but is not, in fact, rehospitalized. The different outcomes of these two cases might be ascribed to their differential ability to control their difficulties in dealing with the reality of their lives; they show different levels of impairment of their social functioning. Would their social competence scores indicate this difference? Clearly not. Though these cases are presented hypothetically, in reality they represent numberless cases from our study. In order to settle this issue, we had to develop other criteria for predicting outcome of acute and chronic schizophrenics based on more comprehensive evaluation of their community life. Such an attempt is presented in detail in Chapter 4.

REFERENCES

1. Aldrich, C.K., and Coffin, M.: Clinical studies of psychoses in the navy. Prognosis. *J. Nerv. Ment. Dis.* **108**: 142–148, 1948.
2. Astrup, C., Fossum, A., and Holmboe, R.: "Prognosis in Functional Psychoses." Charles C. Thomas, Springfield, Ill., 1962.
3. Bender, L.: Schizophrenia in childhood-its recognition, description, and treatment. *Amer. J. Orthopsychiatry* **26**: 499–506, 1956.
4. Bleuler, E.: "Dementia Precox or the Group of Schizophrenias." (Trans. J. Linberi) Int. University Press, New York, 1950.
5. Brown, C.W., Carstairs, G.M., and Topping, G.: Posthospital adjustment of chronic mental patients. *Lancet* **2**: 685–689, 1958.
6. Brown, G.W.: "Schizophrenia and Social Care." pp. 72–91. Oxford University Press, London, 1966.
7. Chapman, L.J., Day, D., and, Burnstein, A.: The process-reactive distinction and prognosis in schizophrenia. *J. Nerv. Ment. Dis.* **133**: 383–391, 1961.
8. Clark, R.E.: The relationship of schizophrenia to occupational income and occupational prestige. *Am. Soc. Rev.* **13**: 325–330, 1948.
8a. Cooper, B.: Social class and prognosis in schizophrenia. Part I. *Br. J. Prevent. Soc. Med.* **15**: 17–30, 1961.
9. Croughan, J.L., Welner, A., and Robbins, E.: The group of schizo-affective and related psychoses. II Studies, *Arch. Gen. Psychiat.* **31**:632–637, 1974.
10. Farina, A., Garmezy, N., Zalusky, M., and Backer, J.: Premorbid behavior and prognosis in female schizophrenic patients. *J. Consulting Psychology* **26**: 56–60, 1962.

11. Frumkin, R.M.: "Occupation and Mental Illness." (September) pp. 4–13. Ohio Public Welfare Statistics, Ohio, 1952.

12. Gabriel, E.: The long term course of schizophrenics as arising late in life, compared versus schizophrenics of all ages. *Psychiatrica. Clinica*, Munich. 7(3) 172–180, 1974.

12a. Garfield, J.L. and Sundland, D.M. Prognostic scale in schizophrenia. *J. Consult Psychol.* **30**: 18–24, 1966.

13. Hammer, M.: Influences of small social networks as factors on mental hospital admission. *Human Organization* **22**: 243–251, 1964.

14. Harris, A., Linker, I., Norris, V., and Sheppard, M.: Schizophrenia. A prognostic and social study. *Br. J. Soc. Prevent. Med.* **10**: 107–114, 1956.

15. Hartmann, W., and Meyer, J.E.: Long-term hospitalization of schizophrenic patients. *Compr. Psychiat.* **10**: 122–127, 1969.

16. Held, J.M., and Cromwell, R.L.: Premorbid adjustment in schizophrenia. *J. Nerv. Ment. Dis.* **146**: 264–272, 1968.

17. Klein, R.G., and Klein, D.F.: Marital status as a prognostic indicator in schizophrenia. *J. Nerv. Ment. Dis.* **147**: 289–296, 1968.

18. Klein, R.G., and Klein, D.F.: Premorbid asocial adjustment and prognosis in schizophrenia. *J. Psychiat. Res.* **7**: 35–53, 1969.

19. Kohn, M.L.: Social Class and Schizophrenia: A Critical Review. *In* "The Transmission of Schizophrenia." D. Rosenthal and S. S. Kety, (eds.), pp. 155–173. Pergammon Press, Oxford, 1968.

20. Langfeldt, G.: The Prognosis in schizophrenia. *Acta Psychiat. Scandinavica* (Suppl. 110) (1–66) 1956.

21. Huber, G., Gross, G., Schuttler, R.: Long-term follow-up study of schizophrenia: psychotic course of illness and programs. *Acta Psychiat. Scandinavica* **52**: 49–57, 1975.

22. Nolan, W.J.: Occupation and dementia praecox. *N.Y. State Hosp. Quart.* **3**: 127–154, 1917. Utica State Hosp.

23. Norris, V.: "Mental Illness in London." Maudsley Monograph No. 6, Chapman & Hall Ltd., London, 1959.

24. Ødegaard, O.: Marriage and Mental Disease. A study in social psychopathology. *J. Ment. Sci.* **92**: 35–39, 1946.

25. Ødegaard, O.: New data on marriage and mental disease. Incidence of psychoses in widowed and divorced. *J. Ment. Sci.* **99**: 778–785, 1953.

26. Ødegaard, O.: A clinical study of delayed admissions to a mental hospital. *Mental Hygiene* **42**: 67–77, 1958.

27. Ødegaard, O.: A statistical study of factors influencing discharge from psychiatric hospitals. *J. Ment. Sci.* **106**: 1124–1133, 1960.

28. Phillips, L.: Social Competence, the process-reactive distinction and the nature of mental disorder. *In* "Psychopathology of Schizophrenia" (J. Zubin and P. Hoch, eds.) pp. 470–481. Grune and Stratton, New York, 1966.

29. Phillips, L., Broverman, I.K., and Zigler, E.: Social competence and psychiatric diagnosis. *J. Abnorm. Soc. Psychol.* **71**: 209–214, 1966.

30. Phillips, L., and Zigler, E.: Social competence. The action-thought parameter and vicariousness in normal and pathological behaviors. *Journal of Abnormal and Social Psychology*, 63, pp, 137–146, 1961.

31. Rose A.M. (ed.): Occupation and Major Mental Disorders. "Mental Health and Mental Disorder." Norton, New York. pp 136–160, 1955.

32. Rosen. B., Klein, D.F., and Klein, R.G.: The prediction of rehospitalization: the relationship between age of first psychiatric treatment contact, marital status and premorbid asocial adjustment. *J. Nerv. Ment. Dis.* **152**: 17–22, 1971.

33. Rosen, B., Klein, D.F., Levenstein, S., and Shanian, S.P.: Social competence and posthospital outcome. *Arch. Gen. Psychiat.* **19**: 165–170, 1968.

34. Serban, G., and Gidynski, C.B.: Significance of social demographic data for rehospitalization of schizophrenic patients. *J. Health Soc. Behav.* **15**: 117–126, 1974.
35. Sherman, L.J., Moseley, E.C., Ging, R., and Bookbinder, L.J.: Prognosis in schizophrenia. *Arch. Gen. Psychiat.* **10**: 123–130, 1964.
36. Shofield, W., Hathaway, S.R., Hastings, D.W., and Bell, D.M.: Prognostic factors in schizophrenia. *J. Consult. Psychol.* **18**: 155–166, 1954.
37. Shofield, W., and Balian, L.: A Comparative study of the personal histories of schizophrenic and nonpsychiatric patients. *J. Abnorm. Soc. Psychol.* **59**: 216–225, 1959.
38. Stephens, J., Astrup, C., and Mangrum, J.C. Prognostic in recovered and deteriorated schizophrenics. *Am. J. Psychiat.* **122**: 116–121, 1966.
39. Turner, J.R., and Zabo, L.J.: Social competence and schizophrenic outcome: An investigation and critique. *J. Health Soc. Behav.* **9**: 41–42, 1968.
40. Walker, R.G., and Kelley, F.E.: Predicting the outcome of a schizophrenic episode. *Arch. Gen. Psychol.* **2**: 492–503, 1960.
41. Wirt, R.D., and Simon, W.: "Differential Treatment and Prognosis in Schizophrenia." Charles C. Thomas, Springfield, Ill., 1959.
42. Zigler, E., and Phillips, L.: Social Competence and outcome in psychiatric disorder. *J. Abnorm. Soc. Psychol.* **63**: 264–271, 1961.
43. Zigler, E., and Phillips, L.: Social effectiveness and symptomatic behaviors. *J. Abnorm. Soc. Psychol.* **61**: 231–238, 1960.
44. Zigler, E., and Phillips, L.: Social competence and the process-reactive distinction in psychopathology. *J. Abnorm. Soc. Psychol.* **65**: 215–22, 1962.

CHAPTER 4

Comparison of Functioning Levels of Schizophrenics and Normals, Implications for Short-Term Prediction of Rehospitalization of Schizophrenics*

There is a general consensus among both clinicians and researchers that the psychosocial functioning of schizophrenics is the main indicator of the level of their adjustment in the community and, at the same time, a predictor of the causes for rehospitalization. As we have seen in Chapter III, the level of social competence, reduced to two dimensions, that of unemployment (or more correctly, Welfare dependence) and marital status alone, are insufficient to account for the social functioning of schizophrenics. Other researchers have looked at other various aspects of psychosocial behavior to determine the level of the schizophrenic's adjustment in the community.

The two most frequently used case history scales are the Wittman Elgin Prognostic Scale (EPS) (30) revised by Becker, and the Phillips Prognostic Rating Scale (PRS) (19). The Elgin Scale scores items pertaining to such diverse categories as body build, personality types, interest patterns, symptomatology, and personal history. The Phillips Scale covers premorbid history in terms of social aspects of sexual life in adolescence and later years, personal relations in general, recent adjustment level in interpersonal relationships, and recent sexual adjustment. Also included are items dealing with precipitating factors and clinical signs of disturbance. Both scales are scored toward the high end of the scale (in the process direction) of the process-reactive continuum.

Research with the EPS showed a positive correlation between scores on the scale and the functioning of schizophrenics from 8 months to 3 years later (30). More recently, the prognostic power of the EPS has been studied in relation to hospital status in a follow-up study spanning a time period of 5 years (20). The EPS predicted the 9 months hospital status and readmissions within the 5 year observation period equally well. It should be pointed out, however, that the predictive power of this instrument was most efficient when applied to subgroups

---

*The data presented in this chapter have appeared in the Article: Serban, G.: Functioning ability in schizophrenic and "normal" subjects: short-term prediction for rehospitalization of schizophrenics. *Comp. Psychiat.*, **16:** 447–456, 1975.

of patients who represented extreme ends in the distribution of the amount of hospitalization. High correlation between the scale scores on the PRS and outcome have also been reported by Farina and Webb *(9)*.

The study reported by Garfield and Sundland *(10)* indicated that a high score on the Phillips Scale appears to be a prognosticator of long periods of hospitalization for schizophrenics. The reverse, however, does not appear to be true, since low scores did not reflect short periods of hospitalization. In the same study, scores on the Elgin Scale appeared to be more strongly related to length of hospitalization. The two scales also appear to differ in terms of classification of good premorbids; the Phillips scale classified two-thirds in the good premorbid category as compared to one-third classified by the Elgin Scale. In an investigation of long-term prognosis in schizophrenia using a 5-year follow-up to determine strictly defined recovered and deteriorated groups of patients. Stephens *et al. (26)* found that, of the 30 items used (20 of the EPS and 10 of the PRS), 27 significantly differentiated the contrasting outcome groups ($p < 0.001$). Subsequent examination of the factorial structure of the prognostic items revealed six factors accounting for 72 percent of the variance. These were: schizoid personality, rigidity, flatness of affect and apathy, insidious onset, inadequate heterosexual relationships, and distortion of reality.

A more recent study by Nuttall and Solomon *(18)* attempted to determine the factorial structure of premorbid adjustment and sought to obtain estimates of the predictive validity of these factors using a sample of 291 male schizophrenic patients. Premorbid adjustment measures consisted of 32 items drawn from the EPS and PRS scales. Application of the principal components analysis produced 7 factors: social withdrawal; adequate vs. inadequate heterosexual relationships; socially desirable vs. socially undesirable ward behavior; rigidity and apathy vs. mood swings and emotionality; type of onset (acute vs. insidious); stubborness vs. self-criticalness and sensitivity; and physical health. The test of the prognostic significance of these empirically derived factors versus the index of chronicity revealed that social withdrawal and lack of interests, inadequate heterosexual relationships and insidious onset were powerful in the prediction of long hosptial stay in low social class patients. The personality traits of stubborness and egocentricity appear to hold prognostic value, primarily in the higher socioeconomic groups. Rigidity tended to be a poor prognostic sign for the lower, but not the upper, socioeconomic groups.

In an attempt to circumvent the problems of using case records as a source of ratings, which are the basis of both the Elgin and the Phillips scales (and may lead to distortion of information, depending on the adequacy and source of the record and the recency of hospitalization. Ullman and Giovannoni *(27)* constructed a true–false measure of premorbid information obtainable directly from the patient. The 24 item scale of premorbid adjustment covers such areas as marital status, employment history, interpersonal relationships, duration of illness, and paranoid symptomatology.

An investigation reported by Held and Cromwell *(12)* suggests that the Ullmann–Giovannoni scale is significantly related to the Phillips prognostic scale, (Part I—Premorbid Adjustment). It appeared, however, that although the scale was adequate in identifying the good and poor prognosis patients, as determined by the Phillips' scale, the items were unrelated to an index of chronicity.

Despite the prognostic value of these scales, they do present certain disadvantages. The Phillips and Elgin instruments rely heavily on case records, which often suffer from incompleteness, lack of comparability from institution to institution, and bias engendered through record-keeping policies of hospitals. The ratings derived from case data of this sort are also subject to rater bias. At the same time, multiple-choice questionnaires administered directly to the patient (of which the Ullman–Giovannoni Scale is an example), depend in large measure on cooperation of patients and their degree of insight into both their current mental state and their fulfillment of social roles.

While a good deal of research activity focused on the delineation of predictive factors in schizophrenia, some investigators emphasized the need for developing measures of the schizophrenic adjustment and social behavior in the community. This area of interest was particularly stimulated by the recent innovations in psychiatric treatment, leading to brief hospitalization. The return of psychotic patients to the community, after a short-term and intensive hospital treatment, has brought into sharp focus the need for measures which may assess the effect of the innovative approaches used in psychiatric institutions and in community-based treatment.

Katz and Lyerly *(14)* developed an adjustment scale addressed primarily to operational definitions of "adjustment" and "social behavior." Of the areas tapped by the scale, the most prominent were: clinical adjustment (level of freedom from psychopathological symptoms as manifested in the patient's complaints and social behavior); adequate social functioning (measured by occupational, social, and family performance relevant to the patient's social role); level of satisfaction in work, social, and home areas; and social behavior (consisting of ways of relating to people). In addition, this scale provides separate measures for expectations. The Katz adjustment scale was designed to assess various aspects of patients' functioning in the community from the point of view of the patients as well as their close relatives. The preliminary validation studies revealed that the scale scores discriminated between well and poorly adjusted groups with the informant scales performing better than the patient scales.

In a later study dealing with adjustment in the community of a variety of discharged psychiatric patients, Michaux et al. *(17)* found that performance of socially expected activities, and the level of the patient's satisfaction with free time activities as derived from the items of the KAS, predicted course of adjustment, relapse, and rehospitalization of the patients.

Despite the apparent comprehensiveness of the KAS as a measure of adjustment in the community, the scale items suffer from too much generalization and vagueness, which may affect the interpretation of the information sought by both the patient and the interviewer. In seeking information from psychotic patients, particularly schizophrenics who exhibit residual thought defects even in remission, it appears crucial to address the items to very concrete aspects of the patients' behavior, expectations, and self-attitudes.

The second shortcoming of the KAS is the omission of inquiry into the extent and quality of interpersonal relationships with different family members, spouse or sexual partner, and other significant members in the patients' social environment, such as friends and neighbors. Employment seeking and dependence on welfare, factors significant in reintegration into the community, are also conspicuous by their absence. In addition, little emphasis is given in the KAS to the quality and quantity of antisocial behavior, which affects, in large measure, the schizophrenics' adjustment to community living and is often a precipitating factor in rehospitalization.

Finally, the Katz scale appears to measure current levels of community adjustment, primarily in the context of the possible discrepancy between level of patients' functioning. A measure of his satisfaction with his community integration, based on the relationship between attempting to meet generally desirable social expectations and the ability to do so, may be construed to be a realistic appraisal of adjustment, but this construct is not really an indicator of the patient's actual functioning level. This is particularly true among schizophrenics for whom levels of expectation tend to be quite different from their actual instrumental and social performance. In this sense, the scale may be measuring, indirectly, the extent of the subject's thinking disorder. Of all the scales of the KAS, only two parts, S_2 and S_4, pertain to functioning and these appear to focus primarily on leisure activities. The expectation level may be interpreted as a measure of aspiration indicative of the patient's motivation and realistic appraisal of his perception of community expectations and demands.

In conclusion, the evaluation of both sets of existing scales, those basically addressing prognostic functioning factors and those measuring posthospitalization adjustment, brings into sharp focus their specific shortcomings. As regards the prognostic scales (Phillips, Elgin, Ullman–Giovannoni), these instruments appear to reflect only well known crude factors allegedly associated with long-term poor and good prognosis, discovered empirically in the course of treatment of schizophrenic patients. These scales were devised before the widespread use of tranquillizing drugs, the use of which has modified the picture of the schizophrenic, particularly that one of early discharge of the chronic patient into the community. The distinction between factors predicting rehospitalization, based on long-term evaluation (of the hospitalized patients), and community living circumstances, became blurred by the stressful social factors associated with functioning in the community which lead to rehospitalization. Such variables as Welfare dependence and inability to relate to parents, friends, living-in partner, and neighbors upon return to the community represent important variables of this nature. The prognostic scales which found application in research do not take these dimensions into account.

With the growing need for tapping community adjustment of schizophrenics, some attempt has been made to include some of the dimensions bypassed by the earlier adjustment measures such as: Ellsworth Adjustment Scale (8); and the Community Adaptation Schedule (21, 22). The Ellsworth scale focused on a combination of instrumental and social functioning and clinical symptomatology, while the CAS, though very comprehensive in scope, unfortunately combined general items measuring functioning with evaluation of expectations and satisfactions with role performance. In addition, they do not measure the stress experienced by the patient in his efforts at integration into the community.

In this context, the author believes that a constructive and meaningful estimation of the psychosocial evaluation of psychotic patients, particularly schizophrenics, should be based on the following criteria: (1) The measure should comprise a comprehensive inventory of individuals' activities in wide psychosocial areas of behavior pertinent to their acceptance by the community after hospitalization. (2) Each of the psychosocial areas should be highlighted by items concrete and specific in nature to minimize misunderstanding, by both the patient and the interviewer, as to the actual instrumental and social performance level each patient exhibits. (3) The items should measure quantitatively and qualitatively the individual's ability to function in that particular area. (4) Since functioning in any of the psychosocial areas could produce varying degrees of experienced stress for the individual, concomitant evaluation of stress is a crucial part of the obtained measurement. Stress, as it affects community functioning, may be best defined as a degree of imbalance between environmental demands for psychosocial performance and the capacity for successful fulfillment of these demands. (5) Adjustment to community life, in the sense of constructive and productive reintegration into the social environment, must be viewed basically as a ratio of functioning over stress; ideally, at least, good adjustment would be represented by adequate fulfillment of one's expected social role without undue anxiety and distress.

The study to be reported applied measurement of psychosocial functioning, which appears to fulfill the criteria discussed above. The measures of psychosocial functioning derived from the Social Stress and Functioning Inventory for Psychotic Disorders (SSFIPD) cover 21 dimensions of behavior, providing a comprehensive survey of interpersonal interaction with family members (parents, relatives, marital or living-in-partner, and children) and other persons in the environment (opposite sex peers, close friends, neighbors, and the community at large). In addition, the inventory permits evaluation of social performance while the patient resides in the community (education received, employment history, management of finances, dependence on public assistance, ability to perform household duties, and general living circumstances), as well as involvement in socially maladaptive activities such as use of addictive and psychedelic drugs and antisocial behavior. The 21 categories of the SSFIPD are fully described in Chapter 2.

A three prong approach was chosen for our study of psychosocial functioning by means of the SSFIPD. The first data analyses were aimed at determining the differences in social and instrumental prehospitalization functioning between the 125 acute and 516 chronic patients comprising the study sample and 96 normals of comparable socioeconomic background. The inclusion of normals in the analyses was dictated by a need to establish a baseline for the other comparisons. The second aim of the data analyses was to identify the significant functioning dimensions for acute and chronic schizophrenics as well as for the normal controls from among the 21 psychosocial variables measured by the SSFIPD. This was done to provide insight into the specific aspects of interpersonal and instrumental behavior exhibited for a period of 6 months to 1 year prior to the current hospitalization of the chronic patients, while they were residing in the community, and to establish the level of premorbid functioning (also covering 6 months to 1 year) of the acute patients. The third approach was devoted to the exploration of the psychosocial factors measured by the SSFIPD which were contributing to the short-term outcome prediction in the two types of schizophrenic patients.

Results of these analyses are reported in the three sections below.

PREHOSPITALIZATION PSYCHOSOCIAL FUNCTIONING OF ACUTE AND CHRONIC SCHIZOPHRENICS IN COMPARISON TO NORMALS

Differences in functioning across the 21 dimensions provided by the SSFIPD and in total functioning scores represent a grand mean of 21 individual dimensions between normals and the two schizophrenic groups.

Examination of Table 1 reveals that in terms of scores representing total psychosocial functioning, the analysis discriminated the groups at a high level of significance.

It appears that in terms of overall level of functioning, the normals obtained the highest scores, acute schizophrenics intermediate scores, and the chronics the lowest scores. These differences were significant at 0.001 level ($F = 77.27$). It is of interest to note that significant differences in functioning were also found between the acutes and normals ($F = 28.24$; $p < 0.001$), chronics and normals ($F = 139.31$; $p < 0.001$), and the acutes and chronics ($F = 35.35$;

Table 1

Analysis of Variance: Comparison of Total D Function Scores for Normals
and Acute and Chronic Schizophrenics*

Normals		Chronics		Acutes	
$\overline{X}$	S.D.	$\overline{X}$	S.D.	$\overline{X}$	S.D.
2.53	0.16	2.23	0.24	2.36	0.23

*Overall $F = 77.27***$; $2/716$ df; Ac/N $F = 28.24***$; Ch/N $F = 139.31***$; Ac/Ch $F = 35.35***$.
***$p < 0.001$.

$p < 0.001$). Normals were found to be functioning at a significantly higher level than acutes (X for normals $= 2.53$ compared to acute X of 2.36) and, in turn, the acutes appear to function on a higher level than do their chronic counterparts (chronic $X = 2.23$). These findings are particularly important, in light of evidence from other research sources, suggesting no significant differences in premorbid functioning of normals from those who become acute schizophrenics (2).

Comparison of the three groups of subjects (normals and acute and chronic schizophrenics) was also carried out for each of the 21 psychosocial functioning dimensions as presented in Table 2.

In terms of overall differences between the groups, only the areas of housekeeping, religious affiliation, alcohol abuse, and use of psychedelic drugs failed to produce reliable differences. This may be partly due to the small number of subjects in these cells. Among the comparisons that are significant, the differences are also in the expected direction, with normals exhibiting higher levels of functioning than acutes, who, in turn, exhibit higher levels than chronics in 14 out of the 21 categories studied. These trends are evident in such variables as education, employment history, dependence on public assistance, living circumstances, relationship with parents, relatives, marital partners and dating behavior, involvement with neighbors and others in the community at large, and use of leisure time. Use of addictive drugs and antisocial behavior, comprising the crucial aspects of socially maladaptive activities, showed a comparable trend in the direction of the differences.

In order to identify more specific differences existing between the three groups of subjects, posthoc comparisons were carried out for normals versus acutes, normals versus chronics and acutes versus chronics. The most discriminating functioning areas for normals and acutes are employment history, relationship with children, dating behavior, sex, and the relationship with friends. As regards the most prominent differences in the comparison of normals and chronics, these appear to center around identical areas except for additional differences in welfare dependence, relationship with relatives and neighbors, alcohol abuse, and antisocial acts.

Table 2

Analysis of Variance: Comparison of D Function Scores for Normals
and Acute and Chronic Schizophrenics for 21 Functioning Categories

Category	Among Groups		Between Groups F Values		
	F	df	n Versus Ac	n Versus Ch	Ac Versus Ch
Education	14.85*	2/716	4.91†	26.36*	7.38*
Job	70.41*	2/716	43.10*	136.56*	16.92*
Housekeeping	0.53	2/676	—	—	—
Welfare	45.76*	2/716	2.56	62.94*	44.54*
Finances	3.29†	2/714	0.02	3.14	4.59†
Living					
circumstances	4.02†	2/378	4.31†	8.02†	0.12
Parents	16.64*	2/704	4.70†	28.88*	9.22**
Relatives	6.52**	2/661	0.61	9.59**	5.73†
Marriage	27.64*	2/368	7.83**	52.61*	9.04**
Children	13.43*	2/255	15.11*	25.80*	0.00
Dating	29.72*	2/597	18.12*	54.44*	10.71**
Sex	18.73*	2/715	15.19*	37.28*	2.29
Friends	25.61*	2/716	4.20†	40.68*	18.76*
Neighbors	6.50†	2/710	0.01	6.53†	8.77**
Others	37.67*	2/716	19.98*	71.75*	11.39*
Leisure	16.38*	2/716	6.25†	29.73*	7.21**
Religion	0.17	2/716	—	—	—
Drinking	2.29	2/716	—	—	—
Addictive drugs	8.77*	2/705	9.08**	17.52**	0.32
Psychedelic drugs	2.66	2/703	—	—	—
Antisocial acts	35.18*	2/713	8.68**	59.67*	21.09*

*$p < 0.001$.

†$p < 0.05$.

**$p < 0.01$.

Comparisons of acutes and chronics revealed more significant differences in educational level, employment history, Welfare dependence, relationship with friends and others in the community as well as involvement in antisocial acts. Although the obtained differences in functioning reflect the varying levels of adjustment of the three groups of subjects in the last 6 months to 1 year prior to the interview, in reality the difficulties of the schizophrenics began a long time ago. An extremely illuminating illustration of the schizophrenics' long-term social difficulties, particularly those in interpersonal relationships is provided for instance by information on sex and dating. As it was previously observed by Phillips *(19)* and Langner *(16)* the expression of the sexual instinct becomes progressively stunted due to the increasing difficulties that schizophrenics experience in coping with the social customs required for its fulfillment. If we take a closer look at supporting data, not included in the functioning section of the dating area, it shows that whereas the groups did not differ in first sexual contact prior to age 10 (chronics 5.63%, N = 13; acutes 7.02%, N = 4 and normals 2.11%, N = 2), during puberty and adolescence (ages 11 through 18) a larger proportion of normals (62.11%, N = 59) than of the chronic (44.16%, N = 102) and acute (45.61%, N = 26) schizophrenics had their first sexual intercourse during this period. Of equal interest is the finding that 20.78% (N = 48) of the chronics and 19.30% (N = 11) of the acutes never had sexual relations as compared to 2.11% (N = 2) of the normals. The differences for the groups of the variable on first sexual contact during adulthood (ages 19–34) were not all that different (Chronics: 22.51%, N = 52, Acutes: 21.05%, N = 12, Normals: 27.35%, N = 26).

Furthermore, the reason for the schizophrenics' inability to express their sexual instinct becomes clearer when one considers the data on the age of the first continuing sexual relationship which had emotional meaning. As may be expected none of the subjects reported having such a relationship during childhood (age 10 or below). During puberty and adolescence, (ages 11 through 18), however, the differences between schizophrenics and normals emerge. Whereas 61 of the chronics (33.52%) and 14 of the acutes (30.43%) reported having their first continuing sexual relationshp during this time, 47 (49.47%) of the normals were so involved. In addition, 46 (25.27%) of the chronics and 10 (21.74%) of the acutes were never involved on a continuing basis with a sexual partner as compared with 3 (3.16%) of the normals. As was the case with the variable of age at first sexual intercourse, the present variable of continuing sexual relationship begun in adulthood (ages 19–34) did not differentiate the three groups of subjects to any significant extent (chronics: 40.11%, N = 73; acutes: 45.65%, N = 21; normals: 47.37%, N = 45).

Distributions of preferences for homosexual, bisexual, and heterosexual relationships among chronic and acute schizophrenics and normal controls indicated that most subjects were interested in heterosexual relationships (chronics: 66.9%, N = 354; acutes: 75.2%, N = 94; and normals: 53.7%, N = 51). Of the 516 chronics, 3.7% (N = 19) preferred homosexual relationships, whereas 1.6% (N = 2) of the acutes and 1% (N = 1) of the normals did so. Among the three groups 6% (N = 31) of the chronics, 4% (N = 5) of the acutes, and 2.1% (N = 2) of the normals indicated an interest in bisexual relationships. It is of interest to note that only the patient groups indicated lack of interest in dating someone [4% (N = 5) of the acutes and 11.8% (N = 61) of the chronics]. It is also of interest to note that we did not find support for the generally held theories that schizophrenics are becoming progressively more homosexually oriented due to their difficulties in relating to the opposite sex. Although we do acknowledge that they do encounter serious and long-standing difficulties in heterosexual relationships as indicated by the above findings in the areas of sex and dating.

In order to determine whether the differences in the 21 functioning scores were affected by age and sex, a regression analysis was performed, and the results indicated that age and sex variables were unrelated to the performance on the 21 social functioning dimensions (as expressed by the total functioning score, summarizing the various aspects of social functioning).

Evaluation of the effect of sex of subject on each of the 21 categories of social functioning was carried out by means of two-way analysis of variance as shown in Table 3.

Table 3

D Functionability: Males and Females by Normals, Chronics, and Acutes: Two-Way Analysis of Variance†

Item	Normal		Chronic		Acute		F test		Sex x Patient
	Male	Female	Male	Female	Male	Female	Sex	Patient	
Education	2.545	2.443	2.227	2.303	2.391	2.348	NS	10.502***	NS
Job	2.688	2.763	2.250	2.250	2.436	2.358	NS	65.348	NS
House	2.702	2.709	2.761	2.581	2.785	2.661	4,654*	NS	NS
Welfare	2.707	2.853	2.137	2.052	2.709	2.498	NS	32.377***	NS
Finances	2.593	2.493	2.438	2.397	2.498	2.624	NS	NS	NS
Living	1.947	1.708	1.422	1.607	1.552	1.516	NS	4,640*	NS
Parents	2.725	2.735	2.487	2.420	2.665	2.523	NS	13.967***	NS
Relatives	2.643	2.667	2.536	2.377	2.672	2.521	NS	5.795**	NS
Marriage	2.677	2.607	2.245	2.224	2.412	2.447	NS	18.327***	NS
Children	2.584	2.530	1.835	2.060	1.734	2.075	NS	14.200***	NS
Dating	2.524	2.496	1.944	1.872	2.159	2.064	NS	29.806***	NS
Sex	2.649	2.841	2.269	2.197	2.408	2.291	NS	19.910***	NS
Friends	2.671	2.659	2.300	2.311	2.542	2.504	NS	18.300***	NS
Neighbors	1.881	1.845	1.631	1.748	1.949	1.788	NS	3.348*	NS
Others	2.486	2.523	1.947	1.930	2.200	2.076	NS	33.629***	NS
Leisure	2.273	2.295	2.074	2.096	2.175	2.166	NS	13.155***	NS
Religion	1.808	1.907	1.774	1.967	1.723	1.898	5.711*	NS	NS
Drinking	2.792	2.655	2.515	2.730	2.520	2.671	NS	NS	3,809*
A. Drugs	3.000	2.977	2.718	2.778	2.780	2.760	NS	8,889***	NS
P. Drugs	2.798	2.631	2.539	2.796	2.320	2.684	4,306*	3.126*	4.945**
Anti-soc	2.971	2.774	2.035	2.548	2.408	2.761	9.971**	22.541***	9.254**

†NS = nonsignificant; * = $p < 0.05$; ** = $p < 0.01$; *** = $p < 0.001$.

The significant effect of sex was found on the variables of housekeeping, religious affiliation, use of psychedelic drugs, and antisocial behavior. In each case, females appeared to function on a higher level on these dimensions, suggesting that the obtained differences were most probably brought about by the cultural role effect, (since females are certainly expected to be more involved with housekeeping than males, and probably exhibit both a stronger religious affiliation and greater inhibition in antisocial activities).

The analysis reported thus far was based on scores which involved basically only that information for which appropriate or relevant answers could be given. These scores were designated as D scores. A second scoring system was also developed which permitted evaluation of functioning based on the inclusion of nonapplicable data. The second scoring method which included the nonapplicable data was designated as E scores. It was devised as an exploratory measure to determine whether or not the inclusion of the inapplicable data might reveal finer nuances of the schizophrenics' functioning, since gaps in certain social and instrumental behaviors may have significant effect on functioning levels. The rationale behind the development of this additional scoring was twofold. On the one hand, it seemed important to determine whether or not "inapplicable" data would change the direction of functioning scores, and on the other hand, the E functioning score provided an opportunity to explore dynamically the areas of functioning where inability to answer the question was due to the irrelevance of the question to one's life situation. For instance, not having children is in itself not particularly indicative of functioning level. Inability to appropriately answer questions regarding relationships with the opposite sex, due to inability to begin or maintain such relationship, however, does influence a realistic estimate of one's functioning in our culture.

Comparison of D and E functioning scoring for normals, acutes, and chronics is presented in Table 4.

Examination of Table 4 suggests that both types of scoring (E and D) tend to provide basically the same information, (although the missing data included in the E score tends to inflate the functioning scores for all groups). Comparisons of normals with chronics revealed that, in terms of significant differences, the addition of inapplicable data washed out the discrimination between groups in the areas of finance management, relationship with relatives, and sex. By contrast, addition of missing data has produced a significant difference in the area of housekeeping for these two groups. Comparisons of acutes and normals in terms of the two scoring systems revealed that the addition of "inappropriate" category has produced significant differences in the areas of housekeeping, use of leisure time, and drinking, which the D score failed to differentiate.

The direction of the differences in the normal–chronic comparisons of the two scoring systems in the area of housekeeping lead us to believe that, when in-

Table 4
Grand Means of D and E Functioning Scores

	$\bar{X}$	6	6^2	N	t C–A*	t C–N*	t A–N*
D functioning							
Chronic	2.192	0.253	0.064	499	7.125	18.799	7.532
Acute	2.357	0.225	0.051	125	$p < 0.001$	$p < 0.001$	$p < 0.001$
Normal	2.547	0.145	0.021	92			
E functioning							
Chronic	3.061	0.165	0.027	499	7.258	11.673	3.221
Acute	3.173	0.150	0.023	125	$p < 0.001$	$p < 0.001$	$p < 0.01$
Normal	3.233	0.122	0.015	92			

*A, acute; C, chronic; N, normal.

applicable data is excluded, the general direction of functioning differences is highest in normals, followed by acutes, with the lowest in chronics. Addition of inapplicable data indicates that chronics earn higher scores than acutes. Closer analysis of the housekeeping area disclosed that a higher amount of missing data represented a higher amount of nonfunctioning, especially for females. For example, question #66: "Do you have difficulty getting things done at home?" 36.8% of the acutes, 50.6% of the chronics and 12.7% of normals found inapplicable. In the next question, which deals with the identification of the main difficulty, the pattern appears to be the same: 60% of the acutes, 72.7% of the chronics, and 43.2% of the normals found the question inappropriate. Obviously, missing data appear to reverse the score, making it appear to measure higher functioning, whereas, in reality, the quality it measures represents nonfunctioning. In still another area, that of finances, when missing data are added it becomes clear how the inapplicable data affects functioning scoring. Question #85 dealing with saving money was found inapplicable for 44% of the acutes, 50.2% of chronics, and 20% of normals. The same trend is maintained in reference to payment of debts. In this category, the missing data appear to refine the score by pointing out the impairment in functioning, although superficially it raises the functioning score. In the area of relationship with relatives, the addition of nonapplicable data appears to reveal the "dead weight" of nonexistent relatives. In the present sample, the findings indicate the acutes have fewer relatives than do normals. For example, 12.8% of the acutes, 14.7% of the chronics, and 11.6% of normals found the question on relationship toward their brothers and sisters inapplicable. In relation to the sex category, the amount of missing data introduced by the acutes and chronics reflects a highly impaired level of functioning, by reversing the trend and making the differences negligible. The question indicative of long-term relationship with the opposite sex (over 6 months or longer) underscores this point further. It appears that 24.8% of the acutes, 28.9% of the chronics and 4.2% of normals found the question inapplicable. It thus appears that qualitative analysis, coupled with the inapplicable data score, reveals and further corroborates the evidence obtained from the scores, based on only relevant information; that is, that normals have the highest functioning level in all areas, with acutes holding consistently the middle position, and the chronics faring the worst. What the missing data seems to indicate is that it can refine the score showing the impairment in functioning through withdrawal from various activities.

EVALUATION OF SIGNIFICANT PSYCHOSOCIAL FUNCTIONING DIMENSIONS FOR ACUTE AND CHRONIC SCHIZOPHRENICS

Comparisons of the two schizophrenic groups with normals throws an interesting light on the functioning levels dispersed through the 21 areas considered in the study. In addition it was deemed important to identify significant dimensions among the psychosocial variables for normals and the acute and chronic schizophrenic groups. To accomplish this and to reduce the overlap, principal components analysis was applied to the 21 psychosocial variables of the SSFIPD, separately for each of the subject groups (acute, chronics, normals). Application of this procedure resulted in the acceptance of 4 principal components factors for normals and acutes accounting for 84.4% and 86.9% of the variance, respectively. Three factors were identified for the chronic group which accounted for 76.1% of the total variance. The variables making up the factors, and their loadings are shown in Tables 6, 7, and 8.

Examination of Table 5 reveals that for normals, factor I, which accounts for 34.8% of the variance, is basically composed of SSFIPD areas dealing with interpersonal relationships with people in general, parents, and friends. Factor II, accounting for 21.2% of the variance, is composed primarily of items dealing with drug use. Factors III and IV, accounting for 16.8% and 11.6% of variance, respectively, appear to be made up primarily of dating behavior and sexual experiences (factor III) and the management of finances (factor IV).

Table 6 represents the extracted factors and their variable loadings for the acute schizophrenic patients. As can be seen, factor I, accounting for 40.9% of the variance, is also primarily a factor tapping interpersonal relationships, particularly with friends, neighbors, and others in the community. Factors III and IV are rather weak factors accounting for only 15.1 and 10.9% of the variance, respectively. Factor III is a mixed factor and Factor IV taps primarily drinking behavior.

Table 5
Principal Components Factor Loadings for Selected
Psychosocial Variables for Normal Controls

Variable	Factors			
	I	II	III	IV
Relationship with others	0.692			
Relationship with parents	0.633			
Relationship with friends	0.482			
Welfare	0.461			
Use of addictive drugs		0.492		
Use of psychedelic drugs		0.492		
Dating			0.599	
Sex			0.445	
Finances				0.510

Table 6

Principal Components Factor Loadings for Significant
Psychosocial Variables of Acute Schizophrenics

Variable	Factors			
	I	II	III	IV
Relationship with others	0.693			
Job	0.608			
Relationship with friends	0.504			
Relationship with neighbors	0.452			
Spare time activities	0.464			
Relationship with family	0.451			
Use of addictive drugs		0.657		
Use of psychedelic drugs		0.765		
Sex			0.453	
Welfare			0.404	
Living circumstances			0.361	
Drinking				0.401

Table 7

Principal Components Factor Loadings for Significant
Psychosocial Variables of Chronic Schizophrenics

Variable	Factors		
	I	II	III
Relationship with others	0.684		
Relationship with friends	0.632		
Job	0.541		
Dating	0.545		
Spare time activities	0.518		
Relationship with neighbors	0.432		
Drinking		0.582	
Use of addictive drugs		0.571	
Antisocial behavior		0.396	
Sex			0.407

The results of the principal component analysis for the chronic schizophrenics is shown in Table 7. Three factors were extracted for this group. Factor I, accounting for 44.6% of the variance, appears again to tap primarily interpersonal relationships. Factor II (18.2% of variance) is composed of items dealing with antisocial behavior and socially maladaptive activities. Factor III, the weakest of the factors (12.2% of variance accounted for), is primarily composed of items dealing with sexual experiences.

PREDICTION OF OUTCOME IN TERMS OF PSYCHOSOCIAL FUNCTIONING

Although the reduction of data achieved by means of the factorial techniques may reduce overlap and minimize the redundancy of the information obtained from the SSFIPD, it was believed that due to the complicated nature of predicting outcome in any psychiatric group (particularly schizophrenics) all 21 areas of functioning covered by the inventory should be included in the analysis. Only on the basis of comprehensive evaluation of social functioning, can one determine the patients' potential for community integration. At the same time, the wealth of functioning data covered by the 21 areas, necessitated some weighting of the contribution of each of the scales, so as to provide a maximum differentiation between the groups of schizophrenics having different prognoses. The statistical method, which permits comparison of the groups with different prognoses on the most discriminating variables alone, and in an increasing combination, with each of the next best discriminators, is the step-wise discriminant function analysis. This procedure was performed separately for 114 readmitted and 91 nonreadmitted chronic patients and 33 readmitted and 37 nonreadmitted acute patients. The independent variables consisted of 21 problem areas as presented in Table 2.

Results of the stepwise discriminant function analyses for acute and chronic schizophrenics are shown in Table 8.

For the acute patients, poor relationship with parents appears to be the most significant single factor leading to readmission within 2 years of original hospitalization. Inability to relate to close friends and members of the opposite sex also appeared to be important variables in failure to adjust to community living. Problems associated with work, living conditions, marriage, and relationship with neighbors tended to contribute less significantly to readmission among acute schizophrenics.

The results indicated that readmission in chronic schizophrenics appears to be associated primarily with antisocial behavior and the inability to maintain lasting sexual relationships with opposite sex peers. Impairments in relating to other persons in the community also appeared to figure significantly in the failure to maintain community tenure. Absence of religious affiliation and poor social relationships with the opposite sex contributed secondarily to relapse necessitating rehospitalization.

Table 8

Stepwise Discriminant Function Analysis: Comparison of Readmitted
and Nonreadmitted Chronic and Acute Schizophrenics on the Best
Discriminating Social Functioning Variables

Variables	Readmitted vs. Nonreadmitted Chronics (F value)
Antisocial acts (AA)	8.07*
Sex (S) + (AA)	7.13*
Neighbors (N) + (AA) + (S)	6.95†
Religion (R) + (AA) + (S) + (N)	6.25**
Dating (D) + (AA) + (S) + (N) + (R)	5.66**

	Readmitted vs. Nonreadmitted Acutes (F value)
Parents (P)	12.43*
Close friends (CF) + (P)	10.34*
Dating (D) + (P) + (CF)	8.25*
Living circumstances (LC) + (P) + (CF) + (D)	7.34†
Job (J) + (P) + (CF) + (D) + (LC)	6.66†
Marriage (M) + (P) + (CF) + (LC) + (D) + (J)	6.20†
Neighbors (N) + (P) + (CF) + (LC) + (D) + (J) + (M)	5.71†

*$p < 0.001$.
†$p < 0.01$.
**$p < 0.05$.

DISCUSSION

The findings of the present study bring into sharp focus the perennial question
regarding the validity of the level of premorbid adjustment and type of onset for
outcome in schizophrenia. The reported results indicate that normals and acute
and chronic schizophrenics do function at different levels. The obtained
differentiation between normals and chronic schizophrenics is not all that
surprising since these samples represent extreme ends of the population distribution of these particular characteristics. However, the level of functioning of the
chronic patients discharged into the community appears to be, in general, too
marginal to deserve a label of extramural adjustment. Furthermore, the finding
which is less expected and deserving of more explanation is the consistently
demonstrated higher functioning level of acutes than chronics; both are lower
than normals. But even this result becomes less puzzling if we consider the link
between psychosocial functioning level and type of onset in schizophrenia.
According to the classical concept, espoused by many psychiatrists and
suggested by some past research, the type of onset generally associated with a
chronic course of the schizophrenic illness is a gradual and progressive process of

emotional and social disintegration beginning many years prior to the manifestation of the florid symptoms of the psychosis. This traditional concept is
supported by the present findings. The results appear to be consonant with those
of Gittleman-Klein and Klein (11) who found, on the basis of the premorbid
asocial adjustment scale, that social withdrawal, inadequacy of peer relationships, limited range of interests, and poor psychosexual adjustment represent a
long term asocial orientation in patients who, on follow-up, exhibit poor
outcomes. Further corroboration is well summarized by Higgins (13) in his
discussion of process-reactive schizophrenia. Our own inquiry into the long-term
problem areas of schizophrenics (some of which date back to youth and
adolescence) presents additional evidence in support of this point (23).

It should be noted, however, that the corollary of this traditional position, that
is, that sudden onset and good premorbid adjustment are associated with
favorable prognosis (15, 25, 28), appears to be less reliably true. In this respect,
Bleuler (3), on the basis of a 23 year follow-up of schizophrenic patients in
Burgholzli Clinic in Zurich, concluded that the course of schizophrenia, as
related to the type of onset, takes more than the two classical predictive
pathways. For instance, in terms of evolution, patients with acute onset might
develop either straight chronic severe psychosis (catastrophic schizophrenia), or
chronic but mild psychosis, or a phasic type (severe or mild) of chronic
psychosis. Chronic onset patients (according to Bleuler's observations) might
progress in their course into the same pattern of straight or phasic evolution of
classic psychosis. Our study presents partial support for these findings. Of
particular importance is the failure of our study to lend support to the conclusion
of Birley and Brown (2), that 50% of schizophrenics studied showed an abrupt
transition from "normal" functioning to schizophrenia as a result of precipitating
stresses experienced within 3 weeks of the patients' hospitalizations. Perhaps in
the Birley and Brown study, as in many others, the results have been
significantly affected by the methodology used. These investigators did not
measure social functioning comprehensively, examined too short a period prior
to hospitalization, and omitted a comparison of findings between psychotic and
normal samples.

The present results are inconsistent with the contention that the majority of
acute schizophrenics function within the normal range, prior to their first
psychiatric admission, and the idea that there are two clearly distinguished types
of clinical onsets predetermining different courses in schizophrenia. The data
suggest that all acute patients, when reliably diagnosed schizophrenic (regardless
of subtypes of schizophrenia they represent), have a long history of difficulties in
coping with everyday life situations which progressively lead to their hospitalization. Our results show differences between them and normals in the areas of
education, employment, relationships with parents and opposite sex peers,
and/or the use of alcohol to relieve anxiety. The discussion of early schizophrenic
decompensation signs presented recently by Donlon and Blacker (6) lends further
corroboration to our findings. According to these authors, true schizophrenics

show, in the earliest phases of the disease (long before they receive the attention of hospital authorities), cognitive and perceptual distortion, affective disturbances resulting in the fear of intimacy with loved ones, a generally hostile–dependent relationship with others, motor retardation, and social withdrawal exhibited most dramatically in frequent job and school changes and other physical relocations, as well as the increasing levels of alcohol and drug abuse. Donlon and Blacker emphasize that these symptoms are present for months, and possibly years, before the overt psychotic episode takes place. Similar observations have been made by Varsamis and Adamson (29) who found such prodromal phenomena to last for an average of 30 months prior to hospitalization. The most prominent long-term problems, among the 44 schizophrenics studied by Varsamis and Adamson, were decreased volition and dysphoria concommitant with the academic and occupational deterioration. In our study, 44.3% of the acute patients, the majority of whom had sudden clinical onset (77.6%) according to the generally accepted criteria, required multiple hospitalizations within a relatively short observation period of approximately 2 years. Moreover, our data fail to support the contention that acute onset is necessarily associated with good prognosis. We have shown a remarkable continuity between past (preschizophrenic stage) problems and current difficulties even in schizophrenics characterized by an acute type of onset (23).

The apparent discrepancy between the more recent findings, including this one, and previous investigations appears to stem from the differences in research methodology. In most previous studies, acute onset refers solely to the florid psychological pathology (delusions, hallucinations) that causes the patient to be rejected by the community. The measurement of premorbid personality was primarily based on the assessment of the functioning of the patients in limited areas of instrumental social performance derived primarily from case history, psychiatric interviews, and social worker reports (19, 11). Although in some cases the assessment of psychosocial premorbid functioning covered a reasonable period of time prior to the onset of florid psychotic symptoms, the obtained information was highly limited in its reliability by the use of data from a variety of sources (different interviewers varying in ability and conscientiousness in obtaining data), and subject to different levels of interpretation in the scoring by various research workers. As far as we know our study is the first one to assess simultaneously both variables of onset and premorbid functioning, obtaining the data directly from the patient and/or his family informant, in an organized and standardized manner, minimizing the variability due to multiple data sources and interview techniques.

The widely held notion that good premorbid adjustment is almost always associated with sudden onset and good prognosis—as well as the converse, that is, poor premorbid adaptation, insidious onset, and thus poor outcome—present some difficulties when they are tested in a more precise manner. By the same token, it is difficult to accept the assertion that some individuals may have a poor premorbid adjustment and be simultaneously considered to be mentally healthy prior to their psychotic break. In order to account for this possibility, after the elimination of cases of mental retardation, minimal brain damage, or any other organicity, one can consider basically only two psychiatric explanations for poor premorbid adjustment. One of these is in the realm of psychopathic behavior, the other one is related to a subtle disturbance of cognition and affect processes, rather specific to the development of schizophrenia. At the point of psychiatric hospitalization, the appearance of acute symptomatology, defining the presence of schizophrenic symptoms, will indicate only that the individual with poor prior social adjustment was actually sick for a considerable time before his psychiatric admission.

It must also be pointed out that poor premorbid adjustment is a relative concept from the social point of view. Judgment as to the quality of this adjustment is generally made with consideration given to the age, social class, innate ability, or sex. In this sense, it has no validity except in comparison with normal social standards applicable to each particular patient's socioeconomic group. In addition, it is possible that some individuals may function relatively well on the instrumental level, (i.e., succeed in holding a job for a considerable period of time), yet at the same time have unusual and long-standing difficulties in various interpersonal relationships, prior to the appearance of florid psychotic symptomatology.

It has become increasingly clear that the presence of truly acute onset in combination with good premorbid adjustment should forewarn the psychiatrist that the diagnosis of schizophrenia may not be appropriate (11). The possibility for the misdiagnosis of schizophrenia increases further when the patient presents a premorbid personality which is not indicative of social impairment of long standing together with overt mental symptomatology frequently associated with schizophrenia (as is often the case in reactive psychosis) (1).

In view of the present findings and the above discussion presenting the profile of the acute schizophrenics, the reservoir group from which the chronics emerge in time suggests a different picture of the acute schizophrenic than that previously described. The acutes as a whole may be best characterized, on the basis of the present data, as a young population functioning on the marginal level for many years prior to their first hospitalization. In comparison with their normal counterparts, they represent a group of individuals who have a confused social role identity and disinterest in the established social values such as employment, self-sufficiency, and high standard of living. As a result of this orientation, they often become drifters, escaping social responsibilities through excessive use of alcohol and psychedelic drugs and exhibiting long-standing difficulties in social and sexual relationships.

The pseudoambulatory chronics (the former process schizophrenics modified by the irregular phenothiazine treatment) (24), on the other hand, appear to shuttle between community living and institutionalization unable to integrate socially.

They function at best on marginal levels. They appear to be socially isolated, unmarried, living alone in halfway boarding houses devoid of meaningful contact with friends and neighbors. In living such a reclusive life, use of drugs and alcohol provides the ambulatory chronic schizophrenics with momentary relaxation. For these patients, the difference between life in the hospital and the aimless existence in the community is almost nonexistent. For most subjects, constant expectation of rehospitalization is a routine anticipation since they are basically socially maladapted and lack the sense of perspective and purpose which would make community integration meaningful.

It is not really surprising, therefore, that the present findings regarding the areas of impaired functioning, leading to readmissions of the chronic patients, are primarily those associated with personal interactions. The readmission predictors reflect the chronic schizophrenic's inability to function in the community due to his tendencies toward antisocial behavior, poor relationships with sexual partners and difficulty in relating to others in halfway houses or other community groups. It should be noted that the predictors identified in the present study represent a shift from the previously described predictive variables, which focused primarily on instrumental social performance, such as gainful employment, adequate occupation, and the status of being married. This shift is all the more understandable if we consider the fact that for the pseudoambulatory chronic, who lives only temporarily in the community between his rehospitalizations, the traditionally assumed predictive indicators comprising social performance lose most of their meaning.

The policy of ubiquitous social Welfare support, in many cases, encourages public assistance dependence as a way of "earning a living" among schizophrenics, diminishing the importance of two of the formerly coveted predictors: employment status and occupation.

For the acute patients, who represent a younger population in comparison with the chronics, rehospitalization is most frequently precipitated by difficulties these patients encounter in adapting to their previous familial and emotional environments. In their transitional phase between the first psychotic episode and eventual chronicity, the problems appear to center around difficulties in emotional relationships with close ones, such as parents, close friends, or boyfriends and girlfriends. All of these represent persons on whom the acute patients have been emotionally dependent, prior to their hospitalization (4).

It should be noted that a structured and standardized assessment procedure designed to cover a wide range of psychosocial functioning components (such as has been used in the present study) permits not only a reliable evaluation of premorbid functioning levels in a comprehensive manner, but also provides data regarding current social functioning, which, when combined with information regarding premorbid adjustment level, serves to predict future outcome.

The data pertaining to the predictive elements of psychosocial functioning obtained in the present study throws new light on the present policy governing the discharge of schizophrenic patients. In this respect, it appears increasingly evident that pseudoambulatory schizophrenics, encumbered by their psychological deficit, are really unable to profit from the presently available community programs. As to the acute patients, it appears that automatic return of such individuals into the folds of their families upon discharge may not represent the wisest choice, since a large proportion of these patients appears to be unable to cope with old emotional ties, particularly those represented by their parents.

Although the impairment in functioning appears to be the most easily detected aspect of the schizophrenic's adjustment, yet, in predicting the adjustment of patients, stress (as a response to the wide range of situational and environmental factors) represents the cause for the schizophrenics' disorganization of behavior.

REFERENCES

1. Astrup, C., Fossum, A., and Holmboe, R.: "Prognosis in Functional Psychosis." Charles C. Thomas, Springfield, Ill., 1962.
2. Birley, J.L.T., and Brown, G.W.: Crises and life changes preceding the onset or relapse of acute schizophrenia: clinical aspects. *Br. J. Psychiat.* **116:** 327–333, 1970.
3. Bleuler, M.: A 23 year Longitudinal Study of 208 Schizophrenics and Supressions in Regard to the Nature of Schizophrenia. In "The *Transmission of Schizophrenia*" (D. Rosenthal and S.S. Kety, eds.) Pergamon Press, Oxford, London, 1968.
4. Brown, W.G., Birley, J.L.T., and Wing, J.R.: Influence of family life on the cause of schizophrenic disorders. *Br. J. Psychiat.* **12:** 241–258, 1972.
5. Burnstein, A.G., Adams, R.L., and Chapman, L.F.: Prognosis in schizophrenia. *J. Nerv. Ment. Dis.* **159:** 137–140, 1974.
6. Donlon, P.T., and Blacker, K.H.: Clinical recognition of early schizophrenic decompensation. *Dis. Nerv. Sys.* **36:** 323–337, 1975.
7. Ellsworth, R.B., and Clayton, W.: Measurement of improvement in mental illness. *J. Consult. Psychol.* **23:** 15–20, 1959.
8. Ellsworth, R.B., Foster, L., and Childres, B.: Hospital and community adjustment as perceived by psychiatric patients, their family and staff. *J. Consult. Clinic. Psychol.* **32:** 1–41, 1968.
9. Farina, A., and Webb, W.W.: Premorbid adjustment and subsequent discharge. *J. Nerv. Ment. Dis.* **124:** 612–613, 1963.
10. Garfield, S.L., and Sundland, D.M.: Prognostic Scales in schizophrenia. *J. Consult. Psychol.* **30:** 18–24, 1966.
11. Gittelman-Klein, R., and Klein, D.: Premorbid asocial adjustment and prognosis in schizophrenia. *J. Psychiat. Res.* **7:** 35–53, 1969.
12. Held, J.M., and Cromwell, R.L.: Premorbid adjustment in schizophrenia. *J. Nerv. Ment. Dis.* **146:** 264–272, 1968.
13. Higgins, J.: Process-reactive schizophrenia. *J. Nerv. Ment. Dis.* **149:** 451–471, 1969.
14. Katz, M.M., and Lyerly, S.B.: Methods for measuring adjustment and social behavior in the community: I. Rationale, description, discriminitive validity and scale development. *Psychol. Rep.* **13:** 503–535, 1963.
15. Langfeldt, G.: The prognosis in schizophrenia. *Acta Psychiat. Scandinavica* (Suppl. 110) (1–66), 1956.
16. Langner, T.S.: "The Mid-Manhattan Study." McGraw-Hill, New York, 1962.
17. Michaux, W.W., Katz, M.M., Kurland, A.A., and Gansereit, K.H.: "The First Year Out." Johns Hopkins Press, Baltimore, Md., 1969.

18. Nuttall, R.L., and Solomon, L.F.: Factorial structure and prognostic significance of premorbid adjustment in schizophrenia. *J. Consult. Psychol.* **29**: 362–372, 1965.
19. Phillips, L.: Case History data and prognosis in schizophrenia. *J. Nerv. Ment. Dis.* **117**: 515–525, 1953.
20. Query, J. Query, W.: Prognosis and Progress: A 5 year study of 48 schizophrenic men. *J. Consult. Psychol.* **28**: 501–505, 1964.
21. Roen, S.R., and Burnes, A.J.: "Community Adaptation Schedule Preliminary Manual." New York Behavioral Publications Inc., New York, 1968.
22. Roen, S.R., Ottenstein, D., Cooper, S., Burnes, A.: Community adaptation as an evaluative concept in community mental health. *Arch. Gen. Psychiat.* **151**: 36–44, 1966.
23. Serban, G., and Woloshin, G.: Relationship between pre- and postmorbid psychological stress in schizophrenics. *Psychol. Rep.* **35**: 507–517, 1974.
24. Serban, G., and Thomas, A.: Attitudes and behaviors of acute and chronic schizophrenic patients regarding ambulatory treatment. *Am. J. Psychiat.* **131**: 991–995, 1974.
25. Stephens, J.H., and Astrup, C.: Prognosis in "process" and "nonprocess" schizophrenia. *Am. J. Psychiat.* **119**: 945–951, 1963.
26. Stephens, J.H., O'Connor, G., and Wiener, G.: Long-term prognosis in schizophrenia using the Becker-Wittman Scale and the Phillips Scale. *Am. J. Psychiat.* **126**: 498–503, 1969.
27. Ullmann, L.P., and Giovannoni, J.M.: The development of a self-report measure of the process-reactive continuum. *J. Nerv. Ment. Dis.* **138**: 38–41, 1964.
28. Vaillant, J.: Prospective prediction of schizophrenic remission. *Arch. Gen. Psychiat.* **11**: 509–617, 1964.
29. Varsamis, J., and Adamson, J.D.: Early schizophrenia. *Ca. Psychiat. Assoc. J.* **16**: 487–490, 1971.
30. Wittman, P., and Steinberg, L.: Follow-up of an objective evaluation of prognosis in dementia praecox and manic-depressive psychosis. *Elgin State Hospital Papers* **5**: 216–227, 1944.

CHAPTER 5

The Measurement of Stress in Schizophrenics and Normals in Community Living*

Modern clinical concepts of schizophrenia have acknowledged the importance of stress as a major factor in the etiology of the schizophrenic process. Yet, in traditional research on predictors of adjustment in psychiatric patients, stress, along with the wide range of situational and environmental factors has received far less scrutiny than have such areas as social class, symptomatic pattern, and duration of illness (29). Perhaps the primary reason for the dearth of research on environmental stress is the difficulty inherent in its objective measurement. The laboratory paradigms of stress with their inherent controls contribute basic knowledge about the effects of stress on individuals, but such studies provide little insight into the nature and dimensions of stress that impinge on patients in their natural and varied habitats.

The seminal work of Selye (35, 36) who conceptualized the general-adaptation-syndrome has contributed greatly to the understanding of the concept of stress as applied to psychopathology. Central to Selye's position is the assumption that stress is basic to all adaptive reactions. However, the same stressor that has adaptive consequences in one case may produce maladaptive responses in another. Four main elements appear to be involved in stress situations according to the Selye model: (1) An antecedent stressor, (2) mediating factors which increase or decrease the impact of the stressor; (3) the "general adaptation syndrome" consisting of nonspecific physical and chemical reactions indicative of the intervening state of stress over time; and (4) consequent adaptive or maladaptive responses, the latter representing a derailment of the mechanisms of adaptation syndrome and appearing as "diseases of adaptation." In an attempt to clarify the nature of social psychological stress in humans, Dohrenwend (7) proposed 8 assumptions about the general nature of relationships among the various elements of the stress response, based on the theoretical underpinnings

---

*The research results presented in this chapter have appeared in the article: Serban, G.: Stress in schizophrenics and normals. Br. J. Psychiat. 126: 397–407, 1975.

brought forth by Selye. In the Dohrenwend formulation, classes of stressors are assumed to be social in nature, and do not involve direct physical harm to the individual. Dohrenwend assumes that stress is a state intervening between antecedent constraint and consequent efforts to reduce the constraint. The probability of maladaptive responses is alleged to vary directly with intensity and duration of stress. This approach, however, was too limited to account for all the facets of the stress phenomena. Several definitions of stress have been proposed in attempts to delineate the conceptual elements underlying the stress framework. One is that these approaches focused on the specification of classes of response as evidence that an individual is under stress. Selye's notion of the general adaptation syndrome exemplifies this conceptual approach, since occurrence of a particular response syndrome defines the occurrence of stress. The main weakness of this conceptualization of stress lies in the difficulty of obtaining similar response clusters to a variety of objective or subjective situations that may or may not be considered as stressful. Additional problems are created since the psychological meaning of the same response pattern may be entirely different, as when increased heart rate results from heavy exercise or a frightening situation. An equally important weakness of this approach is the failure to differentiate between objective and subjective situations, that is self-induced rather than uncontrollable events which cause a particular response pattern.

In an attempt to solve some of the weakness in the response-based approach to stress, some investigators focused on certain classes of stimuli or situations which play a role in creating stress. Conceptualization of stress as stemming from exposure to situations involving certain classes of stimulus properties presents its own problems, however. One of these is created by specification of just what kind of situations with what kind of properties makes for stress. Matters are also complicated by the wide individual differences in response to presumably identical stressors. Broad range of reactions to the same stressful situations has been obtained: from performance enhancement or degradation, (16) to physiological response with or without a concomittant psychological response.

Conceptualization of stress in terms of organism–environment transaction has been proposed to account for some of the weakness inherent in the two approaches discussed above. In this view, stress is conceived as an individual reaction of an organism to environmental events. Central to this position is the assumption that environmental changes lead to the perception of threat by the individual which provides the starting point for the stress experience. Yet, many stress reactions are not necessarily preceded by objectively detectable environmental changes.

The diversity of meanings ascribed to stress reinforces the need for a delineation of the specific element basic to this concept. From a clinical point of view, stress is assumed to occur when there is a substantial imbalance between the environmental demand placed on the organism and his capability to respond to it. Lazarus' (23) contributions are particularly significant in this connection.

He assumes that an environmental demand produces stress only if the individual anticipates inability to cope successfully with it. This phenomenological approach attempts to emphasize that stress is produced by the subjectively interpreted demand and response on the part of the individual. The intervening variable between environmental demand and the stress response, then, involves what Lazarus termed "cognitive appraisal" which produces individual interpretation of an event based on past experience and internal conditions of the responder. Equally important in the formulation of stress is that stress occurs only if failure to meet the demand is perceived to be important. In short, psychological stress implies the anticipation of adverse consequences arising from failure to meet demands.

The nature of demand must also be qualified if a useful framework is to be derived from the "cognitive appraisal" approach. In most conceptualizations, the quality of demand in a stressful imbalance results from overload, or a demand that exceeds the capacities of the individual, or a deficit in demand, particularly social isolation and confinement, may produce stress-like effects (26).

From the clinical point of view, various researchers attempted to extract elements of stress manifested in patients suffering distress. Sifneos (40) for example, emphasized the concept of emotional crisis based on a dynamic descriptive formulation of excessive demands and coping. A more promising framework for a clinically meaningful theory of stress has been derived from experiments with normals (14) who showed the importance of distinguishing between the organism's immediate emergency reaction and his subsequent long term coping with continuing stress. In extrapolating from their research with normals the authors hypothesized that the type of mental illness which the individual develops under stress is predetermined by the type of habitual emergency reaction he displays in his normal state.

A concise, although still tentative theoretical synthesis of recent knowledge of stress in psychopathology, has been made by Tong and Murphy (41). They postulate that conditionable anxiety is the underlying concept in stress, the handling of which results in different maladaptive learning through traumatic escape and traumatic avoidance. They raise important questions as to the nature of stressors (specific or generalized) and the function of anxiety as drive vs. disruptor.

In a more specific consideration of the role of stress in schizophrenia, psychiatric literature abounds with evidence of its crucial effect in the development of this disease. As mentioned in the first chapter, various theories of schizophrenia, and the behavioral theory in particular, have related stress to three predisposing factors: preschizophrenic high anxiety level, hypersensitivity to anxiety, arousing stimuli, and slow rate of recovery from anxiety (10). In this view, schizophrenia is conceived psychophysiologically as an avoidance reaction to anxiety-producing events; the individual's response being dictated by his ability to cope with these stimulus situations. Schizophrenia may thus be understood as a disturbance of adaptation, where accumulated environmental stressors and situational reactions are responsible for the disorganization of personality leading to hospitalization. In this context, Brown and Birley and Wing *(5)* have attempted to demonstrate that schizophrenics are highly sensitive to their social environments and overreact to both positive and negative emotional stimuli in their life changes and crises. It became progressively clearer that acute stress experienced in a crisis situation is understood clinically as a precipitating event while a long term stressor might lead in some individuals to maladaptive coping responses. From this point of view biochemical research can clarify the issue of the individual's reaction to stress.

Investigation of the biochemical correlates of schizophrenia have linked presence of clinical stress with high level of corticosteroid excretions. In fact Sachar *et al. (34)*, Matsumoto *et al. (25)*, and Vertanyan *(43)* found a significant parallel between fluctuations in clinical stress dependent on the phase of the illness and the corresponding amount of ketosteroids (17 OHCS) excreted in the urine of patients. By contrast, acute schizophrenia was associated with increased activity of the creatine phosphokinase (CPK) and aldolase. Chronically psychotic patients, both schizophrenics and depressives, did not show an increase of these enzymes even in periods of exacerbation of their psychotic condition *(27)*. Such enzymes as lactic dehydregenase (LDG), acid phosphatase, alkaline phosphatase, serum glutamic oxalcetic transaminase (SGOT), and serum glutamic pyruvic transaminase (SGPT) were not increased in either category of schizophrenia (acute or chronic) *(27)*. Another group of enzymes, however, appears to be related to schizophrenia. Murphy and Wyatt *(31)*, for instance, found markedly increased platelet MAO activity in schizophrenic patients. Similarly, the metabolism of norepinephrene appears to be affected in schizophrenia as indicated by the presence in urine of catechol-o-metyle transpherase *(1)* and DMPE *(11)*.

At present, studies linking MAO with schizophrenia are still basically inconclusive *(14a)*. Available evidence merely suggests the presence of a relationship between the brain's chemical metabolism and schizophrenic illness.

The only clearly documented and adequately measured interaction between clinical symptoms of schizophrenia and the concomittant chemistry changes appears to be related to epinephrene and other derivatives of 17 KS and OHCS.

Clinically, the measurement of stress met with partial success. Despite some concerted efforts, objective measurement of stress, particularly if extended beyond the concept of precipitating events, to include experienced distress prior to admission to the hospital, has remained an unresolved problem in psychiatry. Although various scales have been created to measure the pressure or intensity of stress *(9, 15, 21, 30, 32, 44)* these instruments basically measure acute stressful change in the individual's life leading to his mental illness or admission to hospital. Most of these scales, because of their construction, measure stress in too general terms or permit the interviewer too much subjectivity in the interpretation of the patient's responses. The need for precise evaluation of stress in schizophrenics becomes particularly significant since its measurement is assumed to facilitate treatment (29), particularly through crisis intervention (37). The first problem in the measurement of stress, as it affects the course of mental illness, is therefore to establish accurate readings of environmental stress as it impinges uncontrollably on the patient. But, several obstacles may be found. It has been shown that stress per se does not necessarily impair performance (19) and, in schizophrenia in particular, deficiency in sensitivity to stress has been observed (28).

The most commonly used approach to the study of stress in the development of schizophrenia focuses on distressing life changes and crises, particularly those occurring just prior to the appearance of florid psychotic symptoms. Precipitating stress, in particular, has figured in the prognostic implications for schizophrenia. Needless to say, precipitating events cannot be considered sufficient conditions for the development of schizophrenia since, according to some investigators, genetic predisposition plays an important role. As Rosenbaum (33) has suggested, precipitating events may combine with genetic factors to produce a schizophrenic state. In a series of studies, Birley and Brown (2, 4) have demonstrated that potentially disturbing events occurred more frequently in the period prior to the acute onset, relapse, and exacerbation of the schizophrenic state. Whether the prognostic value of precipitating events is all that is significant has been questioned by various researchers (6, 37).

One of the important confounding elements in the consideration of crisis events, or precipitating factors, stems from the underlying assumption that events, judged by common sense as being disturbing to an individual (4), necessarily produce emotional disturbance, or that the negative or undesirable quality of certain life episodes is equally stressful to all.

Some measure of improvement in the conceptualization of stressful life events has been represented by the focus on change as the critical factor (13). In this context stressors are "events that disrupt, or threaten to disrupt, the individual's usual activities" (8).

It is implied as well that the stressful events are not only socially undesirable but also require some adaptive or coping behavior in dealing with them (15). As such, stress presupposes the need for readjustment and active coping with unpleasant situations.

Despite some improvements in dealing with precipitating events as indicators of stress in schizophrenic etiology, the focus on precipitating events does not provide a very satisfactory solution to the problem of tapping stress. At best, precipitating events can be considered either a result of long term stress situation or a self-explanatory crisis situation.

In an attempt to deal with stress as it is manifested on the clinical, rather than the experimental level, a different approach may be needed. One such viewpoint of stress in a clinical setting is presented below.

Basic to the position taken here is the assumption, generally accepted by social scientists, that the gratification of human needs is molded by the dictates and structures of the individual's social milieu. Social expectations and demands represent ways in which gratification of needs are sanctioned by society, and as such they may be thought of as stressors, pressures, or environmental forces demanding solutions.

Forced to satisfy his human needs within the framework of prescribed social expectations, an individual undergoes a process of evaluation, consisting of the appraisal, or recognition of a situation involving the satisfaction of his needs within the prescribed social setting. Three separate, but interrelated, elements play an important role in this assessment. The sizing up of the life situation depends in part on the cognitive system which underlies reality testing. Concomittantly, each individual's appraisal is modified by his emotional make-up, determined in part by past learning experiences and reflected in various levels of self-confidence and self-esteem. The third element of equal importance is the person's motivational state, most conveniently conceptualized as an interest in obtaining gratification of a need by the projection of an intentional behavior associated with its achievement.

The separation of these three elements is, of course, artificial in the actual practice of decision-making regarding a life situation or while becoming aware of its implications; the three factors operate in unison to determine the final nature of the problem. It has become more apparent that schizophrenics suffer from a cognitive abnormality in terms of information processing deficit (18). They appear to show a defective "filter mechanism in processing external stimuli events which in turn affects their performance. In this sense the schizophrenic, in order to avoid information input overload, resorts to escape adaptive strategies (3), which in exchange reinforce negative patterns, and induce stress. By the same token, impairments affecting any one of these aspects decrease the ability to evaluate life situations realistically and, thus, negatively influence the response repertoire. In the final analysis, the behavioral response of the individual reflects the extent to which he is able to achieve the perceived goal and to satisfy his needs. Any deficiency in the coping mechanism, whether seen as poor reality testing or as the inability to cope because of the faultily perceived magnitude of the task, will evoke a whole gamut of emotional concomittant states, ranging from mild frustration to high levels of experienced stress.

From the above schema, it becomes apparent that the clinical approach to the evaluation of stress must account for the reaction of an individual patient to his life events. The most fruitful way to accomplish this would be to measure the level of experienced stress in the person's daily interactions, since they represent his attempts to satisfy a variety of personal needs. Although we tend to think of societal demands as representing an "objective" environmental task common to us all, in reality, the manner in which individuals seek fulfillment within the context of their social milieu, is a highly individual one. A situation would become stressful or nonstressful depending on the person's ability to cope with situations, which in turn depends on the degree of threat conveyed to him. The assumption that psychological stress represents a gross imbalance between demand stressors, and response capability of the organism resulting in possible adverse consequences provides a broad conceptual formulation which offers a useful guide for psychopathology related to stress. Therefore, any reasonable measurement of stress, outside of the laboratory, must take into account the personal response toward general events of life, bearing in mind that their effect on the person is influenced by his developmental stage, his interpretation of past experiences, his system of beliefs, and the basic concept he has of himself.

The study of experienced stress, based on the above conceptual formulation, was carried out with the original sample of 125 acute and 516 chronic schizophrenics, as well as 95 normal controls. The measure of stress was derived from the SSFIPD and consisted of 130 items fully described in Chapter 2. Additional information regarding the contributory and major factors precipitating hospitalization, obtained directly from patients in the course of history-taking, was also utilized to elucidate the importance of specific impairments in behavior and social interrelationships in psychiatric admission.

One-way and two-way analyses of variance were used to compare stress scores of the three groups of subjects, and to determine the effects of sex of subject on stress scores, Chi-square tests were applied in comparing distributions of contributory and major factors for admissions of acute and chronic schizophrenics.

Comparisons of the individual means for the 21 stress categories for acutes, chronics, and normals by means of a oneway analysis of variance are shown in Table I.

More detailed intergroup comparisons were handled by the Sheffé method and were used to elucidate which of the subgroup differences have contributed most significantly to the obtained overall differences.

The overall F test for the "among groups" effect was significant for 15 of the 19 stress categories. Lack of data for normals in use of psychedelic drugs and antisocial behavior precluded a reliable test of the differences in these dimensions. The subgroup comparisons, shown in the second half of Table I, indicate that the three groups of subjects—chronics, acutes, and normals—maintained the predicted order. Chronics reported higher levels of experienced stress than the acutes who, in turn, experienced more stress than the normals.

The overall stress score (i.e., the grand mean based on all 19 individual categories) showed a similar pattern.

Comparisons of chronics and acutes with normals show that chronics, when compared with normals, report consistently higher stress in 13 of the 19 categories. Nonsignificant differences were obtained in the area of job and management of finances. Moving on to the comparison of chronics and acutes on the same 19 stress categories, we see that the former have higher stress scores

Table 1

Analysis of Variance: Comparison of D Stress Scores for Normals and
Acute and Chronic Schizophrenic for 21 Stress Categories

	Among groups		Between groups F values		
Category	F	df	N vs. Ac	N vs. Ch	Ac vs. Ch
Education	6.55*	2/716	0.81	9.99*	5.30**
Job	4.83*	2/711	0.36	3.19	7.95*
Housekeeping	2.13	2/417	—	—	—
Welfare	0.75	2/377	—	—	—
Finances	4.90*	2/716	2.06	1.04	9.56*
Living circumstances	6.57*	2/715	0.10	8.05*	7.44*
Parents	13.71†	2/595	1.88	20.82†	11.14†
Relatives	6.72*	2/659	1.55	11.25†	4.31**
Marriage	7.26†	2/367	0.07	10.73*	6.50**
Children	4.72*	2/251	7.03*	8.20*	0.29
Dating	13.81†	2/598	7.71*	24.85†	5.59**
Sex	5.91*	2/716	1.27	9.79*	3.84
Friends	12.27†	2/715	1.51	18.69†	9.93†
Neighbors	4.24**	2/709	5.60**	8.20*	0.00
Others	34.03†	2/716	20.10†	65.71†	8.71*
Leisure	2.14†	2/716	—	—	—
Drinking	3.53**	2/183	3.70**	6.56**	0.88
Addictive Drugs	—	2/116	—	—	—
Psychedelic Drugs	4.26**	2/173	8.50**	6.17**	1.36
Antisocial Acts	—	2/271	—	—	—
Grand Mean	34.06†	2/716	7.25†	56.34†	22.22†

*p 0.01.
†p 0.001.
**p 0.05.

than the latter on 10 categories. The nonsignificant differences pertained to stress experienced in connection with marriage, children, sex, relationships with neighbors, drinking, and the use of psychedelic drugs.

Comparisons of stress levels in acutes and normals revealed that acutes experience more distress than the controls in 6 of the 19 stress categories. These were: relationships with children, neighbors, and others; dating; excessive drinking; and the use of psychedelic drugs.

Tables 2 and 3 report the means and standard deviations of the D-Stress scores for the three groups of subjects: normals, acutes, and chronics. Examination of Table 3 reveals that the direction of differences between the means consistently maintained the expected direction in 11 of the 19 stress categories; normals had lower stress scores than acutes, and acutes lower scores than did the chronics. It is also important to note that the comparison of means between the normal and the chronic schizophrenic groups revealed that the latter experienced more stress than the former in 17 of the 19 categories studied.

Table 2

Means and Standard Deviations of D Stress Scores for Normals and Acute
and Chronic Schizophrenics on the 21 Stress Categories

Category	Normal			Acute			Chronic		
	N	Mean	S.D.	N	Mean	S.D.	N	Mean	S.D.
Education	95	2.35	0.47	124	2.29	0.48	500	2.17	0.51
Job	93	2.62	0.22	122	2.65	0.32	499	2.54	0.38
Housekeeping	74	2.62	0.58	73	2.73	0.56	273	2.55	0.71
Welfare	21	2.41	0.60	44	2.56	0.64	315	2.44	0.63
Finances	95	2.35	0.68	124	2.49	0.62	500	2.27	0.71
Living circumstances	95	2.39	0.68	124	2.36	0.76	499	2.14	0.85
Parents	76	2.55	0.46	106	2.43	0.54	416	2.22	0.61
Relatives	90	2.85	0.26	117	2.77	0.41	455	2.66	0.55
Marriage	71	2.50	0.32	51	2.48	0.36	248	2.33	0.41
Children	43	2.60	0.57	40	2.12	0.89	171	2.20	0.86
Dating	53	2.73	0.30	105	2.54	0.39	443	2.43	0.42
Sex	95	2.67	0.57	124	2.56	0.64	500	2.42	0.72
Friends	95	2.72	0.35	124	2.61	0.59	499	2.41	0.69
Neighbors	95	2.81	0.49	123	2.58	0.74	494	2.58	0.74
Others	95	2.49	0.36	124	2.19	0.45	500	2.05	0.51
Leisure	95	2.52	0.50	124	2.66	0.52	500	2.60	0.54
Religion	89	2.87	0.28	122	2.85	0.30	489	2.83	0.29
Drinking	7	2.69	0.23	31	2.22	0.64	148	2.11	0.58
Addictive drugs	1	0.00	0.00	23	1.97	0.71	95	1.98	0.70
Psychedelic drugs	13	2.69	0.46	36	2.00	0.74	127	2.16	0.75
Antisocial acts	8	1.00	0.00	29	1.21	0.25	237	1.22	0.29
Grand Mean	95	2.60	0.44	124	2.50	0.55	500	2.36	0.59

Examination of particular items within each of the stress categories sheds
additional light on the obtained results by pointing out the specific reasons for the
experienced distress. For example, in the area of education, the acutes and
chronics were chiefly disturbed by the lower level of their educational achievement, when it was compared to that of their families, and their inability to
complete their studies or follow school instructions (acutes $\overline{X} = 2.21$; chronic
$\overline{X} = 2.31$; normals $\overline{X} = 3.00$). A few illuminating observations can also be
made on the reactions of the subjects to work related stress. When asked about
stress due to unemployment, the chronic patients admitted maximum amount of
stress when compared with acutes and normals, most probably because more of
the chronic patients (75%) were jobless for a longer period of time than the acute
patients (57.6%) or the normals (12.6%). The stress mean scores for the three
groups were 2.13, 2.08, and 2.26 for normals, chronics, and acutes, respectively. It is of interest to note that although only a small proportion of the normals
were unemployed (12.6%), as a group they appeared to experience more stress
than did the acute patients, since the latter were less interested in or worried
about work. Similarly, fewer of the acute patients (16%) than the normals

Table 3

D Stress: Males and Females by Normals, Chronics and Acutes
Two-Way Analysis of Variance

		Normal		Chronic		Acute		Sex	Patient**	Sex Patient
Category		Male	Female	Male	Female	Male	Female			
1.	Education	2.374	2.318	2.206	2.111	2.375	2.191	5.358*	5.237*	NS
2.	Job	2.595	2.642	2.541	2.550	2.582	2.719	NS	3.212*	NS
3.	House	2.598	2.661	2.647	2.446	2.703	2.744	NS	NS	NS
4.	Welfare	2.436	2.375	2.508	2.326	2.500	2.627	NS	NS	NS
5.	Finances	2.394	2.299	2.304	2.214	2.461	2.514	NS	3.981*	NS
6.	Living	2.545	2.210	2.215	1.997	2.421	2.288	8.645†	5.011†	NS
7.	Parents	2.582	2.519	2.260	2.146	2.477	2.382	NS	11.052**	NS
8.	Relatives	2.828	2.881	2.716	2.571	2.800	2.732	NS	6.317†	NS
9.	Marriage	2.446	2.577	2.422	2.242	2.575	2.398	NS	5.105†	4.307**
10.	Children	2.538	2.675	2.346	2.075	2.031	2.180	NS	5.530†	NS
11.	Dating	2.715	2.747	2.462	2.376	2.554	2.519	NS	14.307**	NS
12.	Sex	2.622	2.721	2.495	2.301	2.623	2.492	NS	5.726†	NS
13.	Friends	2.709	2.728	2.407	2.409	2.643	2.574	NS	8.656**	NS
14.	Neighbors	2.865	2.744	2.651	2.464	2.677	2.474	6.268^a	5.465†	NS
15.	Others	2.446	2.600	2.044	2.052	2.213	2.168	4.738^a	4.823†	4.744*
16.	Leisure	2.538	2.488	2.651	2.514	2.685	2.644	NS	NS	NS
17.	Religion	2.853	2.892	2.826	2.834	2.842	2.857	NS	NS	NS
18.	Drinking	2.800	2.640	2.129	2.058	2.239	2.173	NS	4.435**	NS
19.	A. Drugs	0.000	3.000	2.090	1.797	1.808	2.141			
20.	P. Drugs	2.800	2.625	2.160	2.167	1.979	2.042	NS	6.086	NS
21.	Anti-soc	0.000	1.000	1.203	1.280	1.227	1.143	NS	NS	NS

*$p < 0.05$.
†$p < 0.01$.
**$p < 0.001$.
NS; non significant.

(37.7%) or the chronic patients (17.2%) were upset by the level of their salaries. The acute group, as a whole, was more upset than the chronic one by the level of functioning in their last job (normals mean = 2.77, acutes mean = 2.68, and chronic mean = 2.50) and by the realization of their progressive decline in working capacity (acute mean = 1.97, chronic mean = 2.17).

Turning to specific stresses associated with housekeeping it appears that the acute patients have more difficulty than the normals, and the normals more than the chronics, in relation to housekeeping (acute mean = 2.15, chronic mean = 2:35, and normal mean = 2.33). The reversal in the stress scores seems to be related to the fact that 45.6% of the acute and 58% of the chronic patients, as compared with 23.2% of the normal controls, found the item about housekeeping inapplicable. Most of the schizophrenic sample was unmarried (64% of the acutes, 59.3% of the chronics versus 26.3% of the controls) and, thus, had little responsibility for housekeeping duties. Even so, the difference between acute and chronic patients was found to be significant at the 0.05 level, due most probably to the fact that the chronic patients, living alone for a more extended period of time than the acutes, were forced to be more involved in housekeeping chores.

Dependence on welfare assistance disturbed the chronic patients and the normal controls to a greater extent than it did the acutes (the mean for normals and acutes was 2.33 and 2.19 for chronics). These results are understandable, in light of the fact that the acute patients were younger individuals and thus largely dependent on their family's financial resources, with the resultant lesser upset caused by Welfare matters; it is interesting to note that only 6.4% of the acutes as compared with 12.5% of the normals reported distress associated with welfare dependence.

As regards stress associated with finances, the normal controls expressed more distress associated with amount of money earned, whereas the chronic patients were disturbed by the long period of time they had to do without income ($p < 0.01$). In this regard the differences between acute and chronic patients were also highly significant ($p < 0.01$).

Turning to stress produced through parental interaction, the groups were differentiated at high levels of significance ($p < 0.001$). The acute patients reported being more upset than the normals, and the chronics more than the acutes, by parental daily interference into their lives, and the familial expectation and demands (the mean stress scores for acutes were 2.24, 2.09 for chronics, and 2.45 for normals). A similar trend was observed regarding stress stemming from interaction with relatives. Acute patients were more upset by their relationships with brothers and sisters than were the normals, but the degree of experienced stress in this area was highest for the chronics (the acute mean = 2.79, chronic mean = 2.64, and normal mean = 2.96 $p < 0.01$). Dealing with relatives appears to be most stress producing to the chronic group as compared with normals, although acutes had more problems in this area than did the controls.

Regarding stress produced by marital interaction, the acutes and the normals appear to experience similar types of problems, whereas the chronic patients seem unable to relate to their mates ($p < 0.01$). It is of interest to note that the acutes found marital sexual incompatability a less significant factor in their marital break-up than did the normals (acute mean = 2.90, chronic mean = 2.73, and normal mean = 2.69). Comparison of relationships upon remarriage revealed that normals tended to relate more successfully to their partners than did the acute patients, apparently because the former group chose more compatable mates.

Differences in stress associated with relationship to children were also found to be significant for the three subject groups ($p < 0.01$). The acute patients expressed greatest distress in this area, most because they were particularly concerned about maintaining meaningful contact and emotional interaction with their offspring. The mean stress scores for the three groups were 2.50, 2.59, 2.91 for the acutes, chronics, and normals, respectively. In summarizing the findings regarding stress produced by familial interaction, it may be said that the chronic patients seem to be most disturbed by it, the acutes exhibited intermediate levels of worry in this regard, and the normals appeared to be least distressed by familial relationships.

Levels of stress associated with social interpersonal relationships particularly with dating and sexual partners differentiated the groups at high levels of significance ($p < 0.01$). Both the acute and the chronic patients felt uneasiness in relating on the emotional level with opposite sex peers as compared to normals (stress means for the three groups were 2.54 for acutes, 2.48 for chronics, and 2.89 for normals.) This problem was especially revealed in the level of frustration experienced in a desire to get married, yet being upset by being unable to do so (acute mean = 2.39, chronic mean = 2.33, and normal mean = 2.56). The groups were also differentiated in terms of levels of difficulty encountered in developing and maintaining sexual relationships with the opposite sex, with the chronics being most upset ($\overline{X} = 2.49$), the acutes moderately so ($\overline{X} = 2.59$), and the normals least of all ($\overline{X} = 2.76$).

Highest levels of stress stemming from inability to make friends were reported by the chronics ($\overline{X} = 2.35$) followed by the acutes ($\overline{X} = 2.56$). As may be expected, normals reported least stress in this connection ($\overline{X} = 2.76$). It should also be pointed out that the chronics showed the highest levels of worry associated with their inability to interact with friends ($\overline{X} = 2.62$ for chronics, 2.82 for acutes, and 2.82 for normals).

In terms of distress stemming from relationships with neighbors, the groups were also clearly differentiated ($p < 0.05$), with the acutes and chronics equally upset by their inability to relate to people in their neighborhoods (the means for acutes, chronics, and normals were 2.58, 2.58, and 2.81, respectively).

In their relationships to authority figures and others in the community, chronics experienced significantly more stress than did the acutes and the normals ($p < 0.001$; $\overline{X}$ for chronics 2.41, $\overline{X}$ for acutes 2.61, $\overline{X}$ for normals 2.69).

The chronic patients were particularly upset by their inability to participate in community activities (the mean stress scores for chronics, acutes, and normals were 1.76, 1.95, and 2.12, respectively) and were especially frustrated by the feelings of total social isolation and absence of social life (chronic $\overline{X} = 2.32$, acute $\overline{X} = 2.50$, and normal $\overline{X} = 2.75$). Religious affiliation did not appear to be a significant source of stress in any of the groups.

Turning to excessive drinking, it was found that chronic patients were the heaviest users of alcohol, as compared with their acute counterparts and the controls (1.41 versus 1.35 for acutes and 1.25 for normals; $p < 0.05$), and as a group they also admitted that their alcohol consumption created serious problems in daily life, exacerbating the experienced stress levels (chronics = 2.25, acutes = 2.38, and normals = 3.00). On the other hand, use of psychedelic drugs represented more of a problem for acutes than for chronics, particularly because of the more frequent number of "bad trips" experienced by the former, creating more anxiety for these patients (the stress means were 1.94 for acutes,

2.09 for chronics, and 2.69 for normals, accounting for the significant difference at the 0.05 levels).

Stress associated with criminal activities and other antisocial behavior could be compared only for the two patient groups, as none of the normals found questions in this area applicable. It was found that acute patients were more distressed by their past antisocial activities than the chronic patients (acute mean = 1.21, chronic mean = 1.22).

Having established stress differentials in the three groups of subjects, it was deemed necessary to establish which problem areas contribute either directly or secondarily to rehospitalization of acute and chronic schizophrenics.

It is of interest to note that careful inquiry failed to reveal clear participating factors for all acute patients. Furthermore, some of the chronic patients gave identical precipitating causes as those identified by acutes. For instance, 47 of the 125 acutes (37.6%) specified one of the 21 stress categories as a major factor in their hospitalization, the remainder, although under high stress upon admission, could not clearly identify any one particular stress category as decisive in their admission. Of the 516 chronics, 198 or 38.4% were able to identify major factors responsible for their readmission. Contributing factors were defined for the purposes of the study as secondary reasons. The distribution of major and contributing factors causing the hospitalization of acute and chronic patients is shown in Table 4.

Examination of the magnitude of percentages for the various major causes in the hospitalization of acute schizophrenics (see Table 4) reveals that the most frequent main reasons for readmission appear to be related to family interaction (marriage 12.0%, parents 9.6%), sexual difficulties (12.0%), and problems with friends (8.8%), follwed by problems associated with a job (4.8%). A different pattern emerges when the chronic patients are considered. For these patients welfare dependence and finances appear to be the most frequent major precipitating events in rehospitalization (1%), with disturbed relationships with parents (11.8%) and friends (10.7%) representing a close second, and disturbances in sexual life, a third most important factor (10.3%).

It must be noted, however, that the major causes of rehospitalization, statistically differentiating acute and chronic schizophrenics when these were compared with areas where no problem was identified, were marriage ($X^2 = 3.92$, $df = 1$, $p < 0.05$: Yates correction applied) and finances ($X^2 = 6.47$, $df = 1$, $p < 0.02$: Yates correction applied). Comparison of the acute and chronic samples on contributing factors revealed that only marriage ($X^2 = 6.67$, $df = 1$, $p < 0.01$ with Yates correction) and job ($X^2 = 4.17$, $df = 1$, $p < 0.05$) significantly differentiated the groups.

The detailed analysis of psychosocial aspects of stress revealed some interesting patterns of subjective reaction to distress in the two schizophrenic subgroups and the normal controls used in the study. It is of particular interest that normals, acute schizophrenics, and chronic schizophrenic patients experience different

Table 4
Contributing and Major Factors Causing Hospitalization of Acute–Chronic Patients

| | Contributing Factor | | | | Major Cause | | | | | | No problem | | | |
| | Acute | | Chronic | | Acute | | | Chronic | | | Acute | | Chronic | |
	N	%	N	%	N	MM	%	N	MM**	%	N	%	N	%
1. Education	21	16.8	72	14.0	1	1	1.6	0	5	1.0	102	81.6	439	86.1
2. Job	32	25.6	178	34.5*	4	2	4.8	14	19	6.4	87	69.6	305	59.1
3. Housekeeping	9	7.2	35	6.7	0	1	0.8	0	4	0.8	115	92.0	477	92.4
4,5,6. Finances	40	32.0	184	35.7	3	2	4.0	45*	27	14.0	80	64.0	260	50.4
7. Parents	36	28.8	120	23.3	8	4	9.6	35	26	11.8	77	6.16	335	64.9
8. Relatives	13	10.4	64	12.4	1	1	1.6	8	7	2.9	110	88.0	437	84.7
9. Marriage	4	3.2	61	11.8†	11	4	12.0	22*	16	7.4	106	84.8	417	80.8
10. Children	11	8.8	60	11.6	0	4	3.2	8	6	2.5	110	88.0	442	85.7
11,12. Sexual Life	31	24.8	132	25.1	11	4	12.0	28	17	10.3	79	63.2	339	64.6
13,14,15,16,17. Social Life	33	26.4	163	31.6	8	3	8.8	38	17	10.7	81	64.8	298	57.8

*p < 0.05.
†p < 0.02.
**Multiple major causes of hospitalization per each patient. Chi square for contributing and major factors vs. no problem for acutes and chronics.

levels of stress in relation to ordinary life demands. Although few would argue that the stress experience of normals, as indicated by the study, requires special comment, the patterns of subjective stress experienced by the two schizophrenic groups are worthy of notice. Contrary to general psychiatric opinion, the chronic schizophrenics in this study reported higher levels of experienced stress than did their acute counterparts when stress was measured in terms of overall grand mean scores encompassing all 21 categories of stressors.

A more detailed examination of specific stress categories reveals that acute schizophrenic patients experience higher levels of stress than do normals in three important areas: relationships with children and opposite sex peers ($p < 0.01$), relationships with neighbors and other significant persons in the community ($p < 0.001$), and maladjusted social behavior evidenced by excessive drinking and use of drugs ($p < 0.05$). It should be mentioned that whereas higher stress for normals was associated only with frustrations associated with the inability to enjoy leisure because of occupational demands and lack of money, for the first admitted schizophrenics, stress centered around problems of coping with close interpersonal relationships which formed the core of their mental ruminations prior to hospitalization. Although the obtained differences in types and levels of stress for normals and acutes are interesting, since they tend to point out the areas of difficulty encountered by schizophrenics prior to their first hospitalization, it is the high levels of stress experienced by the chronic patients that deserve special attention. Contrary to the general findings in the literature (*10, 33*), the present sample of chronic schizophrenic patients reported consistently higher stress. The data strongly suggest that, when compared with normals, the pseudoambulatory chronic schizophrenics find the surrounding world a source of great distress and turmoil. Apparently, any level of involvement with their social environment (except perhaps for instrumental performance, job, and the management of finances, areas which have by now lost much meaning as goals to be pursued) creates, for the pseudoambulatory schizophrenic, a considerable amount of discomfort and anxiety. These patients tend to experience their intercourse with the outside world either in terms of having to deal with insurmountable societal demands, or as always failing in expectations placed on them with the resulting worry and tension.

The discrepancy in stress levels of chronic schizophrenics in our study as compared with those conducted earlier is easily explained if one considers that our sample represented a new type of "pseudoambulatory chronic" schizophrenics, rather than the long-term hospitalized patients who made up the chronic populations in other studies. This new type of chronic schizophrenic is repeatedly discharged into the community as soon as his gross psychiatric symptoms are controlled. He receives episodic phenothiazine treatment when readmitted to a psychiatric hospital or when treated in an ambulatory setting. While residing in the community between hospitalizations, this new chronic schizophrenic is still unable to cope with the minimal social or emotional demands placed on him.

Consequently, he experiences increasing levels of stress associated with the problems of social adaptation.

The comparisons of stress experienced by acute and chronic schizophrenics also reveal some interesting trends. Although both samples of patients represent basically the same type of illness, it is of interest to note that the chronics, with multiple hospitalizations and longer illness experience, report consistently higher levels of stress than do their first hospitalized counterparts, in the areas of educational achievement, work, management of finances, interpersonal relationships with close family members (parents, relatives, marital partners, and children), and others (including friends and other people in the community). In general, the acute patients, the reservoir from which the chronics emerge in time, had less total stress than did the chronic subjects. At the same time, the data strongly suggest that schizophrenics hospitalized for the first time do not really represent persons whose stress experiences are comparable to those of normals. There is ample evidence that acute patients, for a considerable time prior to the appearance of florid schizophrenic symptoms requiring hospitalization, appear to have stressful interactions with their children, opposite sex peers, neighbors, and other persons in the community at large. In addition, difficulties in obtaining and keeping sexual partners seem to be an important source of frustration and worried preoccupation for the acute patients. The present data fail to support the Birley and Brown hypothesis (2) that acute or patients hospitalized for the first time represent persons who, until close to their psychiatric admission, have functioned within normal limits. The consistently observed trends in stress levels obtained in the present study, with least distress manifested by normals, and increasing amounts shown as one moves from acute to chronic schizophrenics, suggest that both qualitatively and quantitatively these populations are different in terms of experienced stress. Apparently, these differences stem from the degree of impairment in coping mechanisms.

A second issue of importance brought out by the study has to do with the significance of precipitating factors in the hospitalization of acute and chronic schizophrenics. The results of the present study strongly suggest the need for a reevaluation of the role of precipitating factors in the etiology of schizophrenia and its importance in relation to the favorable prognosis of this disease (20, 42) The findings of the present research, in conjunction with those reported recently by Birley and Brown (2) throw considerable doubt on the generally accepted association between the presence of clear precipitating factors and type of schizophrenia.

In our study, two major causes of hospitalization (marital difficulties and financial problems) and two contributing factors (marital difficulties and problems associated with work) have emerged as important variables associated with the readmission of acute and chronic schizophrenics. Yet, careful examination of the contributing and major factors presented in Table 4 reveals that the majority of both types of patients were either admitted (acutes) or readmitted (chronics) without any specific major or contributing cause. This finding becomes all the less surprising when one considers the generally high level of global stress among schizophrenics. Whatever may be the major factor, which apparently brings about a particular hospital admission, it is simply an additive to the already high stress level of the patients.

The additional confounding of the role of the major precipitating cause has been brought about by the reported evidence of an increase in the rate of life crises in the three weeks prior to the schizophrenics' hospitalization this finding has been interpreted in terms of causal link by some researchers (2, 4). What these authors have failed to consider is the existent level of stress associated with the low level of the schizophrenics' functioning, which predates the appearance of florid symptoms by a considerable period of time. Precipitating factors, whether major or contributing, should be really interpreted as triggering mechanisms in the readmission of both acute and chronic schizophrenics. This notion appears to be consonant with the emerging literature (17), which has independently questioned the assumption that life events alone bear a direct relationship to the onset in schizophrenia. Recent evidence (24) also points toward the possibility that the causative link may be obscured by the factor of drug therapy maintenance. Schizophrenics released into the community without the benefit of sustained drug therapy present less clear-cut precipitating factors on readmission than do those who are taking drugs. The ''nonmedicated'' patients appear to relapse because of inability to tolerate multivariate stresses occurring in their everyday social situations.

The main implication of this study, supported by the most recent literature, is that precipitating events should really be thought of as pseudocausative agents in readmissions of schizophrenic patients. The real underlying cause of the need for rehospitalization of these patients appears to be associated with the total amount of stress they experience as a result of their impaired psychosocial interactions and disturbed perceptions of reality.

The importance of functioning and stress for the adjustment of the schizophrenics in the community was clearly shown in this and the last two chapters. It appears that the course of these patients in social settings is not fully predicted by either instrumental functioning, precipitating events, or the classical tenets of reactive process or high and low competence classifications.

In order to ascertain directly whether or not the acute–chronic distinction in schizophrenia and the high and low functioning classification (most commonly associated with social competence categorization) are equally efficient in predictive outcome for schizophrenics, we have undertaken a study comparing acute and chronic schizophrenics with their high and low instrumental functioning counterparts in 21 areas encompassing all aspects of daily functioning, and attempted to determine the contribution of each of these approaches to readmission. Results of this comparison and their implications for prognosis are discussed in the next chapter.

REFERENCES

1. Axelrod, J., and Vessel, E. S.: Heterogeneity of N and O metyltranspherase. *Molec. Pharmacol.* **6**: 78–84, 1970.

2. Birley, J.L.T., and Brown, G.W.: Crises and life changes preceding the onset or relapse of acute schizophrenia; clinical aspects. *Br. J. Psychiat.* **116**: 327–333, 1970.

3. Broen, W.E., and Nakamura, C.Y.: Reduced range of sensory sensitivity in chronic non-paranoid schizophrenics, *J. Abnormal Psychol.*, **79**: 106–111, 1972.

4. Brown, G.W., and Birley, J.L.T.: Crises and life changes and the onset of schizophrenia. *J. Health Soc. Behav.* **9**: 203–214, 1968.

5. Brown, G.W., Birley, J.L.T., and Wing, J.K.: Influence of family life as a cause of schizophrenic disorders: a replication. *Br. J. Psychiat.* **121**: 241–258, 1972.

6. Cole, M.E., Swensen, C.H., and Pascal, G.R.: Prognostic significance of precipitating stress in mental illness. *J. Consult. Psychol.* **18**: 171–175, 1954.

7. Dohrenwend, B.P.: The social psychological nature of stress: A framework for social inquiry. *J. Abnormal Soc. Psychol.* **62**: 294–302, 1961.

8. Dohrenwend, B.S., and Dohrenwend B.P.: Class and race as status related sources of stress. In "Social Stress" (S. Levine and N.A. Scotch, eds.), pp. 111–140, Aldine Publishing, Chicago. 1970.

9. Dohrenwend, B.S.: Life events as stressors: A methodological inquiry. *J. Health Soc. Behav.* **14**: 167–175, 1973.

10. Epstein, S., and Coleman, M.: Drive theories of schizophrenia. *Psychosomatic Med.* **32**: 114–141, 1970.

11. Friedhoff, A.J., and Van Winkle, E. A biochemical approach to the study of schizophrenia. *Am. J. Psychiat.* **121**: 1054–1055, 1965.

12. Friedman, E., Shopsin, B., Sathananthan, G., and Gershen, S.: Blood platelet monoamine oxidase activity in psychiatric patients. *Am. J. Psychiat.* **131**: 1392–1394, 1974.

13. Froberg, F., Karlsson, D.G., Levi, L., and Lidberg, L.: Physiological and biochemical stress reactions induced by psychosocial stimuli. *In* "Society, Stress and Disease." pp. 28–295, (L. Levi, ed.), Oxford University Press, New York, 1971.

14. Funkenstein, D.H., King, S.H., and Drolette, M.E.: "Mastery of Stress." Harvard University Press, Cambridge, Mass. 1957.

15. Holmes, T.H., and Rahe, R.H.: The social readjustment rating scale. *J. Psychosomatic Res.* **11**: 213–217, 1967.

16. Horvath, F.: Psychological stress: A review of definitions and experimental research. *In* "General Systems: Yearbook of Social General Systems Research" (L. Von Bertalanffy and A. Rapoport, eds.), vol. 4, pp. 203–230, 1960.

17. Jacobs, S.C., Prusoff, B.A., and Paykel, E.S.: Recent life events in schizophrenia and depression. *Psychol. Med.* **4**: 444–53, 1974.

18. Hemsley, D.R.: Attention and information processing in schizophrenia. *Br. J. Soc. Clinic Psychol.* **15**: 199–209, 1976.

19. Korchin, S.J.: Stress. In "The Encyclopedia of Mental Health" (A. Deutch and H. Fishman, eds.), vol. 6, pp. 1975–1982. Franklin Watts, New York, 1963.

20. Langfeldt, G.: The prognosis in schizophrenia and the factors influencing the course of the disease. Monograph: London. Humphrey Melford, 1937.

21. Langner, T.S., and Michel, S.T.: "Life Stress and Mental Health." The Midmanhattan Study, Free Press, New York, 1963.

22. Lazarus, R.S.: A laboratory approach to the dynamics of psychological stress. *Am. Psychol.* **19**: 400–411, 1964.

23. Lazarus, R.S.: "Psychological Stress and the Coping Process." McGraw-Hill, New York, 1966.

24. Leff, J.P., Hirsch, S.R., Plude, P.D., and Stevens, B.C.: Life events and maintenance therapy in schizophrenic relapse. *Br. J. Psychiat.* **123**: 659–60, 1973.
25. Matsumoto, K., Berlet, H.H., Bull, C., and Heinwich, H.E.: Excretion of 17 hydrocortico steroids and 17 ketosteroids in relationship to schizophrenic syndrome. *J. Psychiat. Res.* **4**: 1,–12, 1966.
26. McGrath, J.E.: A conceptual formulation for research on stress. *In* "Social and Psychological Factors in Stress" (J.E. McGrath, ed.), pp. 10–21. Holt, Rinehart and Winston, Inc., New York, 1970.
27. Meltzer, H., Elkun, L., and Moline, R.A.: Serum-enzyme changes in newly admitted psychiatric patients. Part I. *Arch. Gen. Psychiat.* **21**: 731–738, 1969.
28. Michaux, W.W.: Schizophrenic perception as a function of hunger. *J. Abnormal Soc. Psychol.* **50**: 53–58, 1955.
29. Michaux, W.W., Gansereit, K.H., McCabe, O.L., and Kurland, A.A.: The psychopathology and measurement of environmental stress. *Comm. Ment. Health J.* **3** (Winter: 358–372, 1967.
30. Michaux, W.W., Katz, M., Jurland, A.A., and Gansereit, K.H.: "The First Year Out." The Johns Hopkins Press, Baltimore, 1969.
31. Murphy, L.D., and Wyatt, R.J.: Reduced monoamine oxidase activity in blood platelets from schizophrenic patients. *Nature (London)* **238**: 225–226, 1972.
32. Phillips, L.: Case history data and prognosis in schizophrenia. *J. Nerv. Ment. Dis.* **117**: 515–525, 1953.
33. Rosenbaum, C.P.: Metabolic, physiological, anatomic and genetic studies in the schizophrenias: a review and analysis. *J. Nerv. Ment. Dis.* **146**: 103–126, 1968.
34. Sachar, E.J., Mason, J.W., Holmer, H.S., and Artiss, K.L.: Psychoendocrine aspects of acute schizophrenic reactions. *Psychosomatic Med.* **25**: 510–537, 1963.
35. Selye, H.: "The Physiology and Pathology of Exposure to Stress: A Treatise Based on the Concepts of the General-Adaptation-Syndrome and the Diseases of Adaptation." Acta, Montreal, 1950.
36. Selye, H.: "The Stress of Life." McGraw Hill, New York, 1956.
37. Serban, G.: Relationship of mental status, functioning and stress to readmission of schizophrenics. *Br. J. Soc. Clin. Psychol.* **14**: 201–301, 1975.
38. Serban, G.: Stress in schizophrenics and normals. *Br. J. Psychiat.* **126**: 397–407, 1975.
39. Sheffe, H.: "The Analysis of Variance." John Wiley & Son, Inc., New York, 1959.
40. Sifneos, P.E.: A concept of emotional crisis. *Mental Hygiene,* **44**: 169–179, 1960.
41. Tong, J.E., and Murphy, I.C.: A review of stress reactivity research in relation to psychopathology and psychopathic disorders. *J. Ment. Sci.* **106**: 1273–1295, 1960.
42. Vaillant, G.E.: Prospective prediction of schizophrenic remission. *Arch. Gener. Psychiat.* **11**: 509–517, 1964.
43. Vertanyan, M.E.: Anxiety and the Stress Reaction in Different Forms of Schizophrenia. *In* "Studies of Anxiety" (M.H. Lader, ed.), pp. 28–31. Headley Bros. Ltd., Ashford, Kent, 1969.
44. Wallis, G.G.: Stress as a predictor in schizophrenia. In "Annual Review of the Schizophrenic Syndrome" (R. Cancro, ed.), vol. 3, pp. 497–513. Brunner/Mazel, New York, 1973.

CHAPTER 6

Comparison of Two Classifications of Schizophrenia: Acute-Chronic and High-and-Low Competent on Comprehensive Functioning and Stress Derived From the SSFIPD*

As we have shown in the two previous chapters, the prediction of outcome in schizophrenia in terms of specific psychosocial factors is still debated between the researcher who would like to reduce prediction to its instrumental functioning level and the researcher who would approach it on a global level. A good example of this debate is between the social competence school and the supporters of comprehensive psychosocial functioning in the community. This delemna affects not only the prediction of schizophrenia, but also its classifications.

Since acutes and chronics function at different levels—the acutes at a higher level than the chronics—and the high and low social competence division distinguishes the two groups on the basis of instrumental functioning, we have attempted to find to what extent these classifications are sensitive to the overall problems of schizophrenics living in the community. In addition we have sought to identify the extent to which the acute–chronic and the high and low socially competent classifications tap various deficits in functioning which lead to rehospitalization.

Furthermore, since some researchers *(1, 2, 4)* suggested that there is a correlation between stress and low social status, the classification based on high and low social competencies should also point out the level on which the low socially competent experience stress.

In this context, it appears important to ascertain the extent to which acute–chronic and high and low competence classifications of schizophrenics are comparable in terms of the total amount of stress experienced by the individuals so classified. In particular, it would be interesting to find out whether the low competent group, like the marginally functioning chronic schizophrenics de-

---

*The research results presented in this chapter have appeared in the following article: G. Serban, C.B. Gidynski, and E.L. Melnick: Social performance and readmission in acute and chronic schizophrenics: comparison of two approaches. *Behav. Neuropsych.* 7 (No. 1–12): 6–12, 1975–76.

scribed in the preceding chapter, are also experiencing greater amounts of stress than their more competent counterparts.

With these considerations in mind, the original population of 516 chronic and 125 acute schizophrenics (see Chapter 1) was reclassified on the basis of the four demographic indices of education, occupation, employment, and marital status (forming a cluster of factors defined by Zigler and Phillips *(4)* as indicative of social competence) into high and low competence subjects using above and below mean scores as cut-off points for forming the groups. The acute and chronic schizophrenic subjects remain as originally defined in the sample section of the book (Chapter 2). The 641 schizophrenic subjects divided into acutes and chronics on one hand, and into high and low socially competent on the other, were then compared on 21 functioning categories derived from the SSFIPD. In addition, the two classifications of subjects were also compared in terms of 21 stress scores.

To determine the contribution of instrumental functioning (social competence) and more comprehensive social functioning to readmission, the scores for these variables were submitted to multiple discriminant analysis, run separately for acute and chronic schizophrenics, with readmission status as the dependent variable.

Before comparing the two classifications it might be illuminating to examine the distribution of social competence measures among acute and chronic schizophrenics.

Tables 1, 1a, and 1b reveal that acute schizophrenics differ significantly from their chronic counterparts in terms of social demographic scores ($X^2 = 11.41$, $p < 0.001$). Whereas the largest percentage of acute schizophrenics fall into the two highest score categories (II and III), most of the chronics obtained the lowest scores. Categories I, II, and III, described fully in Chapter 3, reflect three levels of social attainment based on social competence. Category I is indicative of low social attainment; Category II reflects a medium social functioning; while Category III indicates a high level of attainment.

Total functioning scores, based on the 21 functioning dimensions tapped by the SSFIPD for acute and chronic schizophrenics divided into high (above mean)

Table 1

Distribution of Sociodemographic Scores for Acute
and Chronic Schizophrenics

		Sociodemographic Score						
		I		II		III		
Patient	N	N	%	N	%	N	%	X^2
Acute	125	40	32.0	61	48.8	24	19.2	11.41*
Chronic	516	267	51.8	189	36.6	60	11.6	11.41*

$*p < 0.001$.

Table 1a

Distribution of Acute and Chronic Females on the
Sociodemographic Score Grouping*

	Acute		Chronics	
	N	%	N	%
Group I	19	6.6	80	27.6
Group II	28	9.7	78	26.9
Group III	13	5.4	29	10.0
	60	20.7	187	64.5

*The sociodemographic score groupings are discussed in detail in Chapter 3.

and low (below mean) social competence groups, are shown in Table 2. It is of interest to note that 198 (38.3%) of the chronic schizophrenics who have had an average of 3.6 years of hospitalization have received high competence scores. Examination of Table 3 also reveals an interesting trend: the 302 low competence chronic subjects as well as the 51 low competence acute counterparts obtained higher stress scores than did the high competence subjects irrespective of the schizophrenic subtype.

The comparisons of the two classifications, acute–chronic and high and low competence, on each of the 21 functioning and stress dimensions were determined by means of a two-way analysis of variance. Results pertaining to this first comparison, functioning, are presented in Table 4. Of the 21 functioning areas considered, eight significantly differentiated both classifications: acutes from chronics and the high from the low competence schizophrenics. These were: education, job, dependence on welfare, relationship with parents, marital adjustment, relationship with others in the community, spare time interest, antisocial acting out, and the total functioning score encompassing all of the functioning dimensions.

Table 1b

Distribution of Acute and Chronic Males on the
Sociodemographic Score Grouping*

	Acute		Chronics	
	N	%	N	%
Group I	20	4.5	185	41.5
Group II	34	7.6	112	25.1
Group III	11	2.5	32	7.2
	65	14.6	329	73.8

*The sociodemographic score groupings are discussed in detail in Chapter 3.

Table 2

Total Functioning Scores* for Acute and Chronic Schizophrenics
Divided into High and Low Social Competence Groups

Patient	Low Competence			High Competence		
	N	Mean	S.D.	N	Mean	S.D.
Acute	51	2.29	0.245	73	2.44	0.193
Chronic	302	2.18	0.232	198	2.32	0.237

*Total Functioning Scores are based on 21 functioning categories of the SSFIPD (see Chapter 2).

In the area of education, acutes obtained higher functioning scores than chronics ($p < 0.001$) and high competence schizophrenics achieved higher scores than the low competence ones ($p < 0.001$). Regarding employment, acute patients were found to be more frequently employed and reported fewer job-related problems than did chronic patients ($p < 0.02$), as did the high competence schizophrenics when compared with the low competence ones ($p < 0.001$). Similar results were obtained regarding Welfare dependence, with acute patients reporting less experience with public assistance than chronic ones ($p < 0.001$), and high competence schizophrenics relying significantly less on Welfare than the low competence subjects ($p < 0.001$).

The groups were also found to be significantly different on the "relationship with parents" dimension, with the acutes reporting a more adequate relationship with parental figures than chronics ($p < 0.02$), and the more competent patients scoring higher on this dimension than did the low competence individuals ($p < 0.02$). Acutes and high competence subjects also reported more stable marriage histories and more satisfying relationships with their marital partners than did the chronics or low competence schizophrenics as attested to by an F ratio of 7.31 ($p < 0.02$) for the Patient effect and an F ratio of 5.47 ($p < 0.05$) for the Competence group effect. Functioning in terms of relationship with others, including authority figures also differentiated the acute–chronic and the high and low competence groups at high levels of significance. Acutes, as compared with chronics, showed less uneasiness in relating to others and had

Table 3

Total Stress Scores* for Acute and Chronic Schizophrenics
Divided into High and Low Social Competence Groups

Patient	Low Competence			High Competence		
	N	Mean	S.D.	N	Mean	S.D.
Acute	51	2.42	0.254	73	2.55	0.236
Chronic	302	2.34	0.286	198	2.40	0.302

*Total Stress Scores are based on 21 stress categories of the SSFIPD.

Table 4
Two-Way Analysis of Variance: Comparison of Acute and Chronic Schizophrenics and High and Low Social Competence Groups on 21 Social Functioning Variables

| | Patient | | | | | | Patient Competence groups | | | | | |
| | Acute | | Chronic | | | | Low | | High | | | |
Variable	N	X̄	N	X̄	F	DF	N	X̄	N	X̄	F	DF
Education	124	2.37	500	2.25	14.84§	1/620	353	2.16	271	2.40	31.77§	1/620
Job	124	2.37	500	2.27	7.11†	1/620	353	2.19	271	2.45	54.43§	1/620
Housekeeping	118	2.73	466	2.67		1/580	327	2.72	257	2.68	1.05	1/589
Welfare	124	2.55	500	2.17	27.47§	1/620	353	2.05	281	2.67	70.58§	1/620
Finances	124	2.54	500	2.43		1/618	351	2.43	271	2.54	2.78	1/618
Living	60	1.54	278	1.51		1/334	212	1.55	126	1.50	0.31	1/334
Circumstances												
Parents	122	2.59	489	2.47	6.00†	1/608	295	2.47	266	2.59	6.10†	1/608
Relatives	117	2.60	457	2.48	4.72*	1/570	319	2.53	255	5.55	0.23	1/570
Marriage	51	2.60	457	2.48		1/296	181	2.26	119	2.42	5.47*	1/296
Children	38	1.99	175	1.99		1/209	136	1.86	77	2.13	3.79	1/209
Dating	105	2.11	442	1.91	10.60††	1/543	331	2.02	216	2.01	0.02	1/543
Sex	123	2.36	499	2.22		1/619	352	2.35	271	2.23	2.33	1/629
Close friends	123	2.52	500	2.32	13.38§	1/620	353	2.36	271	2.47	3.80	1/620
Neighbors	123	1.87	494	1.68	7.48**	1/614	330	1.75	270	1.81	0.66	1/614
Relationship to Authority	123	2.12	500	1.96	6.53†	1/620	352	1.93	271	2.15	13.18§	1/620
Spare time interests	124	2.17	278	1.51	16.37§	1/620	353	2.05	271	2.21	23.41§	1/620
Religion	124	1.79	500	1.85		1/620	353	1.76	271	1.88	2.92	1/620
Drinking	124	2.58	500	2.61		1/620	353	2.52	271	2.67	6.73**	1/620
Addictive drugs	122	2.75	491	2.76		1/609	346	2.67	267	2.84	9.10††	1/609
Psychodelic drugs	121	2.50	496	2.64		1/613	351	2.57	266	2.57	0.00	1/609
Anti-social acts	123	2.57	498	2.26	14.00§	1/617	352	2.27	268	2.54	10.23††	1/617
Total Functioning	124	2.36	500	2.26	21.71§	1/620	353	2.24	271	2.38	38.93§	1/620

*p < 0.05.
†p < 0.02.
**p < 0.01.
††p < 0.005.
§p < 0.001.

127

fewer problems with authority ($p < 0.001$), and high competence subjects functioned at a higher level along this dimension than did their less competent counterparts ($p < 0.005$). In the use of leisure time, acutes appeared to be more active than chronics ($p < 0.001$), and the high competence subjects appeared more involved in activities than their low competence counterparts ($p < 0.001$).

In their anti-social behavior, acutes seemed to have a record of fewer law violations and arrests than their chronic counterparts ($p < 0.001$) as did the highly competent subjects when compared with the low competent ones ($p < 0.005$).

There were four functioning dimensions which differentiated the acute–chronic patients but failed to discriminate between the high and low competence groups. These were: relationship with relatives, close friends, neighbors, and dating, which measures ability to maintain social relationships with opposite sex and peers. In each case, acutes obtained significantly higher scores than their chronic counterparts ($p < 0.05$, $p < 0.001$, $p < 0.01$, and $p < 0.05$ for relatives, friends, neighbors, and dating, respectively).

Of the 21 categories of functioning studied, the dimensions of drinking and the use of addictive drugs differentiated high and low social competence groups but failed to discriminate between acutes and chronics. For each of these dimensions high competence subjects obtained a significantly higher functioning score (less of these activities) than did their low competence counterparts ($p < 0.005$ for drinking and $p < 0.005$ for use of addictive drugs).

Seven dimensions of the comprehensive functioning measurement failed to discriminate patients in either the acute–chronic classification or the high and low competence grouping. These dimensions were: housekeeping, management of finances, living circumstances, relationship with children, sexual satisfaction, religious beliefs and affiliation, and use of psychedelic drugs.

The two patient classifications were also compared in terms of 21 dimensions of stress by means of two-way analyses of variance. The results are shown in Table 5.

Results indicate that four stress dimensions associated with educational level, income, living standard and disturbance related to poor housing conditions, and spare time activities, as well as the total stress score, representing the sum total of the 21 areas considered, differentiated both the acute–chronic patient types and high and low social competence subjects. In all cases, acutes obtained lower stress scores than their chronic counterparts ($p < 0.001$ for education, $p < 0.02$ for finances, $p < 0.05$ for living circumstances, and $p < 0.001$ for spare time interests), and high competence group reported less stress associated with education than did their low competence counterparts ($p < 0.001$), finances ($p < 0.005$), living circumstances ($p < 0.005$), spare time interests ($p < 0.05$). On total stress score the same trend was observed; acutes and high competence subjects obtained lower stress scores than did the chronic and low competence schizophrenics ($p < 0.001$ for both comparisons).

Table 5
Two-Way Anaylsis of Variance: Comparison of Acute and Chronic Schizophrenics and High and Low Social Competence Groups on 21 Social Stress Variables

| | Patient | | | | | | Competence groups | | | | | |
| | Acute | | Chronic | | | | Low | | High | | | |
Variable	N	X̄	N	X̄	F	DF	N	X̄	N	X̄	F	DF
Education	124	2.28	500	2.17	6.55†	1/620	353	2.07	271	2.37	35.62§	1/620
Job	122	2.64	499	2.55	6.12†	1/617	353	2.58	268	2.62	0.89	1/617
Housekeeping	73	2.72	273	2.55	3.17	1/342	331	2.60	126	2.67	0.72	1/342
Welfare	44	2.57	315	2.45	1.18	1/355	261	2.48	98	2.54	0.34	1/355
Finances	124	2.46	500	2.29	6.11†	1/620	353	2.27	271	2.49	9.44††	1/611
Living	124	2.34	500	2.17	4.18*	1/619	352	2.12	271	2.39	9.97††	1/619
Circumstances												
Parents	106	2.41	416	2.22	8.64††	1/518	295	2.27	227	2.37	2.38	1/518
Relatives	117	2.76	455	2.66	3.60	1/568	319	2.70	253	2.72	0.13	1/668
Marriage	51	2.49	248	2.33	6.35†	1/295	180	2.36	119	2.46	2.95	1/295
Children	40	2.18	171	2.20	0.01	1/207	133	2.09	78	2.29	1.59	1/207
Dating	105	2.54	443	2.42	6.29†	1/544	331	2.50	217	2.46	0.81	1/544
Sex	124	2.57	500	2.41	4.85*	1/620	353	2.54	271	2.43	2.50	1/620
Close friends	124	2.60	499	2.42	7.00**	1/619	352	2.45	271	2.56	2.60	1/619
Neighbors	123	2.59	494	2.58	0.01	1/613	347	2.60	270	2.57	0.26	1/613
Relationship to others	124	2.19	500	2.06	6.59†	1/620	353	2.08	271	2.16	2.34	1/620
Spare time interests	124	2.17	500	2.08	16.38§	1/620	353	2.57	271	2.69	4.69§§	1/620
Religion	122	2.85	489	2.82	0.53	1/607	347	2.84	264	2.83	0.04	1/607
Drinking	31	2.21	148	2.11	0.81	1/175	121	2.18	58	2.14	0.16	1/175
Addictive drugs	23	1.96	95	1.91	0.07	1/114	80	2.05	38	2.83	0.84	1/114
Psychodelic drugs	36	2.02	127	2.20	1.42	1/159	100	2.13	63	2.09	0.81	1/159
Anti-social acts	129	1.22	237	1.22	0.00	1/262	186	1.17	80	1.26	0.90	1/262
Total stress	124	2.36	500	2.26	21.71§	1/620	353	2.38	271	2.48	38.93§	1/620

*Lower values represent higher stress level.

†p < 0.02.

**p < 0.01.

††p < 0.005.

§p < 0.001.

§§p < 0.05.

Stress associated with functioning on a job, in relationships with parents and marital partners, or in social relationships with the opposite sex peers, as well as stress stemming from inability to have satisfactory sexual relationships and disturbed relationships with close friends and authority figures, differentiated acute and chronic schizophrenics, with the acutes obtaining consistently lower stress scores on these dimensions than did their chronic counterparts ($p < 0.02$ for job, $p < 0.005$ for parents, $p < 0.02$ for marriage, $p < 0.02$ for sex, $p < 0.05$ for relationship with close friends, $p < 0.01$ for relationship with authority). No significant differentiation was obtained for the high and low competence groups in these areas.

The last series of analyses attempted to determine the extent of the contribution of social competence and of comprehensive social functioning to the prediction of readmission in acute and chronic schizophrenics. As we have already shown in Chapter 3, the variables underlying the social competence index, which was used to place our subjects into high and low competence classification, were predictive of outcome only in the chronic group of patients. However, it is believed that it is meaningful to determine precisely the extent to which the cluster identifying social competence operates in the prediction of outcome when considering one variable among others from the comprehensive social functioning of SSFID.

To accomplish this, three separate multiple discriminant function analyses were performed. In the first analysis, the social demographic score was combined with the social functioning scores obtained for the 21 psychosocial functioning variables derived from the SSFIPD as predictor variables. The analysis revealed that the combination of the 21 variables correctly identified 75% of the readmission cases in the chronic schizophrenic group, and 94% of the rehospitalized patients in the acute group. In the second analysis, the predictor variables were restricted to the 21 measures of psychosocial functioning derived from the SSFIPD. On the basis of the 21 variables of comprehensive social functioning, 67.8% of the chronic and 91.43% of the acute readmissions were correctly classified. The third and final discriminant function analysis utilized only the sociodemographic score as predictor variable. It was found that this index correctly identified readmission in 68.22% of the chronic patients and in 54.05% of the acute schizophrenics.

The relative importance of the 21 variables predicting readmission in chronic schizophrenics are shown in Table 6, based on a scale of 0.00 to 1.00.

Examination of the table reveals that sociodemographic score, reflecting the level of impaired instrumental functioning, appears to rank highest in importance for identifying the readmitted chronic schizophrenic. Lack of spare time interests and withdrawal from leisure activities, sexual difficulties affecting the ability to relate to the opposite sex, and lack of religious affiliation providing for a form of social cohesiveness with a group appear to be the next most important variables affecting outcome. Impaired relationships with close friends and neighbors, lack

Table 6

Relative Importance of Characteristics Predicting
Readmission of Chronic Schizophrenics

Variable	"Weight"
Sociodemographic score	1.00
Spare time interest	0.58
Sex	0.55
Religion	0.54
Relationship with neighbors	0.43
Relationship with close friends	0.34
Living circumstances	0.32
Anti-social acts	0.29
Drinking	0.28
Job	0.26
Relationship to others	0.23
Use of psychedelic drugs	0.23
Relationship with parents	0.22
Education	0.18
Relationship with relatives	0.15
Dating	0.14
Use of addictive drugs	0.14
Welfare dependence	0.13
Marriage	0.08
Housekeeping	0.06
Management of finances	0.04
Relationship with children	0.02

of steady employment, drinking to relieve anxiety, and anti-social "acting out" tend to contribute moderately to readmission in the chronic group. Relationship with the marital partner and children, housekeeping, and management of finances appear to have little value when differentiating the readmitted and nonreadmitted populations of chronic schizophrenics constituting this sample.

The relative importance of variables predicting readmission in the acute group of schizophrenic patients is shown in Table 7.

In contrast to the chronic group, impaired relationships with close friends and parents, and job-related difficulties appear to contribute most significantly to readmission in the acute group of patients. Relationship with others, living circumstances, management of finances, drinking to relieve anxiety, use of psychedelic drugs, problems with relating socially to the opposite sex peers, and education appear to contribute relatively little when differentiating the readmitted and nonreadmitted samples of acute schizophrenics.

The comparisons of the acute–chronic and the high–low socially competent schizophrenics on a wide range of psychosocial functioning dimensions have significant implications for viewing their psychosocial deficits and for appraising problem areas that interfere with their integration into the community.

Table 7
Relative Importance of Characteristics Predicting
Readmission of Acute Schizophrenics

Variable	"Weight"
Relationship with close friends	1.00
Relationship with parents	0.87
Job	0.77
Relationship with others	0.38
Living circumstances	0.35
Management of finances	0.33
Religion	0.28
Use of psychedelic drugs	0.27
Drinking	0.27
Dating	0.22
Education	0.21
Sex	0.20
Sociodemographic score	0.19
Relationship with relatives	0.18
Marriage	0.17
Relationship with neighbors	0.17
Anti-social acts	0.14
Spare time interests	0.10
Housekeeping	0.09
Relationship with children	0.07
Welfare dependence	0.04
Use of addictive drugs	0.02

Either classification appears adequate for tapping difficulties experienced in relation to instrumental functioning like educational achievement, problems in obtaining and holding a job, dependence on Welfare, and interaction with marital partners. In addition, the chronic patients and the low socially competent schizophrenics can also be identified with problems relating to their parents and other significant figures in the community and with anti-social acting out.

What is of particular interest, however, is the ability of the acute–chronic distinction to provide information about differential functioning in interpersonal difficulties generally associated with early phases of social disintegration, namely, problems with family members, close friends, neighbors, and dating partners. The consistently higher scores of acutes in these areas suggest that once the patient shows a chronic course, with multiple hospitalizations, his interpersonal relationships become more blunted.

It should be noted that the high–low social competence distinction only tapped differential levels of functioning in some interpersonal areas. The fact that this grouping of patients produced significant differences in drinking behavior and the use of addictive drugs is not at all surprising since the classification separated high and low performers, and low performers are known to use alcohol and addictive drugs to deal with environmental pressures. Comparison of the acute–chronic and the high–low competence groups in terms of the 21 stress variables revealed considerable overlap in stress related to education, income, living standards, housing conditions, and spare time activities. In each case, the acutes and the high competence subjects received lower stress scores than did their chronic and low competence counterparts.

The acute–chronic distinction successfully tapped stress in interpersonal interactions, particularly those with parental figures, marital and sexual partners, close friends, and others in the community. This reinforces similar findings along the functioning dimensions. The high–low competence classification appeared to be insensitive to experienced stress. In other words, the division in low and high instrumental functioning cannot separate the true chronic schizophrenic from the acute with a low instrumental functioning. As a result, the chronics who have higher stress were diluted by the acutes who have a lower stress.

As regards prediction of short-term outcome, it appears that the more time consuming evaluation of the broad spectrum of interpersonal and instrumental functioning is justified in that it provides important interpersonal information not included in the briefer competence measure. Although the predictive relevance of the social competence measure for chronic schizophrenics has to be acknowledged, its failure to determine outcome in acute schizophrenics, discussed in detail in Chapter 3, must also be recognized.

The apparent relevance of the social competence discussion in predicting short-term outcome in chronic schizophrenics stems from the fact that for this type of patient, instrumental functioning, as an index of ability to be self-supporting, becomes a more obvious indicator of the chances to find a place in the community upon release. Yet, from a different point of view, one may argue that the predictors encompassed in the social competence index are nothing more than rigid indices of the chronic patient's performance level prior to his hospitalization and certainly not the determinants of the course of his illness. After all, education, marital status, employment history, and occupation reflect either the level of operative social skills which the patient has accumulated in accordance with the expectations of his social class, or the effect of illness on these skills, regardless of social class membership. In fact, onset of illness may well freeze any possibilities for further social development. In some, but not all, patients, the distribution of social competence levels as conceived by Zigler and Phillips (5) supports this position. For example, when acute and chronic schizophrenics are divided into high and low social competence groups, irrespective of the schizophrenic subtype, an interesting phenomenon emerges. Of the 125 acutes studied, 51 (40.8%) were classified as of low social competence, and 198 of the 516 chronics (38.3%), as of high social competence. The findings suggest that a relatively large percentage of chronic schizophrenic patients, who have an average 3.6 years of hospitalization, are still able to maintain high competence levels despite repeated hospitalization.

According to the Zigler and Phillips criteria and findings, the chronic schizophrenics should display uniformly low levels of social competence. Although the low level of social competence appears to be significantly associated with readmission, this association may well be due to the presence of many schizophrenics in that group, most of whom are Welfare recipients unable to manage their finances, unmotivated for work, and generally socially unmanageable (through excessive drinking and involvement with authorities). In this sense, the social competence measure appears to give us only a fairly general picture of the social reintegration possibilities of the discharged patient. This is mainly due to the fact that it is unlikely that the majority of the schizophrenics will improve their skills once rehospitalized. If some do, chances are good that these individuals are not "true schizophrenics," but rather "episodic psychotics." Of those whose social skills do not improve, an index of instrumental functioning will reflect the progressive social deterioration, compounded by repeated hospitalization and community rejection, in the period free from hospitalization. It is possible that the importance of interpersonal relationships has been minimized in the Zigler and Phillips predictive scale on the assumption that interpersonal relationships play a less significant role in the patient's life than does adaptability to societal demands. Perhaps in the era when chronic schizophrenics were largely doomed to spending most of their lives in institutional settings, the gross instrumental indicators had predictive value for the nondeteriorated schizophrenic patients. At that time, our well structured society demanded from its members compliance with a set of expected and cherished values such as marriage, educational attainment, and full employment, and any inability to conform to these demands would presuppose a problem in adaptation inferring mental disturbance. At present, instrumental functioning based on these same considerations is, at best, misleading due to the high rate of divorce, unemployment, and school dropouts independent of any evidence of mental illness in the individual.

Now, factors associated with interpersonal performance take on new predictive meaning in the maintenance of schizophrenics in the community. In this connection, it is of interest that the ability to use spare time constructively, to maintain satisfying relationships with the opposite sex, and to participate in religious activities do figure as important factors in the outcome of chronic schizophrenics, even if they are only the disconnected remnants of their social needs. Obviously, in addition to basic instrumental social skills subsumed under the social competence measure, these psychological factors are also important for the maintenance of a link with the community at large.

The importance of the interpersonal dimension in the prediction of outcome among acute schizophrenics is not difficult to understand, in view of what these patients represent. First of all, upon first hospitalization, there is a sudden worsening in interpersonal relationships, which the comprehensive social functioning measure was designed to tap. This worsening of the interpersonal relationship is produced by the different levels of expectation of family and the patient regarding the organization of the latter's life. This discrepancy leads to conflict, stress, and rehospitalization of the patient. Thus, the acute–chronic distinction in schizophrenia, reflecting primarily psychological deficit, appears to have its clinical merits. In this context, the level of interpersonal impairment in relationships, which affects both functioning and experienced stress, plays a significant role in distinguishing acutes from chronics and thus provides a sounder basis for prediction of outcome than that implied in the social competence classification.

The relevance of the acute–chronic distinction is likely to decrease in the future as the chemotherapeutic treatment of chronic schizophrenics makes long term hospitalizations obsolete and early discharge into the community the prevailing pattern. Through these procedures, eliminating the deleterious effects of prolonged institutionalization, most of the chronics will resemble their acute counterparts with increasing frequency, which will render the old criteria of instrumental functioning irrelevant. Upon discharge, the stabilized schizophrenics are now placed in various rehabilitation programs aimed at increasing employability and the redevelopment of lost skills (i.e., placement programs). It is obvious that these procedures alter their social competence and the significance of the past views of this dimension.

As mentioned in Chapter 1, a multifactorial approach to the understanding of the course of schizophrenia presupposes the evaluation of operant factors responsible for it. One such factor is the genetic factor which assumes chromosomic inheritance of schizophrenia.

The difficulty with the genetic theory of schizophrenia is that it cannot separate clearly the influence of the environmental contribution superimposed on the genetic constitution of the individual. The relationship of these two dimensions is explored in the next chapter.

REFERENCES

1. Clark, R.E.: The relationship of schizophrenia to occupational income and occupational prestige. *Am. Sociol. Rev.* **13**: 325–330, 1948.
2. Clark, R.E.: Psychoses, income and occupational prestige. *Am. J. Sociol.* **54**: 433–440, 1949.
3. Faris, R.E.L., and Dunham, H.W.: "Mental Disorders in Urban Areas: An Ecological Study of Schizophrenia and Other Psychoses." University of Chicago Press, Chicago, 1939.
4. Zigler, E., and Phillips, L.: Social effectiveness and symptomatic behavior. *J. Abnorm. Soc. Psychol.* **61**: 231–238, 1960.
5. Zigler, E., and Phillips, L.: Social competence and the process-reactive distinction in psychopathology. *J. Abnorm. Soc. Psychol.* **65**: 215–222, 1962.
6. Zigler, E., and Phillips, L.: Social competence and outcome in psychiatric disorders. *J. Abnorm. Soc. Psychol.* **63**: 264–271, 1961.

CHAPTER 7

Genetic and Developmental Factors as Related to Stress in Schizophrenia*

One of the strongest factors predicting the occurrence of schizophrenia and its course is genetic inheritance. Yet, clinically, this factor accounts for only 14–16% *(22, 53)* of the schizophrenic cases. On the other hand, environmentalists, supported by family research, claim that deviant family interaction can explain and predict the gamut of schizophrenic reactions. This chapter reviews each hypothesis in terms of the merits it holds for prediction of schizophrenia.

From the purely hereditary point of view, the inconclusiveness of genetic findings has been amply summarized by Penrose. In reviewing evidence on the incidence of schizophrenia in the relatives of the index cases, including identical and fraternal twins *(29, 35, 53)*, parents *(8, 23)*, and siblings *(8, 23, 28, 53)*, Penrose concluded that there was no single gene explanation and at best the genetic contribution consists of a predisposition caused by multiple additive genes. The study of twins has, in general, been rather disappointing from the genetic point of view despite Kallman's consistent claims that schizophrenia could be a recessive trait. A later study by Kallman and Roth *(29)* based on 52 twin index cases suggested that schizophrenia of early onset may be familial. Although a great deal of twin research leads to the conclusion that schizophrenic trait is strongly genetically determined, the variability of the concordance rates of identical twins should serve as a warning that "nothing final about the relative importance of heredity and environment has as yet been established" by the twin method *(21)*. Heston *(25)* found that schizophrenia was more prevalent in children of schizophrenic mothers even if the children were reared in nonschizophrenic homes. Recent research on adopted schizophrenics further

---

*The research results presented in this chapter have appeared in the Articles: G. Serban: Parental stress in the development of schizophrenic offspring, *Comprehensive Psychiat.* 16: 23–36, 1975 and G. Serban, and G.W. Woloshin: Relationship between pre- and postmorbid psychological stress in schizophrenics. *Psychol. Rep.* 35: 507–517, 1974.

suggests that even in the absence of severely disturbed parents, adopted children still develop schizophrenia. From these findings they were inclined to propose a new concept of "schizophrenia spectrum" that would include mental disorders of varying severity that were genetically related *(30)*.

The notion that the hereditary predisposition to schizophrenia is based on metabolic errors has been submitted to numerous investigations. Despite a large research effort the evidence is far from conclusive. For instance, studies of faulty transmethylation of catecholamines with DMPE *(18)* excretion failed to confirm at this time any significant association with schizophrenia *(34)*. Search for the specific metabolite adenochrome *(26)* protein taraxein *(24)*, and protein factor *(20)* has not been profitable either.

Another approach to the search for a biochemical deficiency in schizophrenics has been the investigation of inborn enzyme defects. Bogoch *(7)* found an inverse ratio between the gravity of psychosis and the amount of glycoprotein neuraminic acid in the cerebrospinal fluid of schizophrenics. However, upon recovery, the levels tended to return to acceptable ranges, thus making Bogoch's findings less specific.

Another area of inquiry has focused on sex hormones in schizophrenic patients, but the study of Hoskins and Pincus *(27)*, showing relatively low levels of male sex hormones among schizophrenic men, did not clarify the genetic significance of this finding.

A more recent inquiry into sex chromosomal aberration among psychotics *(23a)*, which might have promising implications for a genetic aspect of schizophrenia, is the emphasis on nondistinction in the paternal and maternal gene cells, but this finding is still too inconclusive *(46)*.

The results obtained by all the different methods of investigation lead to the conclusion that in some cases schizophrenia may be linked to a recessive trait; yet strict Mendelian inheritance has not been proven. It appears that the genetic background may be multifactorial. Inborn biochemical defects may play a role, but their specificity for schizophrenia is far from clear. At this point in time, the most direct inference is that heredity and environment both play a role in the etiology of schizophrenia.

From the point of view of environmental influences, deviant family interaction has been most widely researched. According to Bowen *(9)*, the schizophrenia is a condition resulting from a disturbed process in the family interaction. In his view schizophrenia is a process which develops gradually over two or three generations. The schizophrenic child emerges from a family with a superadequate mother and a detached father, in which he the child is helpless. Lidz and his associates *(33, 34)* speculate that the schizophrenic's serious disturbances in thought and communication stem, in large measure, from disturbance in family interactions. He believes that family disturbances, if pervasive, can impair the offspring's symbolic functioning and his ability to perceive and maintain a discrete and integrated personality; Moreover, they rob him of basic socialization and acculturation. All of these factors make him vulnerable to becoming schizophrenic. One of the most serious examples of family disturbances is disordered intrafamilial communication which distorts the perception of experience and exposes the child to cognitive doublebinds or contradictory messages *(3)*. Wynne and Singer *(58, 59)* and Singer and Wynne *(50, 51)* have documented the amorphous and fragmented styles of communication of parents of schizophrenic children. These styles of communication interfere with the children's language development and their ability to maintain focal attention required for coherent communication. The inconsistencies, contradictory meanings, and denial of the obvious often found in schizophrenic families interfere with the youngster's grasp of the world and prevent a coherent grounding in a system of meanings and logic, making it difficult to attain an ordered perception of life events and relationships *(34)*.

Wynne and Singer *(58, 59)* have characterized the family interactions of schizophrenics in terms of pseudomutuality; that is, a fixed organization of a limited number of engulfing roles which when persistent precludes the child's formation of a personal identity. The disturbances in the family constellation have also been ascribed to marital difficulties among parents of children who later become schizophrenic. Bowen *(9)* characterizes these marital relationships in terms of mutual withdrawal, minimal interaction, and covert hostility, estrangement, and distrust. Cameron *(11)* describes the pseudomutuality of where the facade of adequacy is based on rigid fulfillment of formal roles, mutual denial of hostility, and protestation of love. This facade is maintained despite the fact that many of these relationships later end in divorce or separation.

Since Frieda Fromm-Reichman *(19a)* first described the role of the cold and rejecting schizophrenogenic mother as an important factor in the etiology of schizophrenia, the mothering defect has been subjected to wide scrutiny. It now appears that the main factor contributing to schizophrenia is not so much coldness and rejection as the inconsistency of the mothers who tolerate, but do not actively support the child *(12)*.

In an attempt to test the hypothesis that mothers of schizophrenic patients are more controlling and rejecting than those of normals, Zuckerman *et al. (60)* tested 42 mothers of schizophrenics and 42 control mothers. The authors failed to find support for differences in child-rearing attitudes between the two groups of mothers. As mentioned in Chapter I, it was found that only 25% of the mothers of schizophrenic patients met the classical description of the schizophrenic mother; in the remainder of the cases the presentation of the patient was distorted due to his faulty perception of the relationship *(2)*.

There is accumulating evidence, however, that parental disturbances may play an important role in the psychopathology of the offspring. Waring and Ricke *(55)*, studying the personality patterns and adjustment of parents whose children later became schizophrenic, found in a prospective study that both mothers and fathers of later chronic schizophrenics exhibited severe psychopathology: many of whom were actually psychotics, borderlines with character disorders, or schizoids. The study also lended support to clinical observation of pseudomutual marital relationships (and emotional divorce) among the parents of children who later became schizophrenic. The type of family environment most productive of chronic schizophrenics was found to be a prolonged symbiotic union between parent and child. It is of interest to note that the type of milieu most frequent in families of released schizophrenics was one of extreme rejection and exclusion.

Evidently, the controversy centering on genetic vs. developmental factors in the etiology of schizophrenia is far from settled. Pathological interaction and heredity factors both seem to play a part in schizophrenia. What is needed is the estimation of the degree of risk these factors carry for the development of this disease. Longitudinal studies of those at high risk for schizophrenias (36, 37) are extremely valuable. The final results are as yet inconclusive. The schizophrenic adoption study of Kety, Rosenthal, and Wender (30), although leaning heavily in the direction of genetic transmission of schizophrenia still could not rule out decisively the contribution of environmental factors induced by the adoptee's parents. On the other hand, no causal link could be demonstrated between the anomaly of the family interaction and schizophrenia. No convincing experimental evidence are produced by either group.

Perhaps a more fruitful approach to the search for an etiological basis in schizophrenia than that provided by the heredity versus environment schema would be accepting the powerful intertwining of the genetic predisposition with environmental influences. This approach would focus additional attention on the contribution of a wide variety of psychosocial factors in the genesis of the schizophrenic syndrome. For instance, it is difficult to explain on the basis of only genetic or only environmental factors, the problems experienced by the child, who becomes schizophrenic, during teens or adolescence.

In the past several decades, there has been increasing research interest in the relationship between childhood adjustment and adult schizophrenic status. On the one hand, it suggests that most preschizophrenics are withdrawn, fearful, and share what has been termed "shut-in" personality (4), which suggests the influence of a genetic factor, while on the other hand, it characterizes them as having aggressive anti-social tendencies and other problems (45), pointing toward environmental determinants. Furthermore, the literature in this area, far from clarifying the issue, has difficulty in identifying any type of behavior or personality associated with the development of schizophrenia. However, few loosely defined areas of psychosocial problems have been established. Some of the follow-up studies (38, 40) based on evaluation of guidance clinic records suggest that patients characterized by withdrawal and fearfulness more frequently tend toward neurosis in adulthood than toward psychiatric disturbances. As a matter of fact, another study (41) following up a group of children with aggressive behavior disorders of childhood, found that this group had a high incidence of adult schizophrenia. In this population, a long history of severe aggressive, antisocial behavior was highly correlated with early onset of schizophrenic outcome when compared with other types of psychiatric outcomes of children seen in the St. Louis municipal psychiatric unit. O'Neal and Robins *(43, 44)* and Robins *(48)*, found that the preschizophrenics were characterized by antisocial symptoms, particularly truancy and general antisocial behavior. However, they were less likely than the presociopaths to be arrested. In addition, the preschizophrenics in the Robins studies exhibited neurotic symptomatology as children. Frazee *(17)*, comparing preschizophrenic and prenormal children found more withdrawal symptoms among the preschizophrenics. It should, however, be noted that almost half of the preschizophrenics had been referred for antisocial and acting out behavior. The studies of Fleming *(14, 15)*, conducted at the Judge Baker Guidance Clinic, support the notion that disturbed preschizophrenics exhibit antisocial as well as neurotic symptomatology. The preschizophrenic youngsters have greater emotional disruption in childhood and adolescence with resulting feelings of isolation and vulnerability. About 90% of the preschizophrenics felt helplessly inadequate and a large proportion of them exhibited antisocial behavior as a reaction to their feelings of identity loss. Fleming suggests that feelings of isolation, of alienation, and of general vulnerability may well be the core of the severe breakdown in adulthood. It is of interest to note that the acting out behavior of the preschizophrenic appears to be self-initiated and directed toward the family rather than toward the community *(19, 42)*.

More specific disturbances found among preschizophrenics are abnormal peer relationships *(14, 17, 19, 49)* and academic difficulties *(5, 9, 47, 57)*. Watt *et al.* *(56)* and Friedlander *(19)* for instance, found that 50% of later schizophrenics preferred solitude to being with other people, and Frazee reported that, of his 23 preschizophrenics, 12 had no friends and none showed normal associations with other children. These findings were corroborated by the Fleming study reporting preschizophrenics as unable to form any meaningful peer relationships. In a follow-up study of schizophrenics previously seen in child guidance clinics, Roff reported that significantly more patients than controls had been rated by teachers as having negative peer group adjustment. The preschizophrenics were judged to be generally disliked by their peer group, unable to make and keep friends and being regarded as odd, peculiar or queer. They tended to gain their unpopularity not so much by being shy and isolated as by being aggressive and quarrelsome with other children.

As regards school adjustment, it appears that children who later develop schizophrenia experience more school retardation and failure than do the controls *(17, 19)* and about half of these youngsters fail to graduate from the eighth grade *(48)*. For a long time it has been reported that preschizophrenics as children were often referred to clinics for reasons of backwardness, dullness, and inability in school subjects *(57)*. Recent extensive and documented research indicates that the "sick subgroup" of the high risk group has exhibited more disturbed behavior in school, particularly discipline problems and attention lag than the normals *(36, 37)*.

It appears that the development of mental illness in general, and schizophrenia in particular, is a long-term continuous process in which the child's difficulties with parental figures are extended to and compounded in the social interactions. Just as in childhood his perception of the parents and difficulty in relating to them appears to be the foremost problem; in youth and adolescence his perception of other social objects when affected, distorts the patients' relationship with them, leading to stressful integration. As it was already demonstrated in Chapter IV, the problems which have caused stress in the individual's childhood and adolescence will continue to do so in his adult life.

Taking into account this controversy it was attempted as a part of our research program to address both the factor of genetic predisposition and the factor of environment in the development of schizophrenic illness in order to evaluate the interaction between them. Two studies conducted on the original population of 516 chronic and 125 acute schizophrenics attempted to study the problem from a different perspective. The first study, which will be discussed now, departing from much of the previous research, had the patient recall his own experiences with and reactions to his parents, independent of factual reality. The assumption was that his perception and interpretation of the environment as threatening or stressful became the primary factor leading to his hospitalization.

Stress associated with parental interaction and early adjustment difficulties was assessed by means of the SSFIPD. The actual history of parental illness was verified with the New York State Department of Mental Hygiene. Psychiatric histories were available for patients' mothers only, since it was difficult to identify the biological fathers for the total subject group. However, since the relationship between mother and child has been particularly stressed in the psychodynamic literature, this relationship was made the primary focus of the study. A subset of patients who reported psychiatrically hospitalized fathers were also included.

In the first study, on the basis of genetic history and family-interaction data obtained in the interview, the subjects were divided into four subsamples labeled as groups Ia, Ib, II, and III. These groups represented variations of factual and reported information. The group Ia represented patients who in the interview reported having mothers hospitalized for a similar mental condition and for whom there was no confirming evidence at the New York State Department of Mental Hygiene. Group Ib was comprised of patients who reported hospitalization of their mothers and validation from New York State has been obtained for these cases. Group II consisted of patients who denied having hospitalized mothers, but for whom New York State had hospitalization records. Finally, group III was composed of patients who in an interview reported having hospitalized fathers for a mental illness similar to their own. Both acutes and chronics are represented in these subgroups, although not all of the original sample is included in the four patient categories (see Table 1).

The small size of group Ib is the result of difficulties inherent in tracing drifting schizophrenic populations. Since many of the patients have immigrated

Table 1

Frequencies and Percents of Specified Groups with Relatives Hospitalized for Mental Illness*†**†††

Hospitalized relative	Chronic Mother III Group Ia N	%Ia	%Chr.	Group Ib N	%Ib	%Chr.	Group II N	%II	%Chr.	Father III Group III N	%III	%Chr.	Acute Mother III Group Ia N	%Ia	%Acu.	Group Ib N	%Ib	%Acu.	Group II N	%II	%Acu.	Father III Group III N	%III	%Acu.	Normal sample N	%Nor.
Mother	49	100.0	9.5	13	100.0	2.5	48	100.0	9.3	4	12.9	0.8	5	100.0	4.0	3	100.0	2.4	19	100.0	15.2	0	0	0	2	2.1
Father	3	6.1	0.6	1	7.7	0.2	2	4.2	0.4	31	100.0	6.0	0	0	0	0	0	0	0	0	0	3	100	2.4	2	2.1
Siblings	8	16.3	1.6	3	23.1	0.6	9	18.2	1.7	5	16.1	1.0	1	20.0	0.8	1	33.0	0.8	2	10.5	1.6	0	0	0	2	2.1
Other relatives	7	14	1.4	2	15.4	0.4	4	8.3	0.8	7	22.6	1.4	0	0	0	0	0	0	1	5.3	0.8	0	0	0	5	5.3
Children	0	0	0	0	0	0	0	0	0	0	0	0	0	0	0	0	0	0	0	0	0	0	0	0	0	0
Spouse	0	0	0	1	7.7	0.2	1	2.1	0.2	1	3.2	0.2	0	0	0	0	0	0	0	0	0	0	0	0	0	0

*Mother: Ia × Ib × II*** *(Chronics)* $X^2 = 22.926, p < 0.001$.

†Mother: Acutes Ia × Chronics Ia:Ns; Acutes II × Chronics II*$X^2 = 384, p < 0.05$.

Acutes II × Normals$X^2 = 926, p < 0.01$; Mother: Acutes Ia × Acutes II**$X^2 = 8.16, p < 0.01$.

††(Group Ia = patients who reported on interview that mother was hospitalized; Group Ib = patients who reported the mother was hospitalized on interview and were confirmed on Albany list: Group II = patients whose mothers were hospitalized according to Albany list: Group III = patients who reported on interview that father was hospitalized.

143

to New York City from other parts of the country, psychiatric records for their mothers were not available in New York state. It is also possible that the mental illness of the mother may have occurred before the patient was aware of it, or the mental hospitalization may have been concealed from the patient as a child. It has to be kept in mind that the patient's report of his mother's hospitalization may also represent patient's distortions due to his psychotic condition.

In order to provide a check for the accuracy of the patient reports, the interview was also conducted whenever possible, with a close informant (parents, spouse, sibling, or other person familiar with the patient over an extended period of time). The percent agreement between patients and their informants (N = 228: 182 chronics, 46 acutes) on the SSFIPD items ranged from 94 to 97% except of course, in those cases where either the patient or the informant has only partial knowledge of the relative's illness (see Table 2).

Comparisons of frequencies of hospitalized relatives in the four patient groups and comparable normals (N = 95) are shown in Table 1. The distribution of the arrays were tested, whenever data permitted, by means of chi-square tests of independence.

As can be seen in Table 1 comparison of chronic and acute schizophrenic groups with that of normals reveals that chronic patients had the highest percentages of hospitalized mothers, fathers, siblings, and other relatives. The acute patients showed moderate percent, with the normals showing the smallest frequency in every category of illness. It is of interest to observe, however, that the acute group of patients as compared with the chronic one had a somewhat higher percentage of hospitalized spouses and children (see Table 3). This finding may be due to either a low marriage rate or low fertility rate found among chronic schizophrenics (6).

Of the first three chronic groups, group Ib contained the highest percentage of hospitalized relatives (15.4%) as did group Ib of the acute patients (see Table 1). Group Ib represents the most reliable information on heredity since patient

Table 2
Patients' and Informants' Statements About Hospitalization of Patients' Relatives

Chronic patients who had informants		Chronic informants		Acute patients who had informants		Acute informants	
N	%Chr. Inf.	N	%Chr. Inf.	N	%Acu. Inf.	N	%Acu. Inf.
29	15.9	32	17.5	5	10.9	6	13.0
16	8.7	16	8.8	3	6.5	3	6.5
32	17.5	26	14.2	7	15.2	7	15.2
28	15.3	39	21.4	5	10.9	6	13.0
4	2.1	6	3.2	3	6.5	1	2.2
10	5.4	7	3.7	3	6.5	2	4.4

Table 3
Total Sample of subgroups Ia and Ib for 516
Chronics and 125 acute Schizophrenics

Hospitalized relative	Total chronic sample (Ia&Ib)		Total acute sample (Ia&Ib)	
	N	%Chr.	N	%Acu.
Mother	62	12.0	8	6.4
Father	31	6.0	3	2.4
Siblings	70	13.6	14	11.2
Other Relatives	65	12.6	7	5.6
Children	6	1.2	3	2.4
Spouse	16	3.1	4	3.2

reports and New York state records coincided. These data lend strong support to the assumption that a genetic predisposition was operating in groups Ib and II of our schizophrenic sample.

It may be observed from Table 3 that the percent of state reported hospitalized parents, including fathers not state reported, of chronically ill offspring is 8.0% (15.7% by patient statements).

The obtained percentage in the present sample of chronic schizophrenics is within the limits of Kallman (16.4%), Shields (12%), Essen-Moller (11%) and Alanen (12%) of patients who had mothers diagnosed as schizophrenic, or 23% with functional psychoses included. The ratio corresponds as well to those found in the work of Slater (55), who reported a ratio of two schizophrenic mothers to one schizophrenic father in his sample of schizophrenic patients.

The more important contribution of the present investigation, however, was the study of the patients' emotional responses and their reactions to the interaction with their ill parents, independent of the factual reality of heredity. The extent of disturbance of family relationships caused by the mental illness of a parent was first evaluated by asking a patient whether or not he was upset by the mentally ill behavior of his sick or allegedly sick parents when he was younger. Combining the data from Tables 4A and 4B, it becomes apparent that only 34 of the 39 patients who reported having schizophrenic mothers stated that they were upset about their relationship with them (69.5%), while for the state-list group the percentage was zero. Group Ib showed the highest percentage of patients upset by the hospitalization of a relative (84.6% for mothers). In general, the chronic sample showed the highest percentage of patient disturbance for every category of hospitalized relative, except the father, where group III was highest.

The patients' recent emotional interactions were examined next in an attempt to discover the extent to which the disturbances connected with close family interaction has continued into adulthood. The data pertaining to recent emotional interactions with family were extracted from responses given by the patients to

Table 4A.

Frequencies and Percentages of Specified Groups "Yes" Responses to the Question. "Were you upset by the mentally ill behavior of (relatives specified)?"

Hospitalized Relative	Chronic Sample												Acute Sample												Normal Sample	
	Group Ia			Group Ib			Group II			Group III			Group Ia			Group Ib			Group II			Group III				
	N	%Ia	%Chr.	N	%Ib	%Chr.	N	%II	%Chr.	N	%III	%Chr.	N	%Ia	%Acu.	N	%Ib	%Acu.	N	%II	%Acu.	N	%III	%Acu.	N	%Nor.
Mother	34	69.5	6.6	11	84.6	2.1	0	0	0	3	9.7	0.6	5	100	4.0	0	100	2.4	0	0	0	0	0	0	1	1.1
Father	2	4.1	0.4	1	7.7	0.2	1	2.1	0.2	16	51.6	3.1	0	0	0	0	0	0	0	0	0	3	100	2.4	2	2.1
Siblings	5	10.2	1.0	2	15.4	0.4	7	14.6	1.4	3	9.7	0.6	1	20	0.8	1	33.3	0.8	1	5.3	0.8	0	0	0	3	3.3
Relatives	3	6.1	0.6	2	15.4	0.4	0	0	0	4	12.9	0.8	0	0	0	0	0	0	0	0	0	0	0	0	3	3.3
Children	0	0	0	0	0	0	0	0	0	0	0	0	0	0	0	0	0	0	0	0	0	0	0	0	0	0
Spouse	0	0	0	1	7.7	0.2	1	2.1	0.2	0	3.2	0.2	0	0	0	0	0	0	0	0	0	0	0	0	0	0
Grandparent	0	0	0	0	0	0	0	0	0	0	0	0	0	0	0	0	0	0	0	0	0	0	0	0	1	1.1

Table 4B.
Total of Groups Ia, Ib, and II for Acutes and Chronics

Hospitalized Relative	Total Chronic Sample		Total Acute Sample	
	N	%	N	%
Mother	45	8.7	8	6.4
Father	16	3.1	3	2.4
Siblings	39	7.6	9	7.2
Relatives	20	3.9	1	0.8
Children	2	0.4	0	0
Spouse	10	1.9	1	0.8
Grandparent	3	0.6	0	0

stress scale derived from the SSFIPD. For the purposes of the present analysis, only the categories relating to family interpersonal relationships (with parents, relatives, marital partner, and children) were considered. The obtaining mean stress scores are presented in Table 5. It should be noted that high numerical values indicate low levels of experienced stress. The comparisons in Table 5 include, in addition to data for acute and chronic schizophrenics, the mean scores obtained with the comparable normal sample. Examination of Table 5 reveals that chronics reported higher levels of stress than did the acutes, particularly those subjects in group Ib, which had higher levels in every one of the categories considered. As may be expected the normal sample showed lowest levels of stress in comparison to the patient groups.

The quality of an even more recent interaction with the parents (within the last 6 months prior to the interview) for the three comparison groups: chronics, acutes, and normals is shown in Table 6. It is obvious from Table 6 that group I had a higher proportion of subjects who had difficulty relating to their mothers than did group II, suggesting that the patients' perception of mental illness in his or her mother was based primarily on the quality of the emotional relationships between them. It should be noted that in the chronic group, 24.2% reported getting along "terribly" with their mothers, while 22.6% got along very poorly with their fathers as well. Yet, mental illness of the parents was a stress factor only for group Ib. It is of particular interest that a substantial proportion of every group had only rare contact with their parents at the time the data was collected (23.5%) or they had no contact at all (19.6%).

In order to determine, retrospectively, the effect of absent parent on the environmental climate in which disturbed family relationships could have precipitated a schizophrenic reaction, death of parent during the childhood of the patient was also examined. In terms of parental death, the chronics most often experienced the death of the mother, acutes were intermediate and the percentage was lowest for normals. It should be noted that replacement of the dead mother

Table 5
Mean Stress Scores

	Chronic sample						Acute sample						Significant mean difference by t Test	
Category	Group Ia	Group Ib	Group II	Group III	4 Chronics With Both Parents Mentally Ill	Total Chronic	Group Ia	Group Ib	Group II	Group III	Total Acute	Normal sample	Normal/ chronic	Normal/ acute
Parents	2.16	2.05	2.22	2.01	2.23	2.22	2.22	2.37	2.35	1.80	2.43	2.56	**	
Relatives	2.71	2.71	2.58	2.65	2.50	2.66	2.19	2.00	2.93	2.43	2.76	2.85	**	*
Marriage	2.19	1.90	2.35	2.23	2.58	2.33	1.70	0.00	2.37	0.00	2.48	2.51	**	
Children	2.25	1.50	2.16	2.44	2.43	2.18	1.67	0.00	2.50	1.00	2.20	2.61	**	

**Indicates t value significant at 0.01 level;
*Indicates t value significant at 0.05 level.

Table 6. How Patient Got Along with Mother and Father in Last 6 Months

	Chronic Sample											Acute Sample											Normal Sample	
	Group I			Group II			Group III			Tot Chr		Group I			Group II			Group III			Tot Acu			
Got Along With Mother	N	%I	%Tot	N	%II	%Tot	N	%III	%Tot	N	%	N	%I	%Tot	N	%II	%Tot	N	%III	%Tot	N	%	N	%
Terribly	15	24.2	2.9	8	16.7	1.6	7	22.6	1.4	77	14.9	2	25.0	1.6	1	5.3	0.8	0	0	0	9	7.2	5	5.3
Poorly	8	12.9	1.6	10	20.8	1.9	6	19.4	1.2	75	14.5	4	50.0	3.2	3	15.8	2.4	1	33.3	0.8	14	11.2	5	5.3
Fair	10	16.1	1.9	8	16.7	1.6	5	16.1	1.0	109	21.1	2	25.0	1.6	7	36.8	5.6	1	33.3	0.8	32	25.6	24	25.3
Well	25	40.3	4.8	21	43.8	4.1	11	35.5	2.1	226	43.8	0	0	0	8	42.1	6.4	1	33.3	0.8	66	52.8	61	64.2
INAP	4	6.5	0.8	1	2.1	0.2	2	6.5	0.4	29	5.6	0	0	0	0	0	0	0	0	0	4	3.2	0	0
Total	62	100%	9.7	48	100%	9.3	31	100%	6.0	516	100%	8	100%	6.4	19	100%	15.2	3	100%	2.4	125	100%	95	100%
Got Along With Father																								
Terribly	13	21.0	2.5	5	10.4	1.0	7	22.6	1.4	86	16.7	1	12.5	0.8	2	10.5	1.6	0	0	0	11	8.8	6	6.3
Poorly	7	11.3	1.4	6	12.5	1.2	6	19.4	1.2	69	13.4	2	25.0	1.6	4	21.1	3.2	1	33.3	0.8	23	18.4	6	6.3
Fair	13	21.0	2.5	9	18.8	1.7	5	16.1	1.0	106	20.5	1	12.5	0.8	6	31.6	4.8	1	33.3	0.8	25	20.0	33	34.7
Well	18	29.0	3.5	25	52.1	4.8	11	35.5	2.1	176	34.1	3	37.5	2.4	3	15.8	2.4	1	33.3	0.8	48	38.4	40	42.1
INAP	11	17.7	2.1	3	6.3	0.6	2	6.5	0.4	79	15.3	1	12.5	0.8	4	21.1	3.2	0	0	0	18	14.4	10	10.5
Total	62	100%	9.7	48	100%	9.3	31	100%	6.0	516	100%	8	100%	6.4	19	100%	15.2	3	100%	2.4	125	100%	95	100%

by a mother surrogate apparently had little beneficial effect, especially for patients in group Ib. In this particular group, 45.5% of chronics had mother figures who apparently also suffered from mental illness and appeared to be responsible for the most disturbed family interactions. As regards the death of the father, the same order seems to be maintained that was found for mothers. Chronics have the largest percentage of father loss, followed by acutes, with the normals reporting fewer father deaths in childhood. These data suggest that loss of parent in childhood has a marked effect on the offspring which became chronic schizophrenics in adulthood.

Loss of parents through death during the adolescent years (10–19) was most prominent among the acute patients, followed by the chronic group, with normals showing lowest percentages. This finding is interesting from the point of view of recent trauma (precipitating factor), since acutes are a younger population (54% under age 24) than the chronics.

Obviously, family structure can be disrupted by other causes than death of parent. Either the patients themselves, through socially intolerable behavior, or the parents through divorce, separation, or other reasons, may cause radical changes in the living circumstances of the patient as a child, altering the social climate in which the patient-to-be is raised.

With this in mind, several reasons for family breakup before the patient reached the age of 16 were also examined. The results are shown in Table 7. The major causes of breakup were divorce, separation, or *de facto* division which occurred with the birth of an illegitimate child (who later became the patient). Separation due to the death of a parent, long term imprisonment, or mental illness were considered separately. No significant differences were obtained when separations for acute and chronic schizophrenics were compared with those for normals (14.3% of the chronics suffered loss of parent due to death as compared to 11.2% of the acutes and 10.5% of the normals). While it is reasonable to assume trauma of a broken home as a schizophrenic agent, patients experiencing family as a harmonious social unit, while children, could not be said to be better adjusted than those coming from broken homes.

In order to identify, retrospectively, stressful factors which might have contributed to the development of schizophrenia, childhood problems of the patients were also examined. Table 8 shows the response frequencies to a series of questions dealing with the patients' major difficulties prior to age 18. The same information was obtained from the subjects' informants. The results indicate that the major problem area for both chronic and acute patients was a disturbed relationship with parents prior to age 18. Among the chronic group, 61.3% of groups Ia and Ib, 45.7% of group II, and 71.0% of group III (disturbed by mentally ill father) reported difficulties with parents. The distribution of difficulties with parents of acute patients was 87.5% for group I, 36.8% for group II, and 33.3% for group III. Of the 95 normals studied, 36 or 37.9% reported relationship with parents as a major problem prior to age 18. After age

Table 7
Reasons for Family Breakup before the Age of 16

Reason for family breakup	Chronic sample											Acute sample											Normal sample	
	Group I			Group II			Group III			Total		Group 1			Group II			Group III			Total			
	N	%I	Total	N	%II	Total	N	%OI	Total	N	%	N	%I	Total	N	%II	Total	N	%III	Total	N	%	N	%
Divorce/Separation/ Illegitimacy	26	42.0	5.0	19	39.6	3.7	13	41.9	2.5	161	31.2	1	12.6	.8	6	31.2	4.8	1	33.3	.8	35	28	29	30.5
Long term prison (parent)	1	1.6	.2	0	0	0	0	0	0	1	.2	0	0	0	0	0	0	0	0	0	0	0	0	0
Long term mental illness	6	9.7	1.2	0	0	0	1	3.2	.2	10	1.9	0	0	0	0	0	0	0	0	0	0	0	2	2.1
Death	8	12.9	1.5	8	16.7	1.5	4	13.0	.8	74	14.3	0	0	0	2	10.5	1.6	0	0	0	14	11.2	10	10.5
INAP: Family not broken	21	33.9	4.1	21	43.7	4.1	13	42.0	2.5	250	50.4	7	87.6	5.6	11	57.9	8.8	2	66.7	1.6	76	60.8	54	56.8
Total	62	100%	12.0	48	100%	9.3	31	100%	6.0	516	100%	8	100%	6.4	19	100%	15.2	3	100%	2.4	125	100%	95	100%

Table 8
Major Problems Experienced before Age 18 by Acute and Chronic Schizophrenics and Comparable Normals

Major problem before 18	Chronic Sample											Acute sample											Normal sample	
	Group 1			Group II			Group III			Tot Chron.		Group I			Group II			Group III			Tot Acute			
	N	%I	%Tot	N	%II	%Tot	N	%III	%Tot	N	%Tot	N	%I	%Tot	N	%II	%Tot	N	%III	%Tot	N	%Tot	N-	%Tot
Parents	38	61.3	7.4	21	43.8	4.1	22	71.0	4.3	289	56.0	7	87.5	5.6	7	36.8	5.6	1	33.3	0.8	55	44.0	36	37.9
Opposite sex	30	48.4	5.8	20	41.6	3.9	11	35.5	2.1	206	39.9	4	50.1	3.2	9	47.4	7.2	1	33.3	0.8	36	28.8	15	15.8
Sexual problems	23	37.1	4.5	11	22.9	2.1	6	19.4	1.2	150	29.1	3	37.5	2.4	6	31.6	4.8	1	33.3	0.8	20	16.0	3	3.2
School	27	43.5	5.2	20	41.7	3.9	18	58.1	3.5	223	43.2	4	50.1	3.2	6	31.6	4.8	2	66.7	1.6	56	28.4	38	40.0
Job	20	32.4	3.9	4	8.3	0.8	6	19.4	1.2	83	16.1	0	0	0	3	15.8	2.4	1	33.3	0.8	12	9.6	9	9.6
Friends	29	46.8	5.6	16	33.3	3.1	11	35.5	2.1	182	35.3	3	37.5	2.4	6	31.6	4.8	1	33.3	0.8	34	27.2	15	15.8
People	28	45.2	5.4	17	35.4	3.3	11	35.5	2.1	166	32.2	4	50.1	3.2	4	21.1	3.2	0	0	0	29	23.2	13	13.7
Authorities	17	27.4	3.3	12	25.0	3.3	9	29.0	1.7	104	20.2	1	12.5	0.8	2	10.5	1.6	0	0	0	10	8.0	8	8.4
Personality changes	25	40.3	4.8	6	12.5	1.2	15	48.4	2.9	155	30.0	2	25.1	1.6	4	21.1	3.2	2	66.7	1.6	28	22.4	10	10.5
Drinking/drugs	9	14.5	1.7	5	10.4	1.0	6	19.4	1.2	87	16.9	3	37.6	2.4	2	10.5	1.6	1	33.3	0.8	20	16.0	5	5.3
Physical problems	3	4.8	0.6	6	12.5	1.2	4	12.9	0.8	52	10.1	1	23.1		5	26.3	4.0	1	33.3	0.8	13	10.4	20	21.1
Death	19	30.7	3.7	13	27.1	2.5	9	29.0	1.7	132	25.6	0	0	0	3	15.8	2.4	1	33.3	0.8	26	20.8	24	25.3
Other	9	14.6	1.7	3	6.3	0.6	5	16.1	1.0	45	8.7	0	0	0	1	5.3	0.8	1	33.3	0.8	9	7.2	8	8.4

18, problems with the opposite sex became of primary importance for the patients, although difficulties with parents remained the second most frequently cited problem for the chronic group.

On the basis of these findings, as well as those of others, it becomes obvious that genetic or familial factors alone cannot satisfactorily account for the development of schizophrenia. It seemed important to determine whether or not schizophrenia may be heralded, long before the florid symptoms of the illness appear, by the stressful interaction between the patient and environment which often goes undetected, though manifesting itself by multiple adjustment problems of long standing.

The second part of our study, conducted with the same population, tried to determine whether or not schizophrenics, as compared to normals, experience a greater amount of problems and difficulties in youth and adolescence which carry over into the patients' adult years. By comparing the responses of 95 normals with those of acute and chronic schizophrenics it was possible to determine whether these groups differ to a significant extent in the degree of continuity of problems from youth to adulthood.

For the purposes of the study, the pattern of problems the individuals experienced before and after the age of 18, and the extent of continuity between past and present levels of difficulty was considered for 12 areas of personal and interpersonal behavior. The areas chosen were thought to represent impaired functioning which affected the subjects emotionally and would induce stress when the subject felt unable to meet the needs in these particular areas of interactions. Two of the problem areas (major physical problems and death of someone very close) were not dependent on the subjects' psychological well being or his capacity to function. In all the other problem areas the individual may have played a role in creation of the problem because of weaknesses in his psychosocial functioning. The problem areas employed in the study were: (1) difficulty in getting along with parents; (2) problems in relating to the opposite sex; (3) sexual maladjustment; (4) academic difficulties and impaired intellectual performance; (5) impaired ability to get and hold a job; (6) difficulty in obtaining and maintaining friendships (loneliness); (7) problems in relating to people in general; (8) acting out behavior and problems with authority; (9) dislike of and change in personality; (10) major physical problems; (11) problem drinking and use of drugs; and (12) death of someone very close (parent, sibling, lover, spouse, friend).

The assessment of the 12 problem areas was made on the basis of information obtained from the SSFIPD, a section of which dealt directly with problem areas encountered before and after age 18. The inventory also provided data for the measurement of current stress and functioning in addition to the separate items referring to the subjects' problem areas in the past.

The first part of data analysis concerned establishment of differences for the three groups of subjects (normals, acute, and chronic schizophrenics) on the 12 items referring to difficulties before the age of 18 and those pertaining to problems encountered after the age of 18. The statistical measure used to accomplish this purpose was stepwise discriminant function analysis performed for the 12 items representing major problems before and the 12 items referring to problems after the age of 18. The comparisons were made for acute vs. chronics, acutes vs. normals, and normals vs. chronics. The discriminant function analyses permitted comparison of the groups on the most discriminating of the 12 variables alone, and in an increasing combination with each of the next best discriminators. Results of the analyses are shown in Table 9. Of the 12 pre-18-year items, four made significant contribution to the differentiation among normals and acute and chronic schizophrenics. These were: inability to obtain sexual fulfillment, difficulty in dealing with authority, presence of major physical problems (physical illnesses and/or handicaps) and dislike of, or change in personality. Of the post-18-year items, seven significantly differentiated among the groups; difficulty in obtaining and holding a job, inability to obtain sexual satisfaction, trouble with authorities, problem drinking and use of drugs, difficulty in making and keeping friends, problems in relating to the opposite sex, and death of someone close.

Table 9

COMPARISON AMONG GROUPS ON BEST DISCRIMINATING
PRE-18- AND POST-18-YR. ITEMS

Item	Acute vs Chronic (F)	Acute vs Normal (F)	Normal vs Chronic (F)
Pre-18-yr.			
Sex Problems (SP)	8.51†	5.34*	29.39†
Trouble with Authorities (TA) + SP	9.07†	2.67	18.84†
Physical Problems (PP) + SP + TA	6.19†	4.27†	17.71†
Dislike of Personality (DP) + SP + TA + PP	4.75†	4.01†	15.32†
Post-18-Yr.			
Job Difficulty (JD)	5.68*	16.26†	50.04†
SP + JD	3.71*	14.09†	39.61†
TA + JD + SP	5.86†	9.47†	30.63†
Drinking or Drugs (DD) + JD + SP + TA	4.50†	9.75†	25.74†
Difficulty with Friends (DF)			
+ JD + SP + TA + DD	3.88†	8.52†	22.90†
Relating to Opposite Sex (ROS)			
+ JD + SP + TA + DD + DF	3.26†	9.53†	20.68†
Death of Someone Close + JD			
+ SP + TA +DD + DF + ROS	2.80†	8.11†	18.99†

*$p < .05$.
†$p < .01$.

The next part of the general data analyses focused on a comparision of the subjects' responses on the pre-18-year items with their responses on the post-18-year items. Table 10 presents the percentages of normals and acute and chronic schizophrenics who responded in the affirmative as experiencing the problem for each of the pre-18 and post-18-year items. Examination of Table 10 reveals that in most cases the chronics had the highest percentage of individuals experiencing the problem, followed by acutes, with normals showing the smallest percentages.

In order to determine the relationship between the pattern of problems the individual encountered before and after the age of 18, tetrachoric correlations were computed for the individual's response to pre-18 item and his response to the corresponding post-18-year item. These correlations were computed for each of the 12 pre- and post-18-year items separately for normals and the acute and chronic schizophrenic groups. Table 11 shows the obtained correlation coefficients for each subject sample. All of the coefficients are significant at the 0.01 level, with the exceptions of (1) the problem area pertaining to relationships with the opposite sex for normals, which is significant at the 0.05 level, (2) the problems associated with academic performance for the chronics, and (3) the death of someone close for both the acute and chronic schizophrenic samples, which failed to reach acceptable levels of significance. These results support the notion that the same problems, or lack of problems, which appeared in the past tend to continue into adulthood.

To determine the relationship between the pattern of problems that have created stress for the individual during his childhood and youth and the present

Table 10
PERCENTAGES OF INDIVIDUALS WHO RESPONDED IN AFFIRMATIVE
TO PRE-18-YR. ITEMS

Item	Pre-18-yr.			Post-18-yr.		
	Normal	Acute	Chronic	Normal	Acute	Chronic
Parents	37.9	44.0	56.0	29.7	40.7	45.6
Opposite Sex	15.8	28.8	39.9	37.4	40.7	48.9
Sex	3.2	16.0	29.1	7.7	34.3	43.0
School	40.0	28.8	43.2	6.6	13.2	14.0
Job	9.5	9.6	16.1	11.0	36.4	48.6
Friends	15.8	27.2	35.3	8.8	32.4	42.3
Others	13.7	24.0	32.0	8.8	25.0	34.4
Authority	8.4	8.0	20.2	3.3	8.3	23.3
Personality	10.5	22.4	30.0	11.0	26.9	34.9
Drinking/Drugs	5.3	16.0	16.9	7.7	31.5	36.2
Physical Problems	21.1	10.4	10.1	16.5	14.8	13.7
Death	25.3	21.6	25.4	35.2	24.1	23.0

Table 11

TETRACHORIC CORRELATIONS BETWEEN PRE-18-YR. AND
CORRESPONDING POST-18-YR. ITEMS

Item	Normal	Acute	Chronic
Parents	.72	.78	.83
Opposite Sex	.23	.54	.78
Sex	.49	.74	.83
School	.38	.26	.19
Job	−.97	.97	.46
Friends	.63	.81	.83
Others	.84	.79	.75
Authories	.49	.72	.72
Personality	.85	.60	.64
Drinking/Drugs	.94	.65	.81
Physical Problems	.62	.74	.68
Death	−.54	−.07	.08

conditions of psychological stress he is laboring under, the subjects' responses on pre-18 and post-18-year items were compared with scores on the corresponding categories of areas of stress derived from the SSFIPD. Point biserial correlations were computed separately for the normal and the two schizophrenic groups between the pre- and post-18-year items and stress scores on the corresponding categories from the inventory. The results are shown in Table 12. As can be observed from this table, the correlations for the chronics on the pre-18 items were all significant, except for the problem area of drinking and drug use; the

TABLE 12

CORRELATIONS BETWEEN PRE 18-YR. ITEMS AND MEAN STRESS SCORE FOR
ALL 21 CATEGORIES OF THE STRESS AND FUNCTIONABILITY INVENTORY

Topic	Pre-18-yr. Items			Post-18-yr. Items		
	Normals	Acute	Chronic	Normals	Acute	Chronic
Parents	.28*	.48**	.45**	.51**	.62**	.55**
Opposite Sex	−.16	.31†	.38†	−.12	.40**	.43**
Sex	.00	.27†	.35**	.14	.30†	.39**
School	.40†	.40**	.24**	.23*	−.12	.01
Job	.01	.02	.10*	−.04	.24*	.15†
Friends	.14	.19*	.31**	.19	.35**	.28**
Others	.15	.32**	.32**	.22*	.25†	.43**
Authorities	.00	.10	.18†	.00	.29††	.24†
Drinking/Drugs	−.18	−.13	.09	.14	.01	.09

*p < .05.   †p < .01.   **p < .001.
††Non-significant because of reduced N resulting from missing data.

majority of the correlations for the acute sample were significant (exceptions being items pertaining to job, problems with authorities, and drinking and drugs); it is of interest to note that only two problem areas were significant for the normal control group: problems with parents and education. For the post-18-year items, chronics showed significant correlations for all items except education, relationship with authority, and excessive drinking and use of drugs. Acute schizophrenics showed significant correlations for all items except education, relationship with authority, and drinking and drugs. Three significant correlations were obtained for the normal sample: parents, education, and relationship with others.

To assess the relationship between individual areas of difficulty in the past and the current level of stress the subjects were experiencing, point-biserial correlations were computed for each of the pre-18 items and the mean stress score (derived from sum total of 21 categories of stress measured by the inventory). The correlations performed separately for acutes, chronics, and normal controls are shown in Table 13. The results obtained were similar to those in which the individual categories of stress derived from the inventory were used. The normals showed a few significant correlations of low magnitude; the acute group showed a greater number and larger correlations, which were significant, while the chronics obtained significant correlations for every pre-18-year item, except drinking/drugs, and all of these correlations were significant at a 0.001 level.

Table 13

CORRELATIONS BETWEEN PRE 18-YR. ITEMS AND MEAN STRESS
SCORE FOR ALL 21 CATEGORIES OF THE STRESS AND FUNCTIONABILITY
INVENTORY

Pre-18-yr. Items	Normals	Acutes	Chronics
Parents	.15	.39**	.35**
Opposite Sex	−.04	.34**	.34**
Sex	−.08	.38**	.36**
School	.22*	.29†	.18**
Job	.31†	.06	.17**
Friends	.17	.21*	.41**
Others	.15	.31**	.34**
Authorities	.32†	.04	.15**
Personality	.01	.24†	.26**
Drinking/Drugs	.20*	.12	.06
Physical Problems	−.03	.10	.15**
Death	.05	.09	.17**

*$p < .05$.
†$p < .01$.
**$p < .001$.

As a check on the reliability of the patient's self-report regarding his past difficulties, the responses of the patients were compared with those of informants who also provided the same information about the patient. The informants fell into two categories: (1) close informants such as parents, spouse, child, or sibling and (2) secondary informants, i.e., friends, social workers, distant relatives. There were 228 schizophrenic patients (46 acutes and 182 chronics) for whom complete informant data was available. The reliability of the patients' self-report was determined by the use of chi-square tests testing the distribution of responses given by the patient and his informant on the four pre-18-year items that have been found to significantly discriminate normals, acutes, and chronics (sexual problems, trouble with authority, physical problems, and dislike and change in personality). Results indicated that the patient information about himself was not significantly different from information provided by the informant regarding the four areas of difficulty. It would appear that the use of patient-supplied data serves as a reliable source of information about the patient's past difficulties. (See chapter 10 for details.)

DISCUSSION

It appears that multiple stressful factors contribute to the development of schizophrenia. On the basis of the evidence presented here, it becomes apparent that disturbed family and social relationships rather than purely genetic factors may operate in the etiology of this disease. It is of interest to note that although the effect of a genetic factor cannot be clearly denied, it alone cannot help explain the large number of subjects who become schizophrenic without any clear cut genetic predisposition (i.e., schizophrenic forebears). Our findings appear to support indirectly Bleuler's observations that three-quarters of the children of the schizophrenics were basically healthy (6). At the same time, the results indicate that disturbed family relationships have significance only inasmuch as the patients perceive them as disturbing.

More important is the fact that the patients had difficulty in distinguishing psychologically between a mentally ill parent, as attested to by New York state, and one whom they perceived as disturbed. However, whenever there was an overlap, i.e., a combination of hereditary factors and disturbed family interaction as in Group Ib, the patients reported maximum amount of stress stemming from the familial relationship. It should be pointed out, however, that the patients' perception of the family interaction as disturbed played the crucial role in producing stress, independent of the actual mental condition of the parents (presence or absence of mental illness), as confirmed by the hospital information.

Whatever may be the specific family dynamics leading to stressful family interactions, one fact seems to be undeniable—the schizophrenic appears to have problems in establishing adequate relationships with his parents and society at large (50, 51). With this in mind, we evaluated reactions of acute and chronic schizophrenics to various life experiences. Chronics in Group Ib and Group III (mother perceived as schizophrenic, and attested to being schizophrenic by New York state; father reported as suffering from schizophrenia) reported the highest amounts of stress stemming from disturbed familial interaction.

Two implications emerge from these observations. First, that not only the schizophrenogenic mother, but also the mentally ill father, especially if so perceived by the patient, may contribute to the development of schizophrenia. Second, and equally important, is the perception of disturbance in the parent that creates the stress for the schizophrenic patient. This position finds support in the recent findings of Arieti (2) who claims that only 25% of the mothers of schizophrenics are truly schizophrenogenic, and, in the remaining 75%, disturbances of the mother appear to represent distortions of the mother image by the schizophrenic patients.

The extent of stress created by disturbed family interaction among the schizophrenics becomes all the more apparent when the reactions of these patients are compared with those of normal controls. Chronic schizophrenic patients experienced twice the number of problems in interactions with their mothers and fathers than did the normals. Even in childhood, the chronics had greater difficulty in family relationships than the normals.

Loss of parents through death appears to be the final crucial stress event potentially contributing to schizophrenia. In countradistinction to the general belief that the break-up of the family is one of the major causes of stress in childhood, it appears that death of a parent, with its sense of finality, is a more stressful event for the schizophrenic child. Further support comes from the observation that the highest proportion of deaths of either parent, prior to age 10, is found in our chronic schizophrenic group. For the acute schizophrenics, however, death of the parent when the patient was an adolescent (10–18 years old) appears to have significance.

It should be noted, however, that although death of a loved one in adolescence is assumed to be a precipitating factor in the development of schizophrenia (54) in our sample, this variable did not assume a very significant role with any systematic frequency.

Disturbed parental interactions are by no means the only factors operating in the development of schizophrenia. Other psychosocial problems dating back to childhood and adolescence appear to persist and to lead to hospitalization in adult years. Of the 12 problem areas selected for study, three emerged as potential sources of stress. These were: sexual problems, difficulties with authorities, and dislike and/or change in their personality. The findings are consistent with those obtained by other researchers. Morris *et al.* (41) reported a high incidence of sexual and aggressive acting out behavior among children who became schizophrenic in adulthood. Bower, Shellhamer, and Daily (10) demonstrated that preschizophrenic adolescent boys showed less interest in girls and experienced changes in personality which is congruent with the patient self-reports obtained in the present study. The presence of more antisocial behavior and neurotic symptomatology in preschizophrenics as compared to control groups has also been reported by O'Neal and Robins *(43, 44)*, Robins *(48)*, and Fleming *(14, 15)*.

In general, the experimental studies suggest that adolescent problems with sexuality, authority figures, and dislike or change in personality stand out prominently in the schizophrenics' life histories. It appears that schizophrenics experience two levels of difficulties which may have either additive or interactive effects in the initial process leading to schizophrenia. One of these is an inability of the individual, at the time of his personality formation, to accept himself, resulting in an impaired self-image. The other is an inability to establish socially appropriate behavior patterns leading to a conflict with his milieu.

The individual whose personal image of himself is poor throughout his childhood and adolescence begins to experience difficulties in his first significant social confrontation (outside of the family) with authority figures, and in his relationships with the opposite sex. His sense of inadequacy spreads progressively, like a cancer, to embrace other areas vital to his survival in society (job, friends, etc.), resulting in the adoption of maladaptive defense patterns such as excessive drinking and drug abuse, in an attempt to alleviate escalating stress. It is only a matter of time until the interactive effect of the increasing stress and the emotional response culminates in the disintegration of personality, with the resultant total nonfunctioning.

It is of particular interest that the continuity between past (preschizophrenic) and current difficulties (as supported by the obtained point-biserial correlations between the pre-18 and and post-18-year items), together with the continuity of experienced stress, was found for both chronic and acute patients but not for normals. Moreover, there was little difference between the chronic and the acutes in the maintenance of problem areas over time. This basic trend is particularly important since it indicates that all schizophrenic patients do indeed have a long history of psychosocial problems and disturbances. These findings also hold true for acute schizophrenics (first episode schizophrenia) who had been assumed to function adequately until severe precipitating events caused them to become floridly psychotic.

To the extent to which schizophrenia appears to be characterized mainly by an insidious, gradual impairment of functioning starting in childhood and continuing into adulthood, it presupposes a concomitant distortion of the process of thinking which produces the maladjustment. If it is true that the potential schizophrenic in his developmental years is under stress in his family or environment, then it seems that his coping mechanisms are affected to the point that he responds inadequately to the external input overload. As Miller *(39)* suggested, even "normals" under information overload attempt to adjust by either nonprocessing the information or in one form or another processing them incorrectly. Obviously, the performance is affected, which results in poor adjustment. Then schizophrenia could be considered an illness of gradual distorted adaptations leading in finality to a different modality of adaptation. In terms of normal behavior the schizophrenic appears to be inappropriate, unresponsive, withdrawn, with psychomotorretardation. It is a gradual process that affects his cognition, his appraisal of reality, and his judgment about it. Yet, the mental defect becomes noticeable only when the behavior appears to be socially disintegrating, most likely due to a crisis situation. It is at this time that the diagnosis of schizophrenia is tentatively made.

REFERENCES

1. Alanen, Y.: The family of schizophrenic patients. *In* "The Schizophrenic Syndrome" (J. R. Cancro, ed.) Vol. 1., Brunner-Mazel, New York, 1971.
2. Arieti, S.: An overview of schizophrenia from a predominantly psychological approach. *Am. J. Psychiat.* **131** (3), 241–249, 1974.
3. Bateson, G., Jackson, D., Haley, J., and Weakland, J.: Toward a theory of schizophrenia, *Behav. Sci.* **1**, 251-264, 1956.
4. Beck, S.J.: "The Six Schizophrenias," American Orthopsychiatric Assoc., New York, 1954.
5. Birren, J.E.: Psychological examination of children who later become psychotic, *J. Clin. Psychol.* **39**, 84–96, 1944.
6. Bleuler, M.: Some results of research in schizophrenia. *In* "Annual Review of the Schizophrenic Syndrome" (R. Cancro, ed.), Brunner-Mazel, New York, pp. 3–16. 1971.
7. Bogoch, S.: Cerebrospinal fluid neuranimic acid deficiency in schizophrenia: a preliminary report. *Am. J. Psychiat.* **114,** 172, 1957.
8. Book, J.A.: A genetic and neuropsychiatric investigation of a North-Swedish population with special regard to schizophrenia and mental deficiency. *Acta Genet.* 4, 1, 133–345, 1953.
9. Bowen, M.A.: Family Concept of schizophrenia. *In* "The Etiology of Schizophrenia" (John D. Jackson, ed.), pp. 346–372. Basic Books, New York.
10. Bower, E.M., Shellhammer, T.A., and Daily, J.M.: School Characteristics of male adolescents who later become schizophrenic. *Am. J. Orthopsychiat.* **30,** 712–729, 1960.
11. Cameron, N.: "Personality Development and Psychopathology," Houghton Mifflin, Boston, 1963.
12. Cheek, F.E.: The schizophrenic mother in word and deed, *Family Process* 3, 155–177, 1964.
13. Essen-Moller, E.: Calculation of morbid risk in parents of index cases or applied to a family of schizophrenics. *Acta Genet.* 5, 334–442, 1955. Basel
14. Fleming, P.: Emotional antecedents of schizophrenia. Paper read before the First Conf. on Life History Research in Psychopathology. New York, N.Y. May 2, 1967.
15. Fleming, P.: Prediction of adult psychopathology, their early emotional experiences. Paper read before 2nd conf. on Life History Research in Psychopathology, Univ. of Minn., April 19, 1968.
16. Fowler, R.C., Tsuang, M.I., Cadoret, R.J., and Monnelly, E.: Non psychotic disorders in the families of process schizophrenics. *Acta Psych. Scandinavica* **51**, 153–160, 1975.
17. Frazee, H.E.: Children who later become schizophrenic. *Smith Coll. Studies Soc. Work* **23,** 125–149, 1953.
18. Friedhoff, A.J., and Van Winkle, E.: A biochemical approach to the study of schizophrenia *Am. J. Psychiat.* **121**, 1054–1055, 1965.
19. Friedlander, D.: Personality development of twenty-seven children who later became psychotic. *J. Abnorm. Soc. Psychol.* **40**, 330–335, 1945.
19a. Fromm-Reichman, F.: *Notes on the* Development of Treatment of Schizophrenics by Psychoanalytic Psychotherapy. *Psychiatry* **11**, 263–273, 1948.

20. Frohman, E.C.: "Biochemical Mechanism. in *Lafayette Clinic studies on schizophrenia*" (G. Tourney and J. Gottlieb, eds.) Wayne State University Press, Detroit, pp. 125–157, 1971.
21. Gottesman, I.I., and Shields, J.: Schizophrenia in twins: 16 years consecutive admissions to a psychiatric clinic. *Brit. J. Psychiat.* 112, 809–818, 1966.
22. Gottsman, I.I. and Shields, J.: "Schizophrenics and Genetics," Academic Press, New York, 1972.
23. Hallgren, B., and Sjogren, T.: A clinical and genetico-statistical study of schizophrenia and low grade mental deficiency in a large Swedish rural population. Copenhagen: Munksgaard, 1959. Acta Psychiatrica Suppl 140, 35, 1959.
23a. Hambert, G.: *Males with Positive Sex Chromatin.* Göteborg: Scandinavian University Books, 1966.
24. Heath, R.G., Leach, B.E., and Byers, L.W.: "Taraxein: Mode of Action. Serological Factors in Schizophrenia?" PB Hochner, Inc., New York, 1963.
25. Heston, L.L.: Psychiatric disorders in foster home reared children of schizophrenic mothers. *Brit. J. Psychiat.* 112, 819–825, 1966.
26. Hoffer, A., Osmond, M., and Smythies, J.: Schizophrenia: A New Approach, II, Results of a year's research. *J. Mental Sci.* 100, 29–34, 1954.
27. Hoskins, R.G., and Pincus, G.: Sex hormone relationships in schizophrenic men. *Psychosomatic Med.* 11, 102–109, 1949.
28. Kallman, F.J.: "The Genetics of Schizophrenia." J.J. Augustin, New York, 1938.
29. Kallman, F.J., and Roth, B.: Genetic aspects of preadolescent schizophrenia. *Am. J. Psychiat.* 112, 599–606, 1956.
30. Kety, S.S., Rosenthal, D., Wender, P. and Schulsinger, F.: The types and prevalence of mental illness in the biological and adoptive families of adoptive schizophrenics. *In* "The Transmission of Schizophrenia" (D. Rosenthal and S. Kety, eds.), pp. 345–362. Pergamon Press, Oxford. 1968.
31. Kety, S.S., Rosenthal, D., Wender, P.H., and Schulsinger, F.: Mental Illness in the biological and adoptive families of adopted schizophrenics. *Am. J. Psychiat.* 128, 302–306, 1971.
32. Kuehl, F.A., Osmond, R.E., and Vanderheuval, W.J.A.: Occurrence of 3.4 dimeth oxyphenylactic acid in urines of normal and schizophrenic individuals. *Nature (London)* 211, 606–608, 1966.
33. Lidz, T., Cornelison, A., Fleck, S. and Terry, D.: The intrafamilial environment of the schizophrenic patient: II. Marital schism and marital skew. *Am. J. Psychiat.* 114, 241–248, 1958.
34. Lidz, T., Cornelison, A., Terry, D. and Fleck, S.: Intrafamilial environment of the schizophrenic patient: VI. The transmission of irrationality. *In* "Schizophrenia and the Family." Arch. Neurol & Psychiat., 79, 305–316, New York, 1958.
35. Luxenberger, H.: Untersuchung an schizophrenien Zweillingen und ihren Geschwistern zur Prufung der Realitat von Manifestationschwankungen. Zts. *Neurol. Psychiat.* 154, 351, 1936.
36. Mednick, S.A., and Schulsinger, F.: Factors related to breakdown in children at high risk for schizophrenia. *In* "Life History Research in Psychopathology" (M. Roff and D. F. Rich, eds), Vol. I. pp. 51–93. Univ. of Minn. Press, Minneapolis, 1970.
37. Mednick, S.A., and Schulsinger, F.: Studies of children at high risk for schizophrenia. *In* "Schizophrenias, the First Ten Dean Award Lectures." (S. R. Dean, ed.), M.S.S. Information Corp., New York, pp. 247–293, 1973.
38. Michaels, C.M., Morris, D.P., and Soroker, E.: Follow-up studies of shy withdrawn children. II. Relative incidence of schizophrenia. *Am. J. Orthopsychiat.* 27, 331–337, 1957.
39. Miller, J.G.: Information input overload and psychopathology, *Am. J. Psychiat.* 116, 695–704, 1960.
40. Morris, D.P., Soroker, E., and Burress, G.: Follow-up studies of shy withdrawn children. II. Evaluation of later adjustment. *Am. J. Orthopsychiat.* 24, 743–754, 1954.

41. Morris, H.H., Escoll, P.H., and Wexler, R.: Aggressive behavior disorders of childhood, a follow-up study. *Am. J. Psychiat.* **112**, 991–997, 1956.
42. Nameche, G., Waring, M., and Ricks, D.: Early indicators of outcome in schizophrenia. *J. Nerv. Ment. Dis.* **139**, 232–240, 1964.
43. O'Neal, P., and Robins, L.: Childhood patterns predictors of adult schizophrenia. A 35 year follow up of 150 subjects. *Am. J. Psychiat.* **115**, 385–391, 1958.
44. O'Neal, P., and Robins, L.: The relation of childhood behavior problems to adult psychiatric status: A 30 year follow-up study of 150 subjects. *Am. J. Psychiat.* **114**, 961–969, 1958.
45. Offord, R., and Cross, L.A.: Behavioral antecedents of adult schizophrenia: A Review. *Arch. Gen. Psychiat.* **21**, 267–283, 1969.
46. Penrose, L.S.: Critical survey of schizophrenia genetics. *In* "Modern Perspectives in World Psychiatry" (John G. Howell, ed.), pp. 3–19. Brunner-Mazel, New York, 1971.
47. Pollack, M.: Comparison of childhood, adolescent and adult schizophrenics, *Arch. Gen. Psychiat.* **2**, 652–660, 1960.
48. Robins, L.: "Deviant Children Grow Up." Williams & Williams, Baltimore, 1966.
49. Roff, M.: Childhood Social interactions and young adult psychosis. *J. Clin. Psychol.* **19**, 152–157, 1963.
50. Singer, M., and Wynne, L.: Thought disorder and family relations of schizophrenics III: Methodology using projective techniques *Arch. Gen. Psychiat.* **12**, 187–200, 1965.
51. Singer, M., and Wynne, L.: Thought disorder and family relations of schizophrenics: IV. Results and implications. *Arch. Gen. Psychiat.* **12**, 201–212, 1965.
52. Slater, E.: A review of Earlier Concordance on Genetic Factors in schizophrenia. Proceedings of The Third World Congress of Psychiatry, Vol. 1, p. 15. Toronto Press, Montreal, 1961.
53. Slater, E., and Shields, J.: Psychotic and neurotic illnesses in twins. Medical Research Council Special Report Series, No. 278, London: H.M.S.O. 1953.
54. Vaillant, G.E. Natural history of remitting schizophrenias. Am. J. Psychiat. 120: 366–375, 1963.
55. Waring, M., and Ricke, D.: Family patterns of children who became adult schizophrenics. *J. Nerv. Ment. Dis.* **140**, 351–364, 1965.
56. Watt, N.F., Stolorow, R.D., Lubensky, A.W., and McClelland, D.C.: School adjustment and behavior of children hospitalized for schizophrenia as adults. *In* "Annual Review of the Schizophrenic Syndrome" (R. Cancro, ed.), Vol. 2, pp. 359–383. Brunner-Mazel, New York, 1972.
57. Wittman, M.P., and Steinberg, D.L.: A study of prodromal factors in mental illness with special reference to schizophrenia, *Am. J. Psychiat.* **100**, 811–816, 1944.
58. Wynne, L.C., and Singer, M.T.: Thought disorder and family relations of schizophrenics: I. Research strategy. *Arch. Gen. Psychiat.* **9**, 191–198, 1963.
59. Wynne, L.C., and Singer, M.T.: Thought disorder and family relations of schizophrenics: II. Classification of forms of thinking, *Arch. Gen. Psychiat.* **9**, 199–206, 1963.
60. Zuckerman, M., Oltean, M. and Monashkin, I. The parental attitude of mothers of schizophrenics. *J. Consult. Psychol.* **22**, 4–10, 1958.

CHAPTER 8

The Validity of Diagnostic Signs and Their Prognostic Value in Schizophrenia*

Part I

Mental status evaluations of schizophrenic patients have been traditionally used for diagnosis as well as for prediction of the course of the illness. Needless to say, the use of symptoms for these purposes leads to problems since without proper diagnosis of schizophrenia it is difficult, if not impossible, to make reliable statements regarding the outcome of the disease.

The diagnostic criteria devised by Kraeplin *(28)* and revised by Bleuler *(9)* gained wide acceptance in differentiating schizophrenia from other forms of psychoses. The four crucial symptoms delineated by Bleuler (loosening of association, withdrawal from reality, blunting ambivalence of affect, and autistic thinking) appeared in the beginning to cover quite adequately the core concept of schizophrenia, although subsequent clinical experience failed to corroborate regularly the usefulness of these diagnostic signs. Attempts at refinement of schizophrenic symptomatology are seen in Bleuler's further subdivision of the four crucial symptoms into fundamental and accessory signs, placing hallucinatory and delusional behavior into the latter category. The fundamental signs became blunting, withdrawal from reality, loosening of association, and autistic thinking. Meehl *(33)* later on also included disorders of personal relationships, particularly interpersonal aversiveness and poor rapport with others. Lack of insight, defined as lack of awareness of emotional problems, became another universally used diagnostic sign for identification of schizophrenia.

Further attempts at refinement of diagnostic symptoms and signs have been made by the phenomenological school of Jaspers *(25)* and his followers and by others, notably Langfeldt *(30)*. Langfeldt *(30, 31)*, working within the initial

---

*The research results presented in this chapter have appeared in the article: G. Serban: Relationship of mental status, functioning and stress to readmission of schizophrenics. *Br. J. Soc. Clin. Psychol.* **14,** 291–301, 1975.

concept of schizophrenia formulated by Bleuler, attempted to separate schizophrenia proper from "schizophrenia like" psychoses, emphasizing their different
outcomes. He classified schizophrenia in terms of schizophreniform psychosis
and true schizophrenia identified by process symptom. The former was an acute
schizophrenic episode and/or schizoaffective condition which did not fit the classical identifying Bleulerian concepts. It was observed, concomittantly, that the
schizophreniform cases appear to have generally good prognosis. A further contribution focusing on meaningful diagnostic distinctions within the schizophrenias
has been made by Astrup (6) by his reactive psychosis of good prognosis. Angst
(2) suggested that the schizoaffective type could develop, in time, in any one of
the following three directions: manic-depressive course, remain acute episodic
schizoaffective reactions, or become chronic schizophrenics with a deteriorating
course of illness.

Other clinicians have been preoccupied with the deliniation of various aspects
of primary signs responsible for the course of schizophrenia. Schneider (38)
attempted to reduce the unreliability of diagnosis by determining which symptoms are reversible and are not part of schizophrenia. Since the main difficulty in
this disease appears to be associated with a thinking disorder, Carl Schneider
identified the symptom complexes of the underlying thought disorder of true
schizophrenia in terms of three abnormalities: fusion (combination of unrelated
concepts), derailment (break in train of thought), and irrelevancy (meaningless
concepts of thought), the last abnormality assuming the dominant aspect of the
thinking disorder in the illness under his system. Yet, this description of thought
deficit, although theoretically meaningful, has been difficult to translate into
clinical terms.

Other various aspects of the thought disturbance have been described empirically by numerous researchers in the field, in an effort directed toward the
understanding of the underlying processes leading to the observed deficit. For
example, Goldstein (18) and Vigotsky (53) claimed that inability to form abstract
concepts is the core thinking difficulty in schizophrenia. Inability to understand
figurative language (16) and a tendency to form overinclusive concepts (11) have
also been prominently mentioned. Harrow and co-workers found out that
conceptual overinclusions subside after the acute phase, while idiosyncratic
thinking persists longer. Shakow (41) discussed the importance of the schizophrenic's inability to hold a set specific for psychomotor functioning. Experimental evidence spanning many years of research with chronic schizophrenics
support the existence of cognition defect. Shakow suggests that schizophrenic
patients have difficulty in maintaining "major sets," show slow response time as
reflected in reaction-type situations, and adapt slowly, as demonstrated in both
GSR and heart rate reactions. It has been reported that schizophrenics, as a
group, tend to show a higher degree of unrealistic perceptions as indicated by a
larger percentage of poor responses on the Rorschach Test and make many
common errors in tachistoscopic experiments (3).

Reed *(37)* proposed defect in filtering of both internal and external stimuli as a core problem in schizophrenia. Slowness in processing information *(32)* and a tendency toward personalized thinking, combined with idiosyncratic character suggesting the intrusion of affect disorder into the cognitive activity, have also been noted *(54)*.

However important these findings may be for the understanding of the schizophrenic disorder and for explaining the reasons for some of the adaptive deficit of the schizophrenic, most of this research is based on populations unclearly defined as schizophrenic. There is no clearcut evidence that the subjects would meet any of the strict criteria for identification of schizophrenia. Moreover, this research does not help the clinician or the researcher in discriminating between the true schizophrenic patient and the patient exhibiting schizophrenic-like psychoses. How could all these concepts be integrated clinically to help psychiatrists throughout the world reach agreement as to what is and what is not schizophrenia? Likewise, the accumulated research does not help clinicians in the United States and in England to agree on the differentiation between schizophrenics and manic–depressives. Actually, clinicians in the United States, using looser criteria, favor schizophrenia as a diagnosis while those in England favor affective disorders.

It has long been evident that clearcut diagnostic criteria, based on a strict description of symtomatology, are required to narrow the limits of what is considered schizophrenia. Among the researchers who have attempted to do this is Kurt Schneider, the most disputed one in the United States while being simultaneously better accepted in Europe. On the basis of extensive observation, he has delineated what have become the famous 11 first rank symptoms defining schizophrenia: audible thought, voices that argue with or discuss the patient, voices commenting on the patient's activity, thought insertion, thought with-drawal, thought broadcast, "made" feeling and/or "made" impulses, and "made" volition. These first rank symptoms have the advantage of identifying thought disorder through the clearly specified content of the particular clinical symptoms. Kurt Schneider assumes that these signs occur mainly in schizophre-nia, and are thus generally applicable for diagnosis of the disease. Investigators have attempted to validate the signs only recently *(1, 13, 34, 44)*. Carpenter *et al.* *(13)* found the 11 symptoms in 58% of the schizophrenics, 22% of the manic psychotics, 14% of the depressive psychotics, and only 4% of the neurotics and persons with personality disorders. Furthermore, a recent study in Germany by Koehler and Steingerwald *(27)* still indicates a discrepancy in discriminating schizophrenia from manic–depressive psychosis and psychotic depression by Schneiderian symptoms. It is of interest to note that presence of formal signs of the thought disorder and its severity appear to show only a weak, if positive, relationship to outcome *(12)*. It should be noted, however, that the Kurt Schneider approach to diagnosis became the basis of the IPSE (International Present State Examination) and represents a unifying concept of schizophrenia, which, it is hoped, will bring forth general agreement regarding the clinical manifestation of this illness tested in the International Pilot Project organized under the auspices of the World Health Organization.

Since one of the thorniest problems is posed by whether or not the patient manifests true schizophrenia or a schizophrenia like illness, another formulation of schizophrenic symptomatology classifies symptoms into positive and negative categories. This approach was originated by Jackson *(23)* in an attempt to explain the neurological process underlying the disintegration of behavior and was extrapolated to psychiatry in combination with the original symptomatic clusters of Bleuler. Positive symptoms include such phenomena as delusions, hallucinations, and catatonic motor disturbances that have as a common denominator a flexibility in their manifestation *(45)*. Negative symptoms include blunting of affect, apathy, and blocking. Snezhnevsky characterizes these negative symptoms in terms of inflexibility *(45)*.

Inquiry into antecedents of the positive symptoms revealed that these symptoms may be caused by a variety of factors. In addition they seem to have rather clear-cut onset and resolution *(16, 37a)*. By contrast, negative symptoms are assumed to be caused by the chronicity of "primary disorder" as suggested by Bayard and Pascal's *(7a)* study showing a high correlation between chronicity of illness and presence of blunted affect. An alternative explanation of negative symptoms holds that they reflect a primary disorder which involves the disorganization of complex functions, a point of view supported by the work of Chapman *(16)* who found cognitive and perceptual abnormalities before the onset of delusions and hallucinations.

The permanence of the negative symptom cluster and the relative resolution of the positive symptoms led some investigators to use these classifications in determining prognosis in schizophrenia. In this respect Schneiderian first rank symptoms failed to provide a reliable prognostic guide, mainly because they include hallucinations and delusions which are positive signs and as such without predictive value unless associated with an affect disorder, like blunting of affect which does not belong among first symptoms. In the same vein, formal thought disorder and motor disorder, such as confusion and catatonic motor disorder, do not appear to have any significant predictive powers *(8, 52)*.

Another clinical approach to prediction was the division of schizophrenia into reactive and process types independent of diagnostic subtypes or symptoms. This distinction was based on the belief that there are groups of mental and personality symptoms that are essential in differentiating the acute reactive from the chronic course of illness. From the point of view of mental status, the symptoms indicating favorable prognosis have been delineated by Vaillant *(52)*, who duplicated Langfeldt's work. They are presence of confusion and disorientation as to person and time, clear symptoms of affective psychosis, overt depression, elation, and flight of ideas. Of interest, in this connection, is a study by Priest *et al.* which directly tested the hypothesis that acute schizophrenics are more likely to show affective symptomatology than their chronic counterparts (36). Using Personal Illness and Personal Disturbance scales of the Symptomatic Sign Inventory with 50 schizophrenic inpatients, these authors found that the scores of acutes reflect the presence of primafacie anxiety and depressive symptoms and that affective symptomatology, although present in both acute and chronic schizophrenic groups, predominates in the former. The studies by Stephens et al. (46, 47), examining 54 prognostic variables, corroborated Vaillant's findings that depressive features with ability to express guilt, confusion, and disorientation on admission are associated with recovery. On the other hand, in support of the Bleulerian hypothesis, Stephens et al. also found that emotional blunting is associated with a poor prognosis. Other researchers such as Sherman et al. (43), Pokorny and Faibish (35), and Gross and Huber (19) identified only low levels of psychological and social withdrawal in relation to successful outcome of schizophrenia.

However, a 22-year follow-up study yielded findings contradictory to these of Stephens et al. Huber et al. (22) found that of 502 schizophrenics, 22.1% showed complete psychopathological remission, 43.2% had noncharacteristic types of remission, and 34.7% suffered from characteristic deficiency syndromes. Higher education psychoreactive provocation, depressive traits, perception of delusions, catatonic agitation, and noncharacteristic thought disorders at the onset of schizophrenia were found to carry a favorable prognosis. Conversely, low intellectual level, abnormal primary personality, premorbid disturbances in communication behavior, longer prodromes, disturbances in egoexperience, bodily and acoustic hallucinations were associated, in this sample at least, with unfavorable outcome. Huber concluded that schizophrenia progresses to a certain degree of severity and having reached this plateau remains most often stationary. The existence of "reiner Defect," a noncharacteristic type of remission characterized by less mental energy which appears 12 to 49 years after onset, leads to some improvement in social adaption, which is then ascribed to remission. However, in such remissions residual syndromes are always present.

One of the problems in picking up the negative signs for prognostic purposes is the difficulty in differentiating them from florid symptomatology which often masks the fundamental thought defect in the acute phase of the illness. Yet, the subtle thought defect appears to be the true factor underlying the schizophrenic's inability to interpret reality, to function appropriately in social settings, and to adapt to the demands of daily living (10, 21). In this context, it is not surprising that the researchers who have attempted to identify mental symptoms of true prognostic value have found it easier to identify clinically blunting of affect (46, 47) and withdrawal (43). These variables have already been classified by Bleuler (9) as the fundamental signs of schizophrenia.

If the findings to date reflect the true predictive status of signs and symptoms in schizophrenia, then the mental status of the schizophrenic patient at the time of his psychiatric admission, or at the time of his discharge, cannot predict the evolution of the illness in terms of chronicity. This has been clearly shown in a recent study of 132 schizophrenics evaluated 2 to 3 years postdischarge *(5)*. The authors found that overall psychopathology as measured by the Gurin Mental Status Index, the New Haven Schizophrenia Index, and the Psychiatric Evaluation Form appeared to be independent of such predictive items as age of onset, precipitating factors, and presence of confusion and depression during the index episode. Only when the patient must adjust to community expectations does his behavior reveal the underlying deficit in his thinking. In fact, the behavioral deficit of the patient has started before his acute symptomology as fully discussed in the genetic chapters. It may be added here that subtle signs like shyness, low I.Q., and a high incidence of antisocial behavior in early childhood are sometimes the only clues to the impending schizophrenic process.

After hospitalization, the level of his adjustment reflects realistically his psychological deficit. The patients reaction to problem solving situations indicates his ability to judge, interpret, and solve each situation in his daily existence. This means that any encounter in daily living has a different potential for evoking stress, depending on the patient's level of perception of reality. Viewed in these terms, the patient's adjustment represents an interaction between three factors: his current mental condition, his level of psychosocial functioning, and his tolerance of stress.

In light of these assumptions, a study was undertaken to determine the contribution of functioning, stress, and mental status to the ability of the schizophrenic to maintain or not community tenure. These three factors have been evaluated individually and in combination to provide a clearer picture of their significance for community tenure.

The study was conducted on the original sample of 125 acute (first hospitalization) and 516 chronic (multiple hospitalization) schizophrenics. The Mental Status Evaluation was based on a modified version of the Problem Appraisal Scale (PAS). Assessment of functioning and stress was made by means of the Social Stress and Functionability Inventory for Psychotic Disorders. Details of these measurements have already been described in Chapter II. For the purpose of this study, the items of the modified version of the Problem Appraisal Scale were grouped into 19 categories which represented three subdivisions of psychological dimensions: (1) mental status proper including anxiety symptoms, depression, somatic concerns, persecutory ideation, secondary thought disorder (i.e., delusions, hallucinations and obsessions), primary thought disorder (i.e., disorientation) incoherence, affect disorder, inappropriate behavior, and lack of insight into one's mental condition; (2) Social and interpersonal adjustment including physical and sexual problems, difficulties with family and others, unemployment, and alcohol and drug abuse; and (3) Duration and severity of illness and major contributing stress.

The data were analyzed in two ways. First the procedure consisted of establishing the degree of relationship between the mental status variables and readmission to the hospital within a 2-year observation period. To obtain this information point-biserial correlations were computed to determine which mental status variables were significantly associated with readmission. Second, the data were analyzed to determine the interaction between the mental status variables and the variables of experienced stress and psychosocial functioning. It was believed that the most accurate prediction of readmission would be represented in an equation encompassing these three variables based on multiple correlations. For the purposes of these analyses, the subjects were divided into four subgroups: acute readmitted, acute nonreadmitted, chronic readmitted and chronic nonreadmitted.

Prior to the data analyses specified above, it was deemed important to compare acute and chronic schizophrenics, irrespective of their outcome status, on the significant areas of mental status and supporting social interpersonal adjustment. The results are shown in Table 1. Examination of Table 1 reveals that acute and chronic schizophrenics in the present sample do not appear to differ significantly

Table 1

Comparison of Significant Areas of Mental Status and Social,
Interpersonal Adjustment for Acute and Chronic Schizophrenics

Group Items	Acute			Chronic			t	df
	Mean	St. Dev.	N	Mean	St. Dev.	N		
Anxiety symptoms	3.92	3.4131	124	4.48	3.4220	506	1.64	628
Depression	5.02	4.6256	124	4.59	4.0883	506	0.95	628
Somatic concerns	0.88	1.3727	124	0.81	1.2531	506	0.52	628
Persecutory ideation	6.10	4.2075	124	5.96	3.9710	506	0.34	628
Secondary thought disorder	3.22	2.9000	124	3.40	3.0430	506	0.61	628
Primary thought disorder	3.89	3.4565	124	4.02	3.3282	506	0.38	628
Affect disorder	4.10	2.9166	124	4.34	3.0428	506	0.81	628
Behavioral signs	2.53	1.7345	124	2.68	1.7814	506	0.86	628
Lack of Insight	3.00	1.0992	96	2.96	1.1981	418	0.32	512
Sexual problems	3.81	2.6833	124	4.47	2.7416	506	2.44*	628
Interpersonal adjustment	4.02	3.4043	124	5.03	3.7774	506	2.90†	628
Social adjustment	3.79	2.7734	124	4.32	2.7066	506	1.89†	628
Drugs or alcohol	1.95	2.2236	124	2.44	2.6643	506	2.11*	628
Duration of illness	2.20	1.3852	124	4.51	.8392	506	17.77†	628
Severity of illness	2.39	.7694	124	2.53	.6445	506	1.87*	628
Major or contributory cause	3.39	1.6263	88	3.63	.9567	418	1.34	504

*$p < 0.05$.
†$p < 0.01$.

on anxiety symptoms ($t = 1.64$, $p > 0.05$), depressive symptomatology ($t = 0.95$, $p > 0.05$), somatic concerns ($t = 0.52$, $p > 0.05$), persecutory ideation ($t = 0.34$, $p > 0.05$), secondary thought disorder (hallucinations, delusions, and obsessions) ($t = 0.61$, $p > 0.05$), primary thought disorder (disorientation, incoherence) ($t = 0.38$, $p > 0.05$), affect disorder ($t = 0.81$, $p > 0.05$), behavioral signs of inappropriateness ($t = 0.86$, $p > 0.05$) or insight into illness ($t = 0.32$, $p > 0.05$). The chronics were, however, judged to be more severely ill than their acute counterparts ($t = 1.87$, $p < 0.05$). On problems supporting the mental status, significant differences between the two groups were found in the areas of sexual ($t = 2.44$, $p < 0.05$), interpersonal ($t = 2.90$, $p < 0.01$), and social adjustment ($t = 2.11$, $p < 0.05$), and of course duration of illness ($t = 17.77$, $p < 0.01$). In each of these comparisons chronics obtained significantly higher scores than their acute counterparts.

The relationship between the 19 mental status variables and readmission status was ascertained by means of point-biserial correlations computed separately for acute and chronic patients. Five categories of the PAS were found to be significantly correlated with readmission of the chronic schizophrenic patient. These were affect disorder ($r = -108$, $p < 0.05$), interpersonal adjustment ($r = -0.112$, $p < 0.05$), social adjustment ($r = -0.198$, $p < 0.001$), drug or alcohol abuse ($r = -0.134$, $p < 0.05$), and severity of illness ($r = -0.115$, $p < 0.05$). Although these correlations are significantly different from zero, they are of low magnitude; the highest of the obtained correlations (0.198) accounts for only 3.9% of the variance. The results obtained for the acute group of patients (n = 70) showed the same trend. Of the 19 mental status categories considered, only one, duration of illness, showed a significant ($r = 0.309$, $p < 0.01$) association with readmission status.

In order to determine the contribution of the variables of mental status, stress and psychosocial functioning in prediction of short term readmission, an intercorrelation matrix was set up for these four variables and a regression analysis performed with stress (mean D stress score), functioning (mean D functioning scored), and mental status (means of the items referring to mental status proper) regressed on the readmission status variable. The obtained intercorrelations showed that total stress score did not correlate significantly with any of the other three variables. Total functioning score was found to correlate significantly with mental status ($r = 0.254$, $p < 0.001$) and readmission ($r = -0.129$, $p < 0.05$) for the chronic patients and with mental status only ($r = 0.380$, $p < 0.01$) for the acute schizophrenic subjects. Mental status alone was found to correlate significantly with readmission ($r = -0.107$, $p < 0.05$) only for the chronic group. The regression analyses showed that the combination of functioning and mental status improved the prediction of readmission, resulting in a higher coefficient than when either of these variables were taken alone (for chronics $r = 0.149$, $p < 0.05$). No such findings were found to hold for the acute sample. It should be remembered, however, that although the variable of total mental status correlated significantly with readmission in the chronic group, the correlation coefficient was low, and in fact accounted for only 1 percent of the variance. Total mental status score appeared to be unrelated to readmission in the acute patients. The variable of stress appeared to have no utility in predicting readmission for either the chronic or the acute group.

It, thus, appears that the dimension of patient psychosocial functioning seems to be the most useful variable for predicting short term readmission, since of all the variables taken singularly, total functioning scores showed the highest correlation with rehospitalization. At the same time, the study throws considerable doubt on the value of mental status as a predictor of readmission for schizophrenic patients. This appears to be so despite some evidence that the presence of affective symptoms may serve as a sign of positive outcome (in terms of readmission) among chronic schizophrenics, except when combined with blunting of affect (7, 26). It should be noted, however, that although the correlation between the presence of affective reaction and readmission was statistically significant for this group, it accounted for only 1% of the variance.

The findings regarding the predictive value of mental status for acute schizophrenic patients corroborate the findings obtained for the chronic subjects, since only duration of illness showed a significant correlation with readmission status in the acute group.

In general then, the present findings fail to support the contentions of Vaillant (52) and Stephens (47) who assumed, on the basis of their investigations, that mental status is useful in predicting outcome in schizophrenia. It should be noted, however, that these investigators found only moderate correlations between the mental status variables of confusion and depression and outcome status. None of the mental status variables accounted for more than 28% of the variance in those studies. In addition, important flaws in the methodology used by these authors may have affected the obtained results. Vaillant (52), for example, used samples of patients who were evaluated retrospectively, and also employed first year residents as judges of mental status. Although his studies were based on both long and short-term periods of observation, no attempt was made to use first-hand information in the follow-ups. Instead the data came from indirect sources and questionable mental status reports.

The study of Stephens et al. on the other hand, used two groups of subjects differing widely from one another. One group consisted of severely psychotic patients hospitalized throughout the follow-up period; the other group consisted of alleged schizophrenics, supposedly recovered, who escaped hospitalization for the entire 5 year follow-up period. It is difficult to compare these groups in terms of diagnosis and severity of illness where mental status was assessed. Aside from these considerations, it should be noted that, according to Bleuler (9), confusion and depression, as mental status variables, are not primary signs of the schizophrenic syndrome. One may, therefore, contend that their presence in the schizophrenic sample throws considerable doubt on the appropriateness of the diagnosis.

The present study is by no means the only one indicating a minimal relationship between mental status variables and schizophrenic outcome. Cancro *(12)*, using various indicators of thought disorder in prediction of outcome obtained low level correlations accounting for only 16% of the total variance. Sherman *et al. (43)* reported no significant correlations between thought disorder variables and outcome. Of the variables used to predict recovery, only withdrawal symptoms produced significant results, accounting for 9% of the variance.

The controversy about the predictive value of mental symptoms at admission would be less puzzling if one considered that these variables reflect the patient's nonspecific mental response to his inability to cope with his environment. Within the confines of the hospital, the mental condition subsides to the previous levels. At discharge, on the other hand, the patient is assumed to function independently despite the presence of some residual psychological defect. It is, therefore, only when the schizophrenic patient reenters his environment and is, in due course, unable to tolerate the stresses of daily living, that he becomes gradually or suddenly mentally disorganized which could be considered as a nonspecific reaction to stress, leading to hospitalization. Since mental status and stress could not be objectified, only the individual's level of functioning remains as the salient indicator of the course of his integration in society. This notion has been fully explored in Chapter IV and supported by the study of Brown *et al.* ( ) who showed that even a more narrow range of functioning, restricted primarily to work impairment, is highly predictive of relapse.

The relationship between functioning, stress tolerance, and mental status variables, and outcome in schizophrenia is complex. The multiple factors do not necessarily have an additive effect. The complexity of prediction has been aptly illustrated in our study in the results of the multiple correlation where functioning and mental status were tested in relation to readmission of chronic schizophrenics. The individual correlations for functioning and mental status with readmission were 0.13 and 0.11, respectively. Simultaneous consideration of these two factors (functioning and mental status) tested by means of multiple correlations resulted in the multiple r of 0.15, a somewhat larger coefficient than that produced by considering each of the factors individually. The low magnitude of this correlation does not preclude an assumption that readmission may well be a multidetermined event. Other factors not directly tested here may weight heavily in the outcome prediction equation, such as medication use and acceptance of the patient by the community *(5)*. It is also possible that some of the predictors identified in the present study are reliable only for short-term follow-up. This would be particularly true for the predictive variables established for the acute segment of the schizophrenic sample. This population, as mentioned, may contain individuals whose final and correct diagnosis of schizophrenia will emerge only in time. It must be remembered that, even with the most careful diagnostic procedures, one cannot always separate acute schizophrenic episode cases from those representing true schizophrenia.

REFERENCES

1. Abrams, R., and Taylor, M.: First-rank symptoms, severity of illness, and treatment response in schizophrenia. *Compr. Psychiat.* **14**, 353–355, 1973.
2. Angst, J.: "Zur Atiology und Nosologie Endogenor Depressiven Psychosen." Springer-Verlag, Berlin-Heidelberg, 1966.
3. Angyal, A.F.: Speed and pattern of perception in schizophrenic and normal persons. *Charac. Personal.* **11**, 108–127, 1942.
4. Arlow, J.A., and Brenner, C.: The psychopathology of the psychoses. A proposed revision. *Int. J. Psychoanal.* **50**, 5–14, 1969.
5. Astrachan, B.M., Brauer, L., Harrow, M., and Swartz, C.: Symptomatic outcome in schizophrenia. *Arch. Gener. Psychiat.* **31**, 155–160, 1974.
6. Astrup, C., Fossum, A., Holmboe, R.: "Prognosis in Functional Psychosis, Clinical, Social and Genetic Aspects." Charles C. Thomas Publisher, Springfield, Illinois, 1962.
7. Astrup, C., and Noreik, K.: "Functional Psychoses: Diagnostic and Prognostic Models." Charles C. Thomas, Springfield, Illinois, 1966.
7a. Bayard, J., and Pascal, G.: Studies of prognostic criteria in case records of hospitalized mental patients. J. Consult. Psychol. 18, 122–126, 1954.
8. Bellak, L.: "Dementia Praecox." Grune and Stratton, Inc., New York, 1948.
9. Bleuler, E.: "Dementia Praecox or the Group of Schizophrenias." International Universities Press, New York, 1950.
10. Broen, W.E., and Nakamura, C.Y.: Reduced range of sensory sensitivity in chronic non-paranoid schizophrenics *J. Abnorm. Psychol.* **79**, 106–111, 1972.
11. Cameron, N.: Reasoning, regression and communication in schizophrenics. *Psychol. Monogr.* 50, No. 1 Whole No. 221, pp. 1–34, 1938.
12. Cancro, R.: Clinical prediction of outcome in schizophrenia. *Compr. Psychiat.* **10**, 349–354, 1969.
13. Carpenter, W.T., Strauss, J.S., and Muleh, S.: Are there pathognomic symptoms in schizophrenia? An empirical investigation of Schneider's first-rank symptoms. *Arch. Gener. Psychiat.* **28**, 847–852, 1973.
14. Carpenter, W.T., and Strauss, J.S.: Cross-cultural evaluation of Schneider's first-rank symptoms of schizophrenia. A report from the International Pilot Study of Schizophrenia. *Am. J. Psychiat.* **131**, 682–687, 1974.
15. Carpenter, W.T., Strauss, J., and Bartko, J.J.: Part I. Use of signs and symptoms for the identification of schizophrenic patients. *Schizophrenia Bulletin,* Issue No. 11, Winter, 1974.
16. Chapman, J.: The early symptoms of schizophrenia. *Br. J. Psychiat.* **112**, 225–251, 1966.
17. Chapman, L.J., Burstein, A.J., Day, D., and Verdone, P.: Regression and disorders of thought. *J. Abnor. Soc. Psychol.* **63**, 540–545, 1961.
18. Goldstein, K.: Methodological approach to the study of schizophrenic thought disorder. *In* "Language and Thought in Schizophrenia" (J. S. Kasanin, ed.), W. W. Norton, New York, 1944.
19. Gross, G., and Huber, G.: Prognosis in schizophrenia. *Psychiat. Clinic.* **6**, 1–16, 1973.
20. Gurland, B.J., Fleiss, J.L., Cooper, J.E., Sharpe, L., Hendall, R.E., and Roberts, P.: Cross national study of diagnosis of mental disorders: Hospital diagnoses and hospital patients in New York and London. *Compr. Psychiat.* **11**, 18–25, 1970.

21. Harrow, M., Harkavy, K., Bromet, E. and Tucker, G.J.: A Longitudinal Study of Schizo-phrenic Thinking. *Arch. Gen. Psychiat.* **28**, 179–182, 1973.
22. Huber, G., Gross, G., and Schuttler, R.: A long-term follow-up study of schizophrenia: Psychiatric course of illness and prognosis. *Acta Psychiat. Scandinavica* **52**, 49–57, 1975.
23. Jackson, H.: Remarks on evolution and dissolution of the nervous system. *J. Ment. Sci.* **33**, 25–48, 1887.
24. Jansson, B.: The prognostic significance of various types of hallucinations in young people. *Acta Psychiat. Scandinavica* **44**, 401–409, 1968.
25. Jaspers, K.: "General Psychopathology." University of Chicago Press, Chicago, 1963.
26. Kind, H.: Prognosis. *In* "The Schizophrenic Syndrome." (L. Bellak and L. Loeb, eds.), Grune and Stratton, Inc., New York, pp. 714–734, 1969.
27. Koehler, K.G., and Steingerwald, F.: Consistency of Kurt Schneider-oriented Diagnosis over 40 years. *Arch. Gener. Psychiat.* **34**, 51–55, 1977.
28. Kraeplin, E.: "Dementia Praecox and Paraphrenia." Livingstone, Edinburg, 1919.
29. Lane, E.A., and Albee, G.: Intellectual antecedents of schizophrenia. *In* "Life History Research in Psychopathology" (M. Roff and D. F. Ricks, eds.), Vol. I. pp. 189–207. University of Minn. Press, Minneapolis, 1970.
30. Langfeldt, G.: The prognosis in schizophrenia and the factors influencing the course of the disease. Monograph: Humphrey Melford, London, 1937.
31. Langfeldt, G.: Schizophrenia, diagnosis and prognosis. *Behav. Sci.* **14**, 173–182, 1969.
32. Marchbanks, G., and Williams, M.: The effect of speed on comprehension in schizophrenia. *Br. J. Soc. Clinic. Psychol.* **10**, 55–60, 1971.
33. Meehl, P.E.: *Schizotaxia, Schizotypy, Schizophrenia.* Paper presented at the 70th Annual Convention of the American Psychological Association, St. Louis, Mo., September, 1962.
34. Mellor, C.S.: First-rank symptoms of schizophrenia. I. The frequency in schizophrenics on admission to hospital; II. Differences between individual first-rank symptoms. *Br. J. Psychiat.* **117**, 15–23, 1970.
35. Pokorny, A.D., and Faibish, G.M.: Criteria of outcome in schizophrenia. *Hosp. Commun. Psychiat.* **(November)**, 341–347, 1968.
36. Priest, R.G., Shariatmadari, M.E., and Tarighati, S.H.: Affective states in schizophrenia. *Br. J. Soc. Clin. Psychol.* **12**, 283–288, 1973.
37. Reed, J.L.: Schizophrenic thought disorder: a review and hypothesis. *In* "The Annual Review of the Schizophrenic Syndrome" (Robert Cancro, ed.), Vol. 2, pp. 135–171. Brunner-Mazel, New York, 1972.
37a. Fromm-Reichman, F.: Notes on the development of treatment of schizophrenics by psychoanalytic psychotherapy. *Psychiatry* **11**, 263–273, 1948.
38. Schneider, C.: "Die Psychologie der Schizophrenen" Thieme, Leipzig, 1930.
39. Schneider, K.: "Clinical Psychopathology." (5th Ed.). Grune and Stratton, New York, 1959.
40. Schooler, N., Goldberg, S., Bocthe, H., and Cole, J.: One year after discharge: Community adjustment of schizophrenic patients. *Am. J. Psychiat.* **123**, 986–995, 1967.
41. Shakow, D.: Segmental set: a theory of the formal psychological deficit in schizophrenia. *Arch. Gen. Psychiat.* **6**, 1–17, 1962.
42. Shakow, D.: Psychological deficit in schizophrenia. *Behav. Sci.* **8**, 275–305, 1963.
43. Sherman, L.J., Moseley, E.C., Ging, R., and Bookbinder, L.J.: Prognosis in schizophrenia. *Arch. Gen. Psychiat.* **119**, 945–951, 1964.
44. Skoda, C.: On differential diagnostic value of Kurt Schneider's First Rank Symptoms. Paper presented to the Scientific Work Session of the Psychiatric Society of Czechoslovakian Medical Society, Prague, Czechoslovakia, March, 1973.
45. Snezhnevsky, A.V.: The symptomatology, clinical forms and nosology of schizophrenia. *In* "Modern Perspectives in World Psychiatry." (J. G. Howells, ed.), pp. 425–477. Oliver and Boyd Ltd., Edinburgh, 1968.

46. Stephens, J.H., and Astrup, C. Prognosis in "process" and "nonprocess" schizophrenia. *Am. J. Psychiat.* **119**, 945–951, 1963.
47. Stephens, J.H., Astrup, C., and Mangrum, J.C.: Prognostic factors in recovered and deteriorated schizophrenics. *Am. J. Psychiat.* **122**, 1116–1121, 1966.
48. Strauss, J.S., and Carpenter, W.T.: The prediction of outcome in schizophrenia. I. Characteristics of outcome. *Arch. Gener. Psychiat.* **27**, 739–746, 1972.
49. Strauss, J.S., and Carpenter, W.T.: Prediction of outcome in schizophrenia. II. Relationship between prediction and outcome variables. *Arch. Gener. Psychiat.* **31**, 37–42, 1974.
50. Strauss, J.S., Carpenter, T., and Bartko, J.J.: Part III. Speculation on the processes that underlie schizophrenic symptoms and signs. *Schizophrenia Bulletin,* (Winter) issue No. 11, 61–69, 1974.
51. Swartz, C.C., Myers, J.K., and Astrachan, B.M.: Concordance of multiple assessments of the outcome of schizophrenia. *Arch. Gener. Psychiat.* **32**, 1221–1227, 1975.
52. Vaillant, G.E.: Prospective prediction of schizophrenic remission. *Arch. Gener. Psychiat.* **11**, 509–517, 1964.
53. Vigotsky, L.S.: Thought in schizophrenia. *Arch. Neurol. Psychiat.* **31**, 1063–1077, 1943.
54. Whitbeck, C., and Tucker, G.J.: Thought disorder: Implications of a new paradigm. Unpublished manuscript, 1972.

Part II*

If the signs and symptoms of mental-status evaluation of schizophrenia at admission or discharge appear to have minimal prediction power for the course of the illness, then it will be of interest to determine their value in terms of the patient's adjustment to the community.

The first question that arises concerns the severity of psychological impairment of the schizophrenic discharged into the community. In this respect, Astrachan, Harrow et al. found that post-discharge schizophrenics, followed up for three years, continued to have mental symptoms despite treatment given in the community (4). Although these data support the findings of Huber (12) previously mentioned, they do not provide any decisive evidence for the diagnosis of schizophrenia, particularly since thinking disorder is not specific to schizophrenia (11). This means that for the alleged schizophrenics discharged into the community, it still remains to establish diagnostic criteria that would be valid in identifying them as schizophrenics.

To what extent are the mental signs and symptoms, when used alone, able to discriminate the schizophrenics and the non-schizophrenics in the community? The issue becomes more complex when we consider that after the acute symptomatology has subsided, a significant number of schizophrenics suffer from depression for a period estimated from three to 16 months as demonstrated by McGlashan and Carpenter (14), Roth (18), and Kayton (13). Furthermore, the conditions of living in the community, with its demands, place new stress upon schizophrenic ex-patients that produces high levels of anxiety and additional depression.

Taking into account these facts, it is reasonable to assume that the adjustment of schizophrenic patients in the community would be decided by the interaction of their residual thought disorder with their circumstances of living. Basically, the patient's perception of reality, with its distortions, will decide his response in meeting the societal demands in an adaptive or maladaptive manner, resulting in either the maintenance of mental and social functioning or its disintegration. Since the residual mental deficit plays an important role in the patient's community integration, it would be meaningful to find out whether the diagnostic subclassifications play an additional part in it. In this respect, present research indicates that paranoids have a more favorable prognosis than other schizophrenics, due to their more integrated ego functioning (21). In the same context, episodic schizoaffectives have a more favorable prognosis than all other types, as supported by various research Angst (3), Astrup (5), Hay and Forrest (10).

---

*The research results presented in Part II have appeared in the following articles: G. Serban, and C.B. Gidynski: Relationship Between Cognitive Defect, Affect Response, and Community Adjustment in Chronic Schizophrenics. *Brit. J Psychiat.*, June, 1979 and G. Serban: Mental Status, Functioning, and Stress in Chronic Schizophrenic Patients in Community Care. *Amer. J. Psychiat.*, **136, 7**, 948–952, 1979.

For clarifying the issue about the contribution of mental status of patients to the adjustment of the schizophrenics in the community, a second study was undertaken in NYU-Bellevue Medical Center. This focused on: (1) the significance of Schneider's First Rank Symptoms in the diagnosis of ambulatory schizophrenics; (2) the interaction between various signs and symptoms of mental status and the level of functioning and experienced stress in schizophrenics living in the community; (3) the relationship between the diagnostic subclassifications and the degree of functioning and stress of the patient; and (4) the prognostic value of specific cognitive, affective, and behavioral impairments for schizophrenics' community adjustment.

One hundred outpatient chronic schizophrenics of both sexes, representing consecutive volunteers who had been receiving aftercare treatment at Bellevue Outpatient Department and Fountain House, for a minimum of one year prior to participation in this study, served as subjects. Eighty-seven of the subjects had an average of 3.94 hospital admissions within the last ten years, while the average amount of hospitalization was 8.61 months for each subject. Eight of the subjects had been treated only as outpatients for approximately five years.

All patients were diagnosed as schizophrenic in the treatment facilities in accordance with DSM II criteria (APA, 1968) (2). The diagnosis was reconfirmed independently by the project psychiatrist by means of the Psychiatric Assessment Interview (PAI); Carpenter (7), and Schneider's First Rank Symptoms (20). In addition, the Feighner et al. (8) criteria for chronic schizophrenia were used as guidelines. Alcoholics, drug addicts, and the mentally retarded with a secondary diagnosis of schizophrenia were eliminated from the sample.

Of the 100 schizophrenic subjects, 50 were diagnosed as undifferentiated, 26 paranoid, 22 schizoaffective, and two latent. The average age of the subjects was 38.66 years; mean educational level was 11.31 years. Fifty-one were male and 49 female; 67 were white, 23 black, and ten Puerto Rican. In terms of marital status, 59 were single, 34 separated or divorced, eight married, and nine widowed. In terms of original occupation, 44 were blue-collar workers, 21 white-collar employees, ten had semi-professional and administrative occupations, 18 were housewives or students, and seven had no known occupation. At the time of the study, 69 of the subjects were on welfare assistance, four were never employed, four were housewives, and four were students on family support. Three of the subjects were employed full-time, 12 in part-time supplemental work, and four held regular part-time employment. All subjects were treated with major tranquilizers while participating in the study.

The mental status of the patients was evaluated by means of the Psychiatric Assessment Interview (PAI) derived from the eighth edition of the Present State Examination (PSE) (WHO, 1973) by Strauss and Carpenter (7). This structured interview consists of three scales: (1) Signs and symptoms based on 117 questions covering 39 symptom areas: concentration, somatic symptoms, variation in feeling, sleep, irritability, social withdrawal, sexual feelings, slowed functioning, indecisiveness, depressive mood, suicidal tendencies, self-mutilation, tension, subjective and autonomic anxiety, situational anxiety and phobic avoidance, dangerous behavior, elated mood and hyperactivity, obsessional and compulsive symptoms, derealization, depersonalization, auditory, visual, tactile, gustatory, olfactory and somatic aberrations, experiences of thought control, thought dissemination, ideas of control of behavior or will, ideas of reference, of persecution and of self-depreciation, nihilistic ideas, ideas of grandeur, religious, fantastic and sexual ideas, insight and memory; (2) Psychiatrist's evaluation of aberrant perceptual and bizarre ideational experiences of the patient; and (3) Ratings based on 83 items of behavior observed during the interview period. These cover the patient's personal appearance; retardation of motor activity; agitation or excitement; bizarre behavior; behavioral expression of affect; abnormalities in pitch and modulation of voice; and quantity of speech, non-social speech, and idiosyncracies of speech. A fourth scale, developed for the purpose of this research, was total mental status which represented average rating across the three sections of the instrument described above. The PAI evaluations cover a one-month period.

Each item of the PAI was scored 1.0 when the manifestation was absent, 1.5 when questionably present, 2.0 when present but not severe, and 3.0 if present and continuously severe.

The patients' current community adjustment was assessed by the SSFIPD. The raw ratings obtained for the two instruments were converted into mean scores (by adding the item values for each subtest of each instrument and dividing them by the number of items actually rated). The mean scores were then used in all subsequent statistical analyses. The PAI yielded four scores: signs and symptoms score; psychiatrist evaluation of perceptual and ideational aberrations; observed behavior; and total mental status score based on average ratings across the three sections of the instrument. Two scores were derived from the SSFIPD: total social functioning score, representing a mean score based on ratings obtained on 21 dimensions of psychosocial functioning; and total stress score, also representing a mean score of ratings obtained on 21 stress dimensions.

RESULTS

The data indicated that Schneiderian First Rank Symptoms (FRS) were present in 66% of the sample of schizophrenics. In 34 cases, FRS were not present, although in 32 of these we found thought disorder identified as idiosyncratic speech. The scores for FRS derived from the PAI range from 1 to 3 points. In our sample, the scores ranged from 1.00 to 2.02 points. Using a cut-off point at three successive (33%) points in the distribution, we found 32 cases to have high FRS scores, 33 moderate FRS scores, and 34 low FRS scores.

In order to determine whether presence of FRSs is associated with the diagnostic subclassification of schizophrenia, we divided the FRS scores at the median into high and low scores and tested the arrays in three diagnostic subclassifications (undifferentiated, paranoid, and schizoaffective). The chi-square test failed to differentiate the groups ($X^2 = < 1$, df 2, p > .05).

To answer the second question posed, we attempted to define the relationship between mental status variables and the various adjustment indicators. Pearson's Correlation Coefficients were computed as shown in Table 1. Examination of Table 1 reveals that self-reported mental status correlated significantly with all

Table 1

Correlations of PAI Mental Status Scores with the SSIAM
and the SSFIPD Adjustment Scores

SSFIPD	Mental status (Reported)	Psychiatrist's evaluation	Observed behavior	Total score
Total functioning	−.425**	−.293†	−.130	−.417**
Total stress	−.476**	−.244*	.021	−.407**

*p < .05
†p < .01
**p < .001

adjustment measures. The SSFIPD measure of functioning correlated −.425 (p < .001) with current signs and symptoms. This negative correlation is due to the fact that mental status and functioning are in inverse relationship in indicating pathology. This is also true for the correlation between stress and mental status. The SSFIPD total stress score correlated −.476 (p < .001) with mental status. These findings indicate that the presence of symptomatology interferes significantly with the community adjustment of schizophrenics in the areas of both functioning and stress.

Based on these findings, we have attempted to identify the particular areas of the 21 categories of functioning and stress that are significantly correlated with the mental status of the patient. Tables 2 and 3 give a detailed presentation of this relationship. A brief examination of the tables shows that the interaction among the components of functioning, those of stress and self-reported mental status follow the same trend with regard to mental status.

The relationship between the psychiatrist's evaluation of the patients' perceptual and ideational aberration, and the various indices of adjustment is less impressive. Both functioning and stress scores derived from the SSFIPD correlated significantly with the psychiatrist's ratings (r = −.293, p < .01 for functioning and r = .244, p < .05 for stress). The results indicate that the

Table 2
Correlations Between Functioning Dimensions of SSFIPD and Mental Status of PAI

Functioning dimension	Mental status (reported)	Mental status (Total score)
Education	−.264†	−.278†
Job	−.166	−.211*
Housekeeping	−.328†	−.274*
Welfare	.072	.036
Finances	−.301†	−.305†
Living circumstances	−.106	−.030
Parents	−.243*	−.209*
Relatives	.146	.093
Marriage	−.508**	−.398*
Children	.208	.168
Dating	−.325†	−.277†
Sex	−.177	−.144
Social life/Friends	−.288†	−.263†
Neighbors	−.062	−.070
Other people	−.386**	−.387**
Religion	−.017	−.034
Drinking	−.033	−.050
Addictive drugs	−.042	−.028
Psychedelic drugs	.002	.039
Antisocial behavior	−.197*	−.219*

*$p < .05$
†$p < .01$
**$p < .001$

psychiatrist's evaluation, although significant, contributes modestly to the projection of existent impaired functioning and increased levels of experienced stress of the patient.

However, the total mental status score, encompassing signs and symptoms sections, the psychiatrist's ratings, and the observed behavior, correlated significantly with all measures. (See Table 1). The total functioning score of the SSFIPD ($r = -.417$, $p < .001$), the SSFIPD total stress score ($r = .407$, $p < .001$) were highly correlated with mental status.

To determine the predictive contribution of the specific signs and symptoms to the schizophrenic's level of functioning and experienced stress, stepwise regression analyses were performed using the following mental-status-symptom clusters as independent variables: depression, anxiety, derealization, delusions, auditory/visual hallucinations, other hallucinations, insight, mania, somatic symptoms, ideas of reference, memory, thought control, and behavior observed in the interview. Total functioning and stress scores derived form the SSFIPD were used as dependent variables. Results of the analyses are shown in Tables 4 and 5.

Table 3

Correlations Between Stress Dimensions of SSFIPD and Mental Status of PAI

Stress dimension	Mental status (reported)	Mental status (Total score)
Education	−.380**	−.272†
Job	.011	.051
Housekeepiing	−.560**	−.435**
Welfare	−.168	−.144
Finances	−.116	−.099
Living circumstances	−.222*	−.174
Parents	−.219	−.241*
Relatives	−.137	−.126
Marriage	−.033	.046
Children	−.313	−.372
Dating	−.294†	−.218*
Sex	−.237*	−.192
Social life/Friends	−.283†	−.215*
Neighbors	−.235*	−.210*
Other people	−.466**	−.372**
Religion	−.083	−.082
Drinking	−.011	−.174
Addictive drugs	.0	.0
Psychedelic drugs	−.013	.109
Antisocial behavior	.225	.251

*$p < .05$
†$p < .01$
**$p < .001$

Examination of Table 4 reveals that anxiety seems to be the most significant predictor of experienced stress, accounting for 35.7% of the total variance. Addition of somatic symptoms variable to the prediction equation resulted in an increase of 3.3% to the variance. Other signs and symptoms including; ideas of reference, auditory and visual hallucinations, other hallucinations, and derealization together account for 1.5% of the additional variance, with the remaining mental status variables contributing less that 1% to the prediction equation. All 13 clusters of signs and symptoms accounted for 40.8% of the total stress variance.

With regard to prediction of total functioning (See Table 5), depression has the most significant position, accounting for 17.1% of the total variance. The addition of observed behavior variables and anxiety explained 25.1% of the variance. The symptoms of derealization and delusions also appear to influence functioning, but to a lesser degree. Lack of insight, manic symptoms, and auditory and visual hallucinations make a minimal contribution to the prediction of functioning (less than 2% of the variance). All 13 clusters of signs and symptoms account for 30% of the total functioning variance, which is well within acceptable levels.

Table 4
Stepwise Regression Statistics for Predicting Total Stress*

Variable	Multiple R	Multiple R²	Increases in R²
Anxiety (A)	.597†	.357	
Somatic symptoms (SS) + (A)	.624†	.390	.033
Ideas of reference (IR) + (SS) + (A)	.629†	.395	.005
Auditory/Visual hallucinations (AVH) + (IR) + (SS) + (A)	.633†	.401	.006
Other hallucinations (OH) + (AVH) + (IR) + (SS) + (A)	.635†	.403	.002
Derealization (D) + (OH) + (AVH) + (IR) + (SS) + (A)	.636†	.405	.002

*$N = 100$
†$p < .001$

Table 5
Stepwise Regression Statistics for Predicting Total Functioning*

Variable	Multiple R	Multiple R²	Increases in R²
Depression (D)	.413†	.171	
Behavior (B) + (D)	.470†	.221	.050
Anxiety (A) + (B) + (D)	.501†	.251	.030
Derealization (DE) + (A) + (B) + (D)	.514†	.264	.013
Delusions (DS) + (DE) + (A) + (B) + (D)	.524†	.275	.011
Insight (I) + (DS) + (DE) + (A) + (B) + (D)	.533†	.284	.009
Mania (M) + (I) + (DS) + (DE) + (A) + (B) + (D)	.539†	.290	.006
Auditory/Visual hallucinations (AVH) + (M) + (I) + (DS) + (DE) + (A) + (B) + (D)	.543†	.295	.005

*$N = 100$
†$p < .001$

DISCUSSION

The strict diagnosis criteria used in the sample, based on Schneiderian First Rank Symptoms (FRS), indicate that 66% of the subjects previously diagnosed as schizophrenic continue to present FRS during community tenure, as indicated by Schneider's formulation, while 24% appear to be free of gross perceptual or ideational aberrations. However, only two cases of the 24 who did not manifest FRS were also free of idiosyncratic speech, defined as thought disorder by C. Schneider (19) and Fish (9). It is interesting that patients living in the community for at least one year continue to manifest ideational and perceptual disturbance of various degrees and that 33% of these had high scores on the FRS variable. These findings suggest the association of FRS with chronic schizophrenia, as indicated by Robins and Guzze (17) who found a correlation between FRS and poor prognostic signs. Other investigators were unable to validate these findings (1); Mellor found in his sample that schizophrenics without FRS had been ill for a long time, presupposing a more unfavorable course (16).

The second part of the results powerfully document the close relationship between the mental status of the patient and his ability to function socially. Mental status correlated strongly with functioning, stress, and total adjustment.

Total adjustment, as expected, correlated with total mental-status score, derived from the PAI. Furthermore, total adjustment differentiated diagnostic subclassifications of schizophrenia (undifferentiated, schizoaffective, and paranoid) while Schneider's FRS failed to discriminate them, indicating a similar distribution of FRS scores in all three subclassifications. Noteworthy, chronic paranoid schizophrenics, who are considered by some (Zigler and Levine, 1973) to have a higher level of cognitive development than other types of schizophrenics, in our sample, responded more poorly to stress and appeared less well adjusted than the schizoaffectives.

The analysis of the interaction between mental status and various dimensions of functioning and stress showed an interesting pattern. The nine areas of psychosocial functioning are those in which the patient still attempts to reorganize his life. The areas of non-interaction are either those in which the patient is inactive, such as job, or isolated, as from his relatives or children. Other dimensions are unaffected, such as welfare and religion. Drinking does not correlate because of the biased sample due to the elimination of schizophrenic-alcoholics. A similar pattern of interaction is present between the dimensions of stress and mental status, with the exception of three areas: living circumstances, sex, and relationship with neighbors. In these areas of living, regardless of the level of functioning, due to the difficulty in the interpersonal relationship, the subject experiences stress related to his mental status.

The significant association found between mental status and social adjustment led us to further investigate the unique contribution of the various components of mental status to the patient's psychosocial functioning. Depression appeared to be the most potent predictive variable for functioning. This finding suggests that schizophrenics in the community tend to be depressed, and not, as classically assumed, indifferent to their social condition. Their depression seems to differ somewhat from depression identified in the literature as post-psychotic depression by McGlashan, and Carpenter (15), since they were less characterized by feelings of emptiness and disinterest in doing things, and more by a sense of helplessness and a bleak future outlook.

Other mental status aspects, such as observed behavior, contribute much less to the prediction of functioning, due to the fact that the patient appears to be less aware that his inappropriate behavior influences his social performance. This poor insight is further demonstrated by the low predictive value of other symptoms and signs such as derealization, delusions, insight, and hallucinations.

This suggests that the patient is incapable of making an association between these symptoms and his difficulty in functioning.

As regards the mental status signs and symptoms predicting stress, anxiety leads, by far, all other mental status predictors. This suggests that the subjectively experienced stress incurred in the patients' daily activities finds its counterpart in anxiety signs and symptoms of the mental status. Although the association between stress and anxiety has been frequently noted and taken for granted in explaining and/or defining stress, it was not demonstrated through a correlational analysis, due to the lack of a direct measurement of clinical stress. Anxiety, although basically responsible for disrupting behavior and poor functioning, is experienced by the patient as stress, since he experiences it in the process of appraisal of a situation with which he thinks he cannot cope. This means that the patient will experience anxiety in response to coping with daily events of his life, and depression, when he sees the results as unsatisfactory.

The second variable of mental status predicting stress is that of ''somatic symptoms'' which have always been related to stressful situations of internalization of anxiety.

Other clusters of mental signs, perceptual and ideational aberrations, appear to be much less adequate in explaining the stress variance due to the same low level of insight manifested by the patients.

The contribution of these findings to the understanding of the adjustment of the schizophrenic in the community cannot be denied. The close interaction between his mental status, his functioning and stress appears to represent the key factor responsible for his level of integration into the main stream of community life.

Closely interacting with the mental state of the schizophrenic, affecting his functioning and reaction to stress, is the psychological dimension of motivation.

REFERENCES

1. Abrams, R., and Taylor, M.: First Rank Symptoms, severity of illness, and treatment response in schizophrenia. *Comprehen. Psychiat.* **14**, 353–355, 1973.
2. American Psychiatric Association: *Diagnostic and Statistical Manual of Mental Disorders.* 3rd Ed., DSM II. Washington, D.C.: American Psychiatric Association, 1968.
3. Angst, J.: *Zur Atiologie und Nosologie Endogener Depressiven Psychosen.* Berlin-Heidelberg: Springer-Verlag, 1966.
4. Astrachan, B.M., Brauer, L., Harrow, M., and Swartz, C.: Syptomatic outcome in schizophrenia. *Arch. Gen. Psychiat.* **31**, 155–160, 1974.
5. Astrup, C., and Fossum, A. et al.: *Prognosis in Functional Psychosis.* Springfield, Ill.: Charles C. Thomas, 1962.
6. Carpenter, W.T., Strauss, J.S., and Bartko, J.J.: The diagnosis and understanding of schizophrenia. Part I. Use of signs and symptoms for the identifcation of schizophrenic patients. *Schizophren. Bull.*, Issue No. II, **Winter, 1974.**
7. Carpenter, W.T., Sacks, M.H., and Strauss, J.S. et al.: (1976) Evaluating signs and symptoms. Comparison of structured interview and clinical approaches. *Brit. J. Psychiat.*, **128**, 397–403, 1976.

8. Feighner, B.W., Robins, E., and Guze, S.B., et al: Diagnostic criteria for use in psychiatric research. *Arch. Gen. Psychiat.*, **26**, 57–63, 1972.
9. Fish, F.: *Schizophrenia*. John Wright, Bristol, 1962.
10. Hay, A.J., and Forrest, A.D.: The diagnosis of schizophrenia and paranoid psychosis; an attempt at clarification. *Brit. J. Med. Psychol.*, **45**, 233–341, 1972.
11. Harrow, M., and Quinlan, D.: Is disordered thinking unique to schizophrenia? *Arch. Gen. Psychiat.*, **34**, 15–21, 1977.
12. Huber, G., Gross, G., and Schuttler, R.: A long-term follow-up study of schizophrenia: Psychiatric course of illness and prognosis. *Acta Psychiatrica Scandinavica*, **52**, 49–57, 1975.
13. Kayton, L.: Good outcome in young adult schizophrenia. *Arch. Gen. Psychiat.*, **29**, 103–110, 1973.
14. McGlashan, T.H., and Carpenter, W.T.: Postpsychotic depression in schizophrenia. *Arch. Gen. Psychiat.*, **33**, 231–239, 1976a.
15. McGlashan, T.H., and Carpenter, W.T.: An investigation of the postpsychotic depressive syndrome. *Amer. J. Psychiat.* **133**, 14–18, 1976b.
16. Mellor, S.C.: First Rank Symptoms of schizophrenia. *Brit. J. Psychiat.*, **117**, 15–23, 1970.
17. Robins, E., and Guze, S.B.: Establishment of diagnostic validity in psychiatric illness: Its applications to schizophrenia. *Amer. J. Psychiat.*, **126**, 983–987, 1970.
18. Roth, S.: The seemingly ubiquitous depression following acute schizophrenic episodes, a neglected area of clinical discussion *Amer. J. Psychiat.*, **127**, 51–58, 1970.
19. Schneider, C.: *Die Schizophrenen Symptomverbande*. Berlin: Springer, 1942.
20. Schneider, K.: *Clinical Psychopathology*. Translated by M.W. Hamilton. New York: Grune & Stratton, Inc., 1959.
21. Zigler, E., and Levine, J.: Premorbid adjustment and paranoid-nonparanoid status in schizophrenia: a further investigation. *J. Abn. Psychol.*, **82**, 189–199, 1973.

CHAPTER 9

Motivation in Schizophrenics and Normals*

The integration of schizophrenics into the community presupposes the presence of a level of motivation on the part of the discharged patients that enables them to fulfill societal demands and/or their personal needs.

The schizophrenic appears to assess unrealistically his present abilities and future possibilities as an expression of his needs. Whereas the normal individual is able to project his future achievements from his present level of abilities, the mentally ill, particularly the schizophrenic because of his residual thinking and/or emotional defect, appears unable to do so. The normal motivational pattern suggests a continuum between past accomplishments and future goals, while clinical experience indicates that for the schizophrenic there is a breakdown in this linear or ascending motivational orientation which results in a gradual lowering of the patient's social competence.

Since schizophrenics suffer from a deficit in motivation, particularly lack of goal direction (11), their current motivational patterns have important implications for their future life organization. Keeping these considerations in mind, the main remaining problem is the measurement of motivation itself and the development of an instrument to measure the difference between the motivations of schizophrenics and normals and to indicate specific areas of discrepancy between them.

First, it is necessary to define the motivational concept underlying existing tests of motivation. In general, motives are conceived as "latent dispositions which strive for a particular goal–state or aim, e.g., achievement, affiliation, power'' (2). Expectancy is defined as the anticipation that the performance of an act is instrumental to the attainment of the goal associated with the motive (2).

Based on this general framework, motivation can be measured by tests based on self-report (6) or by objective evaluation of the individual's behavior in

---

*Statistical work done by Edward Melnick, Ph.D., Associate Prof. of Statistics, New York University. The results section of this chapter was written by Dr. Melnick.

particular situations. Some researchers *(10a, b)* believe, however, that both these methods are faulty, due to either spuriously high relative validity and reliability created by nonmotivational variables (e.g., acquiescence factors) or to their inability to tap the unconscious factors of motivation. As a result, they turned to indirect forms of measurement, such as the behavioral measure of motivation as organized fantasy using the TAT and the FTI. Yet these investigators encountered the same difficulties in terms of internal consistency, reliability, and validity of the test instrument when compared to performance criteria.

Furthermore, these difficulties became apparent when tests attempting to assess the achievement motives by self-report showed a low correlation with projective tests, indicating that they were not measuring the same aspects of motivation *(14)*.

Regardless of these shortcomings, researchers tend to agree that what should be stressed in the testing of motivation is the drive, direction, and selectivity of motives as activators of a particular behavior toward a goal. While adhering to this concept, and at the same time trying not only to reduce the above mentioned difficulties but also to tap other components of motivation besides the drive for achievement, the senior author devised a test (M.A.A.I.S.) in which motivation is defined mainly as an intentional state of readiness, which is actualized when the individual becomes committed to its execution *(12)*. This concept of motivation is based on the phenomenological view espoused by Ach *(1)* and developed by Lewin's field theory *(9, 10)*. Both conceptualized motivation as an intentional act and a striving tendency carried out in the cognitive sphere of activity. Lewin's theory of the psychological field, which emphasizes the behavioral act as a function of the individual's phenomenal field, presents a realistic and convenient starting point for the analysis of motivational behavior. In this context, motivation can be considered as a resultant of the tension produced by a set of internal and external forces exerting on the individual a state of readiness for a behavioral act which if executed, leads to word reduction or resolution of the initial tension. In Lewin terms, when an individual performs tasks, each of these tasks presupposes the presence of an intention which implies in its mechanism of activation a force–tension concept similar to that found in the Hullian energy model or the instinctual drive concept of the Freudian approach. Within the framework of the phenomenological approach, the acknowledged intention becomes the crucial energizer of motivation. Since intention appears to be the basis of motivational activity, let's analyze it in terms of its psychological components as proposed by Ach. He assumes that intention presupposes the presence of four elements. The first element is a state of tension which is defined as an accumulated state of discomfort associated with nonfulfillment of a particular set of needs. These needs may be instinctual or social values. The state of tension energizes seeking behavior and continues to be present, at various levels, until the need is fulfilled. The second element is related to mental representation of an eventual act. The third component is understood as a determination or desire on the part of the person to perform an act. The fourth element is behavioral striving for achievement. In this context, the most significant element is the state of tension created by the need to be eventually gratified through the performance of an act. For Lewin, intentional activity is defined as a mental representation of a goal which has equal power to any human "primary needs," and, as such, it instigates behavior. The support for this approach comes from his work on interrupted tasks, tasks prevented from completion, which lead to tension. This experiment brings into sharp focus the importance of intention as a driving force directed toward its full realization in that act. Other experiments with various tasks and across a wide range of populations have shown that subjects experience irritation when interrupted in their completion of a task and tend to resist interference with the fulfillment of their intentions. Any commitment to a task gives directional force to that task for its final execution.

From a phenomenological understanding of motivation as an intentional act we may proceed now to defining its other major components. In this sense, implicitly admitted in the definition of motivation is its temporal direction in realization. Motivation, as observed at any point in time, has its antecedents in the past as well as projections into the future. The foundation of the intentional motivation behavior lies in the past experiences of the individual which determine, to a certain degree, the direction that intentional act will take. Part of the past experiences consist of past learning experiences, attitudes, and feelings which color the individual's present appraisal of his possibilities in the pursuit of gratification of his needs. The second temporal dimension of motivation rests on the individual's current self-appraisal or evaluative projection of the task. They represent the person's self-concept and enter into the motivational equation primarily as his estimate of his capacity to learn, or to perform tasks within the context of his concomitant interest which serves as an energizer for action. The third temporal dimension is related to the projection of this possibility and need in the future and expressed as aspirations for achievement. In short, then, an intentional act is based on tapping knowledge of the past," appraising the possibility for action in the present, and projecting it into the future as a need for achievement.

As a working hypothesis for a new motivational test (M.A.A.I.S.) (see Chapter II, Part II and Appendix A), it was considered that motivation should be investigated in terms of the above mentioned components: (a) as a mental construct of an anticipatory act; (b) as a striving force, leading to the achievement of the act (the drive factor); and (c) as a determinant of future behavior based on past and present experience.

The temporal direction of motivation is related to a person's past level of achievement, his present self-appraisal, and future projection for actualization. It is assumed to be a continuum interaction between these factors though the strength of motivational emphasis varies with time. This is supported by the fact that any person has to reevaluate himself continuously when presented with new situations in which he has to project new sets of expectancies towards life. These potentialities are perceived within his socioeconomic environment, which determines as such his choices for the act. In this sense, motivation is viewed as initiating and maintaining organized behavior. Clinically, it means that any measure of motivation will assess only the potential purposive behavior as it is construed on a conscious level.

The M.A.A.I.S. attempts to broaden the measure of motivation based on the above discussed motivational components beyond self-report of general interest tendencies (6, 8), or need for achievement (2, 10a). Furthermore, attention was directed toward those intracomponents of motivation which we assumed may be impaired by the psychotic disorganization.

In this context, the senior author considered it insufficient to measure only the high or low level of need for achievement without also attending to particular components of motivation responsible for skewed motivation. Practically, M.A.A.I.S., by taking the past performance of the individual as the base line, and the estimation of his present self-appraisal in learning as a launching basis for behavior, it attempted to find the direction of his future aspirations for performance.

As mentioned at the beginning, the hypothesis to be tested by M.A.A.I.S. was that the normally motivated individual will show a continuity between past achievements and future goals based on a realistic assessment of his present abilities and interest as an expression of his needs. Conversely, it was assumed that any mental condition which impairs motivation will change either the expected direction of temporal continuity or the interaction of its components.

The study of differential organizational patterns of motivation in schizophrenics and normals was conducted at Bellevue Hospital during the years 1970–72. The patient population consisted of 515 schizophrenics of whom 317 were male (61%) and 198 female (38.5%). Their ages ranged from 17 to 52 years with 142 (27.6%) below the age of 24, 329 (63.9%) between 25 and 44, and 44 (8.5%) above age 45. In terms of education, 209 (40.6%) had less than an eleventh grade education, 188 (36.5%) had completed high school and 118 (22.9%) had higher education. The marital status of the patient population was as follows: 314 (61%) were single; 136 (26.4%) were previously married; and 65 (12.6%) were married at the time they took the test. Employment status was as follows: 185 (35.9%) were on welfare; 184 (35.7%) were unemployed; 29 (5.6%) worked part-time; and 117 (22.7%) were either employed, full-time students, or housewives.

In addition, 104 "normals," never hospitalized or treated for mental illness, with comparable sociodemographic characteristics volunteered to take the test. They were selected from social agencies within the hospital Catchment Area. According to the Hollingshead and Redlich socioeconomic Classification Index; the sample fell mainly in groups 4 and 5.

Motivational patterns of both schizophrenic and control groups were tested with the M.A.A.I.S. (fully described in Chapter II). Briefly, the test attempts to assess specific areas of motivation, that is, goals, drives, vocation, profession, and status in terms of present and future time continuum, intentional learning, interests, and future aspirations. The M.A.A.I.S. permits evaluation of past achievements across the five motivational areas, the determination of self-concept based on the assessment of the ability to learn a particular activity, the level of preparedness for reaching goals in the near future, and the aspiration level regarding tasks the subject feels committed to achieve at some point in the future.

The test was individually administered to all subjects in the hospital setting. The patients were tested within the first four days after admission to the project. At the time of testing they were considered by the hospital staff to be in good contact. Throughout their hospitalization, the schizophrenic subjects were receiving thorazine as part of routine treatment.

The statistical analysis of the responses to M.A.A.I.S. included:

(i) Factor analysis of patients' scores in order to describe the correlation patterns of the responses in terms of a minimal number of latent random variables called factors.

(ii) Factor analysis of scores from nonhospitalized individuals. The results were compared to the analysis in step (i).

(iii) Standardization of scores (patients and nonhospitalized subjects) for the control (sociodemographic variables: type of vocation, years of schooling, intelligence, and age-sex characteristics.

(iv) Construction of a linear discriminate function to classify an individual as either patient or nonpatient.

(v) Construction of a quadratic discriminate function to classify individuals. Unlike the assumption for the linear function, the quadratic function does not require common covariance matrix for the two populations.

(vi) Summary of the effectiveness of the quadratic discriminate function based upon a second sample of individuals. This indicates the validity of MAAIS.

(vii) Reliability of the questionnaire is determined by comparing covariance matrices of the 4 factor scores from 2 independent samples of patients.

(viii) Internal consistency of the factors is tested with the Kuder–Richardson Formula 20.

DATA ANALYSIS

Factor Analysis of M.A.A.I.S.

The 200 M.A.A.I.S. items were classified into the 20 subclasses defined in the Description section of this Chapter. These subclasses were intercorrelated and, based on responses from 97 patients at Bellevue Hospital, squared multiplied correlations were used as communality estimates to extract 4 principal component factors. These factors were rotated orthogonally by the varimax procedure. Oblique rotation (promax) of 4 principal components yielded an essentially identical structure. The cumulative proportion of total variance explained by the 4 factors were: (1) 52%, (2) 71%, (3) 85%, and (4) 92%. The factor loading matrix is in Table 1.

Factor scores were formed by selecting those subclasses with maximum loadings on the respective factors. All loadings were 0.30 and, excluding D_1 and D_2, the remaining loadings were 0.68. To obtain an individual's factor scores, each subclass was only scored on the factor with which it had the largest loading.

Table 1

Factor Loading Matrix for 97 Schizophrenics,
Oblique Rotation (Promax)

	Subclasses	Factors			
		I	II	III	IV
D2	Drive—intentional learning	−0.32	0.00	−0.48	0.34
G3	Goal—interest	−0.96	0.06	−0.37	0.51
G2	Goal—intentional learning	−0.89	0.04	−0.54	0.47
D4	Drive—aspiration	−0.86	0.11	−0.20	0.39
D3	Drive—interest	−0.81	0.17	−0.51	0.45
G4	Goal—aspiration	−0.79	0.52	−0.38	0.45
J4	Job—aspiration	−0.07	0.96	−0.17	0.25
P4	Profession—aspiration	−0.19	0.96	−0.27	0.20
S4	Status—aspiration	−0.16	0.85	−0.37	0.16
P3	Profession—interest	−0.41	0.25	−0.82	0.48
P2	Profession—intentional learning	−0.57	0.18	−0.81	0.57
S2	Status—intentional learning	−0.31	0.12	−0.81	0.35
S3	Status—interest	−0.36	0.25	−0.81	0.24
J2	Job—intentional learning	−0.26	0.22	−0.79	0.37
J3	Job—interest	−0.15	0.25	−0.68	0.20
S1	Status—achievement	−0.62	0.07	−0.29	0.74
P1	Profession—achievement	−0.27	0.17	−0.40	0.73
J1	Job—achievement	−0.70	0.10	−0.49	0.72
G1	Goal—achievement	−0.66	−0.03	−0.26	0.72
D1	Drive—achievement	−0.11	0.09	−0.18	0.46

Since D_1 and D_2 could not be clearly classified as elements of any of these factors, they were placed into factors based upon psychological considerations. However, when factor scores were computed, their influence was reduced by weights reflecting their factor loadings relative to the loading weights of the other subclasses in the factor. The four factor scores were computed as:

Factor 1: $Y_1 = 0.4\,D_2 + D_3 + D_4 + G_2 + G_3 + G_4$
Factor 2: $Y_2 = J_4 + P_4 + S_4$
Factor 3: $Y_3 = J_2 + J_3 + P_2 + P_3 + S_2 + S_3$
Factor 4: $Y_4 = 0.6\,D_1 + G_1 + J_1 + P_1 + S_1$

The four factors were labeled: (1) Personality Self-Appraisal and Improvement Factor reflecting present and future strivings of the subject in terms of drives and goals $(D_2, D_3, D_4. \ . \ . \ .)$; (2) Vocational Aspiration Factor comprised of job, profession, and status conditions which subject is committed to achieve in the future $(J_4, P_4, S_4. \ . \ . \ .)$; (3) Vocational Self-Concept Factor reflects present learning ability and interest related to job or profession as perceived by subject $(J_2, J_3. \ . \ . \ .)$; (4) Past Achievement Factor pertinent to past accomplishments $(D_1, G_1. \ . \ . \ .)$.

The separation in the temporal conditions of motivational components appears to be delineated by the factor analysis. In addition, sample correlation matrix for these factors were computed:

Factors	1	2	3	4
1	1.00	0.39	0.71	0.49
2	0.39	1.00	0.57	0.26
3	0.71	0.57	1.00	0.55
4	0.49	0.26	0.55	1.00

The same four factors were also obtained from an orthogonal factor model.

The test was also administered to the 104 normal subjects. Based on their responses, a factor analysis was computed using squared multiple correlations as communality estimates. Oblique rotation (promax) of four principal components resulted in the factor loading matrix in Table 2. The cumulative proportion of total variance explained by the 4 factors were: (1) 52%; (2) 69%; (3) 82%; and (4) 90%.

They were labeled: (1) Vocational Self-Appraisal Factor clusters past and present job and professional motivations; (2) Personaltiy Self-Appraisal Factor contains the self-evaluating ability to learn and the interest to reach for a set of personality improvement drives and goals; (3) Job Interest and Aspiration Factor defines the interest and future striving for achievement as related to job and present status: (4) Temporal Motivational Integration Factor reflects striving for

Table 2

Factor Loading for 104 Normal Subjects

Oblique Rotation (Promax)

	Subclasses	I	II	III	IV
		\multicolumn{4}{c}{Factors}			
J2	Job—intentional learning	−0.88	0.15	0.05	−0.26
P2	Profession—intentional learning	−0.75	0.00	0.02	0.08
P1	Profession—achievement	−0.66	−0.19	−0.17	0.31
J1	Job—achievement	−0.63	−0.29	0.13	0.03
P3	Profession—interest	−0.51	0.18	0.35	0.02
D3	Drive—interest	0.07	0.82	0.13	−0.07
D2	Drive—intentional learning	−0.00	0.81	0.06	−0.10
D4	Drive—aspiration	0.00	0.55	0.08	0.27
G3	Goal—interest	0.08	0.48	0.09	0.25
G2	Goal—intentional learning	−0.12	0.47	−0.26	0.42
S2	Status—intentional learning	−0.37	0.40	−0.07	0.22
J3	Job—interest	−0.20	0.15	0.77	−0.34
S3	Status—interest	0.10	0.22	0.63	0.05
J4	Job—aspiration	0.15	−0.24	0.60	0.01
G4	Goal—aspiration	0.17	0.27	−0.08	0.76
G1	Goal—achievement	−0.09	−0.03	−0.37	0.73
P4	Profession—aspiration	0.01	−0.31	0.23	0.51
D1	Drive—achievement	−0.11	−0.02	0.03	0.44
S4	Status—aspiration	0.09	0.12	0.34	0.42
S1	Status—achievement	−0.23	0.10	0.17	0.36

competency where past achievement of drives, goals, and status are linked to future need for self-improvement. Thus, the normals relate their drives and goals over a continuum beginning in the past and extending into the future. The schizophrenics, on the other hand, consider their drives and goals starting only with the present and extending into the future. Their past activities, disconnected from the present, are grouped into an independent factor.

A further analysis was done in order to compare the number of identical variables comprising the two sets of factors computed from the hospitalized and nonhospitalized individuals, which are presented below. The factors are numbered from 1 to 4 where 1 represents the factor accounting for the greatest

Patient Factors	Nonpatient Factors			
	1	2	3	4
1	0	4	0	1
2	0	0	1	2
3	3	2	2	0
4	2	0	0	3

percentage of explained variation and 4 represents the factors accounting for the smallest explained variation.

The objective of this analysis was to study universal motivation drives by comparing the two different sets of factor scores. No known statistical tests for performing this analysis have appeared in the statistical literature. However, two types of indices have been proposed for relative comparisons of pairs of factor scores. Their constructions were derived from the computation of correlation coefficients of Tucker's coefficient of congruence and Ahmavarra's T. These indices are:

(i) [2] Ahmavaara's T

$$T = (A_1{}^T A_1)^{-1} A^T{}_1 A_2 \tag{2}$$

where A_1 represents the factor matrix from the patient's scores (dimensionality 20×4); A_2 represents the factor matrix from the nonhospitalized individual's scores (dimensionality 20×4); and $A^T{}_i$ represents the transpose of matrix A_i.

(ii) [3] Tucker's coefficient of congruence

$$\text{Opq} = \frac{\sum\limits_{j=1}^{n} {}_1 a_{jp} = a_{jq}}{\sqrt{\left(\sum\limits_{j=1}^{n} {}_1 a^2{}_{jp} \right) \left(\sum\limits_{j=1}^{n} {}_2 a^2{}_{jq} \right)}} \tag{3}$$

where $i^A{}_{jp}$ is the jth loading factor for factor p from population i and n represents the number of common variables in factors p and q from the two populations.

If $n = 1$, then Opq will be 1; and if $n = 0$, then Opq will be zero.

These numbers are not correlation coefficients, although they range between $+1$ (Ahmavarra's T can fall in an interval slightly larger than $[-1,1]$). $A +1$ represents perfect agreement between the two factors scores (-1 represents perfect inverse agreement). A zero value represents no similarity between factor scores. As there is no known probabilistic distribution for either of these numbers, they can only be interpreted in a relative sense (e.g., does $Opq = 0.8$ represent high or low similarity?)

Ahmavaara's T is computed from the factor loading matrix so that the loadings for *all* variables for each factor affect the computations. Thus, if two factors are poorly defined (the variables could go into either factor because of similar loadings), the T statistic may be larger than a number computed for each factor separately. Since the M.A.A.I.S. factors were well-defined, this situation is of little interest. On the other hand, if the identical variables in the two factors are quite similar, but the other variables have dissimilar loadings, then T will be lower than a number based solely upon the variables comprising the factors.

Based on our sampled data, Ahmavaara's T statistic is:

$$T = \begin{pmatrix} -0.10 & -0.59 & 0.01 & -0.28 \\ -0.39 & 0.26 & 0.22 & 0.31 \\ 0.39 & -0.43 & -0.26 & -0.00 \\ -0.47 & -0.52 & 0.12 & 0.35 \end{pmatrix}$$

Tucker's coefficient of congruence is only influenced by the common variables in the two factors. Since our factors are clearly defined, this might be more informative if there were not such a small number of variables for four factors. The computed coefficients are

Patient Factors	Nonpatient Factors (Opq)			
	1	2	3	4
1	0.0	-0.97	0.0	-1.00
2	0.0	0.0	1.0	1.00
3	0.99	-0.90	-0.99	0.0
4	-0.99	0.0	0.0	0.98

Scoring M.A.A.I.S

This study is primarily concerned with the motivational patterns of schizophrenic patients. Responses to the M.A.A.I.S. from 97 patients were used to test a multivariate regression model. The matrix of dependent variables (97 × 4) had four columns representing: (i) type of vocation [ocren job scale: Labor Department Occupation Scale (   )]; (ii) years of schooling, based on a scale 1–10; (iii) intelligence (16PF E Form); and (iv) age–sex characteristic. The matrix of independent variables for the null hypothesis model (97 × 4) had four columns representing the four derived factors. The matrix of independent variables for the alternative hypothesis model (97 × 20) had 20 columns representing the 20 original variables used in factor analysis. The statistic for testing the null hypothesis was:

$$\frac{(E_A - E_N)/(80-16)}{(T - E_A)/(97 - 80)} \tag{4}$$

where E_A was the explained variation from the alternative hypothesis model; E_N was the explained variation from the null hypothesis model; and T was the total variation in the data.

When the null hypothesis is correct, this statistic has an F distribution with 64 and 17 degrees of freedom. Since the computed value was less than 1.2, there was no evidence to reject the null hypothesis. This test provided further confidence in the factor analysis of the data.

Once the model was established, the raw scores for the four factors were adjusted for the secondary variables (analysis of covariance). This meant regressing the secondary variables upon the raw scores and testing the residuals (sign test and Durbin–Watson statistic) for the assumptions underlying the linear model. No tests led to a rejection of the model and so the raw scores Y. $i=1$, . . ., 4 were adjusted to have zero means. Thus, the standardized formulae were:

$$Y^s_1 = Y_1 + 0.056 X_1 - 0.721 X_3 - 42.971$$
$$Y^s_2 = Y_2 - 13.013$$
$$Y^s_3 = Y_3 - 0.949 X_2 - 35.947$$
$$Y^s_4 = Y_4 + 0.04 X_1 = 0.891 X_2 - 0.744 X_3 - 173 X_4 - 22.560$$

where X_1 = ocren job scale; X_2 = years of schooling: X_3 = intelligence: and X_4 = age-sex characteristic where X_4 = 1, . . ., 10 represents an age category (see first page of MAAIS) for a male and X_4 = 11, . . ., 20 represents an age category for a female.

Validation of M.A.A.I.S.

The main concept underlying the development of M.A.A.I.S. is that schizo-phrenics and individuals living functional lives have different motivational patterns. The validity of this test is measured by its discriminatory power to classify an individual pattern of motivation as psychotic or functional. This property of the test was determined from a sample of 224 patients and 104 nonpatients meeting the same economic-demographic characteristic as the patients. The analysis was performed with a linear discriminate function obtained from the four adjusted factor scores.

The sample means for the patients were

	Y_1	Y_2	Y_3	Y_4
p^T = (0.10	0.15	0.17	0.4)

where the elements of vector $-^T{}_p$ are the adjusted average scores for factors 1 through 4, respectively. The adjusted nonpatient scores for the four factors were represented by the vector

$$\underset{N}{T} = (3.04 \quad -3.60 \quad 3.14 \quad 1.05)$$

Hotelling's T^2 statistic was used to test the null hypothesis that the two groups of responses were generated from a population with a common mean vector. The test statistic was

$$T^2 = \left(\frac{n_1 \quad n_2}{n_1 + n_2} \right) \left(\bar{p} - N \right)^T S^{-1} \left(\bar{p} - \bar{N} \right) \tag{5}$$

where $n_1 = 224$ and $n_2 = 104$ are the sample sizes and S^{-1} is the inverse of the pooled estimate of the common variance–covariance matrix defined

$$\frac{1}{n_1 + n_2 - 2} (V_1 + V_2)$$

where

$$V_1 = \sum_1^n (P_j - \bar{P})(P_j - \bar{P})^T$$

and

$$V_2 = \sum_1^{n_2} (N_i - \bar{N})(N_i - \bar{N})^T$$

The quantity $F =$

$$\frac{n_1 + n_2 - 5}{n_1 + n_2 - 2)4} T^2$$

has the F distribution with degrees of freedom 4 and $n_1 + n_2 - 5$. Since the computed T^2 statistic was 15.3 and the associated F was 3.8, the probability of exceeding such an F value is less than 0.005 and therefore the hypothesis of equal means is rejected at the conventional 1 percent level.

Under the assumption of equal variability for the two populations, the linear discriminate function was:

Classify a respondent as motivationally schizophrenic if

$$Z \le 0.00189$$

and classify a respondent functional if

$$Z > 0.00189$$

where $Z - 0.00024\, Y^s{}_1 - 0.00072\, Y^s{}_2 - 0.000011\, Y^s{}_4$ \hfill (6)

The magnitude of the coefficients in equation (6) represent the relative importance of each factor for classifying the test respondents. Thus, for example, factor 2 (vocational–aspiration factor) is 3 times more important than factor 1 and factor 4 has hardly any value for discriminating among populations. The value of the left-hand side of equation (6) represents a single number score for the test. This discriminate function correctly classified the population 71% of the time.

Recognizing the questionable assumption that normals and schizophrenics have the same variability around their average responses, a quadratic discriminate function has been computed. Define the variance–covariance matrix for the four adjusted factor scores of the patient population as $\Sigma_1 = \dfrac{1}{n_1} V_1$ and the variance–covariance matrix for the nonpatients as $\Sigma_2 = \dfrac{1}{n_2} V_2$ Then, if an individual's four factor scores are represented by the vector W, the discriminate function classifies an individual as a patient if

$$(W-\bar{N})^T \sum_2^{-1}(W-\bar{N}) - (W-\bar{P})^T \sum_1^{-1}(W-\bar{P}) > 0.3 \tag{7}$$

Based upon this test, 79% of the respondents were correctly classified. Testing a second group of 293 Bellevue patients using equation (7), 84% of the patients were correctly classified as patients. A statistical test for studying the hypothesis that the classification occurred by chance is the chi-square variable.

$$\frac{(m-2n)^2}{n} \sim x^2 (1) \tag{8}$$

where m represents the total number of observations and n represents the number of correctly classified persons. Based upon these results it is virtually impossible that this classification could have occurred by chance, since the calculated X^2 was greater than 60 and $P\ (X^2_{(1)} > 8) = 0.005$.

Reliability of M.A.A.I.S.

We have tried as well to measure the accuracy (consistency and stability) provided by the test by testing its reliability. It is determined by computing the variability of an individual's scores when obtained under identical conditions.

Obviously, this is not possible in psychological testing, since an individual and his environment are always changing. To circumvent this problem, two analyses have been performed. In the first analysis the interrelationships of scores are compared based upon independent random samples. The second analysis measures the internal consistency of the questionnaire. All results are based upon responses from patients at Bellevue Hospital.

In the first analysis, 484 test results were randomly placed into two groups containing 263 scores and 221 scores, respectively. Then a correlation matrix was computed for each group based upon the four factor scores. The matrix for the first group was

$$\begin{pmatrix} 1.00 & 0.43 & 0.70 & 0.42 \\ 0.43 & 1.00 & 0.52 & 0.33 \\ 0.70 & 0.52 & 1.00 & 0.50 \\ 0.42 & 0.33 & 0.50 & 1.00 \end{pmatrix}$$

and the matrix for the second group was

$$\begin{pmatrix} 1.00 & 0.42 & 0.68 & 0.45 \\ 0.42 & 1.00 & 0.54 & 0.29 \\ 0.70 & 0.52 & 1.00 & 0.54 \\ 0.42 & 0.29 & 0.54 & 1.00 \end{pmatrix}$$

A maximum likelihood ratio test was used to test the null hypothesis that the two groups represent samples drawn from populations with a common-variance matrix. The chi-square test statistic is

$$X^2 = C \left(\sum_1^2 n_i n |\Sigma| - \sum^2 n_i n |\Sigma_i| \right) \tag{9}$$

where $C = 0.99$, $n_1 = 263$, $n_2 = 221$, Σ_i is the sample variance-covariance matrix for sample, i, $|A|$ is the determinant of A, Σ is the pooled variance-covariance matrix defined

$$\Sigma = \sum_i^2 \frac{h_i \Sigma_i}{\Sigma n_i} \tag{10}$$

and $X^2_{(10)}$ is a chi-square random variable with 10 degrees of freedom. In this analysis, $X^2_{(10)}$ was 8.9, which is smaller than the percentage point $X^2_{.50; \ 10} = 9.34$, we accept the reasonableness of the null hypothesis that the two matrices are samples from the same population which implies that the test is very reliable. This finding is consistent with the higher discriminatory power noted in the discriminate analysis conducted on scores from Bellevue patients.

A second procedure for testing reliability of a questionnaire is to divide the questions into two sets and then compute a correlation between the scores (split half correlations). The problem with this technique is that the statistic is dependent upon the manner by which the questionnaire is divided. A solution to this difficulty is the Kuder–Richardson Formula 20. This formula corresponds to the average correlation over all possible split-half coefficients. The results are:

Factor	Kuder–Richardson
1	0.999
2	0.973
3	0.998
4	0.997

These analyses indicate a high degree of reliability on the M.A.A.I.S. Test. These computations reflect the well-defined factors determined from the factor analysis of the data.

DISCUSSION

Based on the structure of this test it was possible to have covered all the components of motivation from the intentional purpose to the final decision for performance. This approach had two merits.

First, the test proved to have substantial discriminating power for it has been estimated that in the "normal" population, with sociodemographic characteristics similar to the Bellevue patients, the base rate for discrete mental disorders is about 20% while the base rate of possible misdiagnosed schizophrenics due to psychotic reactions similar to schizophrenia is about 15%.

The test discriminated between the schizophrenic sample and the normal sample at the 0.005 level of significance. It also discriminated between their patterns of motivational orientation. Although the test was not designed specifically to measure motivational disorders in mentally ill patients, it differentiated the motivational organization of schizophrenic patients from that of normals. The normals were uniformly higher in motivational organization of personality than the schizophrenic patients. This finding supports the assumptions of motivational disorganization espoused by Shakow *(13)*.

While both schizophrenics and normals differentiated their present vocational abilities and interests, the schizophrenics in contradistinction to normals, lumped together their entire past motivational experience in factor 4, seeing it totally separate from future potentialities. The normals saw a logical continuity between past and present experiences and present interests and future aspirations. Moreover, for normals, past goals and drives were seen as related to future goals and status. For schizophrenics, the past was seen as consummated experience unrelated to the future as expressed in factor 2 (vocational aspiration). The relative inability of schizophrenics to represent vocation, goals, and drives over a continuum of time represents an interesting nondiscriminative function on the part of schizophrenics, which has major implications for their interpretation of reality.

While for the normals, the factor with the highest loading in oblique rotation is factor 1, which comprises past and present vocational orientation, for schizophrenics it is factor 2: vocational aspirations and jobs. This indicates that the normals identify their highest level of motivation as related to their present occupational success, while the schizophrenics deny their present social condition, projecting themselves in an undefined future.

In addition, the schizophrenic group's concept of future is seen only on a concrete level (in terms of employment) and is thus totally separated from goals and drives, which, in reality, would represent the striving force for future self-realization. This raises the question to what extent this disorganization of motivation is due to the schizophrenic thought impairment or to deviant motivational organization of behavior. According to Fontana's study (8a), the schizophrenic deficit is a function of his self-presentation which is interpreted as serving goals different from those of normals. Our data agree with his findings, but we consider disorganization of motivation to be related to the psychological deficit as a part of the schizophrenic process.

In conclusion, there appear to be clear differences in motivational organization between normals and schizophrenics. Schizophrenic motivation is principally past and present oriented: it is related to gratification of immediate needs. Normal motivation is basically present and future oriented; it is oriented to aspirations. In addition, the motivational time perspective of schizophrenics appears to be broken. These findings imply that successful therapeutic intervention has to focus also on the reorganization of the motivation of schizophrenics.

REFERENCES

1. Ach, N.: "Uber Die Willensakt und das Temperament." Leipzig: Quelle & Meyer, 1910.
2. Atkinson, J.W., and Reitman, W.R.: Performance as a function of motive strength and expectancy of goal attainment. *In* "Motives in fantasy, action, and society" (J.W. Atkinson, ed.), pp. 278–287. Van Nostrand Co., Princeton, New Jersey, 1958.
3. Barron, F.: An ego strength scale which predicts response to psychotherapy. *J. Consult. Psychol.* **17**, 327–340, 1953.
4. Brainard, P.P., Brainard, T.R.: "Brainard occupational preference inventory." The Psychological Corporation, New York, 1956.
5. Cattell, R.B.: "16 PF Form E." Institute for Personality and Ability Testing, Champaign, Illinois, 1968.
6. Cattell, R.B.: "Motivation Analysis Test, MAT" The Institute for Personality and Ability Testing, Champaign, Illinois, 1964.

7. Edwards, A.L.: "The Social Desirability Variable in Personality Assessment and Research." Dryden, New York, 1957.

8. Edwards, A.L.: The assessment of human motives by means of personality scales. *In* "Nebraska Symposium on Motivation," pp. 135–162. Lincoln University of Nebraska Press, 1964.

8a. Fontana, F.A., Klein, B.E.: Self Presentation and The Schizophrenic "Deficit." *Journal. Consult. and Clin. Psychol.* **32,** 250–256, 1968.

9. Lewin, K.: Vorsatz, Wille und Bedurfnis. *Psychol. Forsch.* **17,** 330–335, 1926.

10. Lewin, K.: "The Conceptual Representation and the Measurement of Psychological Forces." Duke University, Durham, North Carolina, 1938.

10a. McClelland, D.C., Atkinson, J.W., Clark, R.A. and Lowell, E.L. The Achievement Motive Appleton, Century-Crofts, N.Y., 1953, pp. 8–95, 300–570.

10b. McClelland, D.C. Methods of Measuring Human Motivation. In "Motives in Fantasy, Action, and Society" J.W. Atkinson, ed., p. 1–8, Van Nostrand Co., Princeton, New Jersey, 1958.

11. Rodnick, H.E., and Garmezy, N.: An experimental approach to the study of motivation in schizophrenia. *Nebraska Symposium on Motivation.* University of Nebraska Press, 1957.

12. Ryan, T.A.: "Intentional behavior." pp. 3–28. Ronald Press Co., New York, 1970.

13. Shakow, D.: Psychological deficit in schizophrenia. *Behav. Sci.* **8,** 275–305, 1963.

14. Shaw, M.C.: Need achievement scales as predictors of academic success. *J. Educ. Psychol.* **52,** 282–285, 1961.

15. U.S. Department of Labor: Work Experience of the Population, 1969. Special Labor Force Report 127, Bureau of Labor Statistics, Washington, D.C., 1971.

Adjustment of Schizophrenics in the Community*

As we have seen throughout this volume, the rehabilitation and readjustment of schizophrenic patients entering extramural life is affected by a multitude of factors. Some of these are inherent in the patients' condition; others are basically environmental in nature. In the first category are the effects of deterioration of the patient brought about by lengthy institutionalization, a matter which has received wide currency in recent literature. The residual thought defect, even in the absence of florid psychotic symptomatology, is another factor affecting outcome in the community since it interferes, to a significant extent, with readjustment efforts by distorting the perception of the social expectations of the community milieu, and by impairing the ability to deal with social roles.

Several factors are of particular importance in the rehabilitation of the schizophrenic patient in the community. One of these is the support of and the quality of interaction with family members in whose care many of the patients are released. Closely related to this variable are the attitudinal expectations of the family regarding the patient's social functioning, specifically his ability to fulfill social roles as a productive member of the community. The third crucial factor is the continuation of treatment on an outpatient basis and the following through on the recommended medication program. The fourth variable of great importance in the rehabilitation procedure is determined by the patient's level of awareness of his difficulties in coping with the community demands, and of his deviant

*The research results presented in this chapter have appeared in the following articles: Serban, G., Gidynski, C.B., and Zimmerman, A.: Role of informants in community oriented mental health programs for schizophrenics. *Diseases of the Nervous System* 36, 215–291, 1975; Serban, G., Gidynski, C.B., and Zimmerman, A.: Informants' post-discharge expectations of the schizophrenic's community adjustment. *Psychiatry Digest* (Original Article) Sept., 14–19, 1976; Serban, G., and Thomas, A.: Attitudes and behaviors of acute and chronic schizophrenic patients regarding ambulatory treatment. *American Journal of Psychiatry* 131, 991–995, 1974; Serban, G., and Gidynski, C.B.: Schizophrenic patients in community: legal misinterpretation of "Right to Treatment." *New York State Journal of Medicine* 74, 1977–1981, 1974.

behavior which affects his willingness and motivation to seek help voluntarily before the stresses experienced in extramural living culminate in another enforced hospitalization. In the studies reported in this chapter we have attempted to assess the significance of each one of these factors in relation to rehospitalization of the schizophrenic population based on a 2 year follow-up period.

Among the environmental factors of considerable importance for the readjustment of former patients, all too often ignored in the enthusiasm of rehabilitative efforts within the community settings, is the interest and availability of the family as a supportive force in the readaptation of schizophrenics.

Deykin (9), for instance, studying the readjustment efforts of 14 chronic schizophrenic patients each with approximately a 5-year hospitalization in a Boston State Hospital, found that 64% of the patients made an adequate community adjustment as a function of high family and community tolerance of their deviance, combined with low levels of expectations regarding them. Deykin suggests that, of the many factors contributing to successful discharge of chronic schizophrenics, family and community supports are crucial.

Whether the continued presence in the community of many marginally adjusted schizophrenics is due to the tolerance of deviance, particularly by parental families, or is a reflection of the understanding and support which delays the need for rehospitalization, is still an unresolved issue. However, evidence is accumulating which indicates that tolerance of deviance is critical to the fate of schizophrenic patients (33). The authors found that the performance level of the patient bears a direct relationship to the expectations of family members. Patients with the highest performance levels tended to cluster in families where relatives held either high or at least moderate levels of expectations during the first 3 to 6 months after the patient's return to the family. These findings are consonant with the position taken by Hammer (17) who suggests that married chronic schizophrenics are more likely to be accepted back after discharge by the family unit, and may be more motivated to assume their role responsibilities than are single patients for whom such role expectations are less well defined. Further evidence regarding the importance of expectations is cited by Ellsworth (10, 11) who found that rehabilitation of psychiatric patients occurred less often when the patients were placed in a setting tolerant of their marginal adjustment.

Whatever the underlying reason, the effect of the social' milieu on the community progress of the discharged schizophrenic appears to be of great importance (22). It should not be forgotten, however, that contact with close relatives at home may also have a deleterious effect upon some schizophrenic patients particularly if the home environment contains, in addition to the patient, a seriously disturbed relative (3). Another factor which may contribute to the nonbeneficial family interactions upon discharge is the lack of concordance between the expectations of patients and those of their close relatives. Folkard (14), for instance, reported that the expectations of chronic patients regarding prospects at discharge were more optimistic than those expressed by their relatives. This very discordance in viewing adjustment prospects by the patients and their close ones may well be responsible for the prevalent attitude of family members of schizophrenics that the latter benefit from extensive hospitalization (1). The authors found that as many as 48% of the families studied would like to keep their relatives hospitalized for the remainder of their lives.

According to Brown, Birley, and Wing (6) the optimal social environment for patients who remain handicapped by a thought disorder, as in the case of schizophrenics, is that of a structured and mentally stimulating one but devoid of situations requiring complex decision making. To be avoided at all costs are emotional overinvolvement with the patient, criticalness and hostility since these factors have been found to be significantly associated with symptomatic relapse. If the Brown *et al.* assumptions are correct, then it would seem that adequate readjustment of schizophrenics to the community would depend, in large measure, on the understanding of their illness by significant persons in their immediate social environment.

This approach will permit us to know not only whether the informant could be useful as a source of factual information for the psychiatric evaluation on patients' admissions, but also as a potential therapeutic agent for his maintenance in the community. The previous research in this area is controversial (11, 34, 35). For instance, Stevenson (35) indicates that informants can provide information about the premorbid level of functioning or precipitating events which lead to the hospitalization of the patient, while Ellsworth (11) found few significant correlations between patients' psychosocial self-report and that reported by the family.

In order to clarify these issues we first examined the degree of agreement between schizophrenic patients and their close family members regarding the former's premorbid adolescent problems, reasons for admission, social functioning, and experiences of stress before hospitalization.

The study was conducted with 228 schizophrenic patients of both sexes and their informants. Of the 228 patients studied, 46 were first hospitalization (acute) and 182 multiple hospitalizations (chronic) cases admitted to Bellevue Psychiatric Hospital in New York City. The informants were categorized as close (spouses and other primary family members) and secondary (aunts, uncles, and cousins as well as friends, neighbors, clergy, and social workers who were acquainted with the patient for at least 2 years prior to hospitalization). Of the 182 chronic patients studied 148 had close informants and 34 had secondary informants. Of the 46 acute patients 34 had close informants and 12 had secondary informants. The informants were selected by the patients themselves. The selection was dictated by both informant availability and the patients' closeness to them. Before the selected informant was accepted for the study, he or she was interviewed (either at the Hospital or at home) by a clinical psychologist or a specially trained social worker who determined the extent of the informant's knowledge of the patient. To further verify parts of the data obtained from informants, parents and spouses were used concomittantly since each informant contributed information not available to the other. In all cases, the informants were asked to refrain from giving any information of which they were not absolutely sure. The same inventories were given to the informants and to the patients.

The patient history data used for this study was derived from the SSFIPD administered independently to the patient and the informant. Factors under consideration could be divided in four areas: (1) difficulties the patients have encountered in their youth and adolescence such as sexual problems, difficulties with authorities, dislike of and/or change in personality, and major physical problems were also selected for the study in an attempt to examine the extent of agreement between the patients and their informants regarding the developmental problems of patients; (2) reason and type of admission (voluntary versus nonvoluntary); (3) community functioning and experienced stress as derived from the scores of SSFIPID. (4) finally, items tapping attitudes toward post hospitalization after care and community adjustment such as the need for and the use of tranquilizing medication, outpatient treatment, change in living conditions, relationship with spouse and other important persons, job procurement, and dependence on welfare assistance were also included. The degree of agreement between patients and their informants about the former's functioning in the community was tested by means of the Pearsonian zero order correlations and the chi square tests of independence.

Patients and Informants Areas of Agreement: Psycho Social Problems of Adolescence

The results pertaining to problems encountered by the patients during their adolescence disclosed a close agreement between both types of patients and their informants. Reports regarding existence of sexual problems among chronics were not significantly different from those obtained from their informants ($X^2 = 0.87, df\, 1, p > 0.05$), nor were there any discernable differences between acutes and their informants in this area ($X^2 = 3.69, df\, 1, p > 0.05$). Both types of patients and their informants also agreed closely on difficulties with authorities (chronics: $X^2 = 0.56, df\, 1, p > 0.05$; acutes: $X^2 = 1.1, df\, 1, p > 0.05$), information regarding change in or dislike of personality (chronic: $X^2 = 1.72, df\, 1, p > 0.05$; acute: $X^2 = 0.59, df\, 1, p > 0.05$), and evidence of physical problems (chronic: $X^2 = 0.06, df\, 1, p > 0.05$; acute: $X^2 = 0.41, df\, 1, p > 0.05$). Examination of factual data revealed few areas of disagreement between both types of patients and their informants. Inquiry into length of unemployment, ranging from less than 1 month to longer than 5 years, revealed no significant differences between the acute patients and their informants ($p > 0.05$). For the chronic patients, however, the informants ascribed to the patients a longer unemployment interval than did the patients' self-reports ($X^2 = 0.22$, df 3, $p < 0.05$). In terms of Welfare dependence, the two types of patients and their informants agreed closely ($p > 0.05$).

As regards the two items tapping interpersonal relationships (involvement with a steady boy–girl friend and number of previous marriages) the two groups of patients and their informants were in agreement ($p > 0.05$) for both items.

Inquiry into drinking behavior revealed that whereas acute patients and their informants were in close agreement ($p > 0.05$) the chronic patients tended to underestimate their drinking behavior as compared to that reported by their informants ($X^2 = 14.5$, df 4, $p < 0.02$). No significant disagreements were found between patients and informants as regards the use of addictive drugs ($p > 0.05$).

Reason for Admission

The patients (both acute and chronic) and their informants were also similar in reporting the type of agent responsible for the patients' admission ($p > 0.05$) and in identifying persons with whom the patients were living prior to their hospitalization ($p > 0.05$).

Information pertaining to the patient and informant view of the latters' admission factors is presented in Table 1. Since acute and chronic patients did not differ significantly on the admission variables considered, the analysis was based on the combined group of subjects. As indicated in Table 1, except for the confusion category, the informants reported a significantly greater proportion of admissions due to antisocial acts ($p < 0.05$), inappropriate behavior ($p < 0.05$), bodily problems ($p < 0.05$), drug and alcohol abuse ($p < 0.001$), and depression ($p < 0.001$) than did the patients themselves.

Table 1

Response Agreement between Patients and Their Informants
on Reasons for Admission

Reason for admission	Patients				Informants				
	Yes		No		Yes		No		
	N	%	N	%	N	%	N	%	X^2
Antisocial acts	38	16.7	190	83.3	55	25.1	164	74.9	4.84*
Confusion	168	73.7	60	26.3	158	72.5	60	27.5	0.08
Inappropriateness	130	57.0	98	43.0	146	67.0	72	33.0	4.68*
Bodily problems	53	23.3	175	76.7	88	40.6	129	59.4	15.38†
Drug and alcohol abuse	27	11.8	201	88.2	54	24.9	163	75.1	12.85†
Depression	69	30.3	159	69.7	108	49.3	111	50.7	16.95†

*$p < 0.05$.
†$p < 0.001$.

Community Functioning and Stress

In order to obtain a more complete picture regarding patient and informant view of comprehensive social functioning and experienced stress on admission, zero-order correlations were computed for the 21 areas of functioning and stress derived from the SSFIPD, comparing responses of both types of patients with those of their close and distant informants. The obtained correlation coefficients for chronic patients and their close and distant informants on the 21 functioning variables are shown in Table 2.

Examination of Table 2 reveals that the highest correlations were in the areas of drug abuse (addictive drugs $r = 0.74$, $p < 0.001$; psychedelic drugs $r = 0.65, p < 0.001$); relationship with children ($r = 0.62, p < 0.001$); alcohol abuse ($r = 0.55$, $p < 0.001$); Welfare dependence ($r = 0.59$, $p < 0.001$); antisocial acts ($r = 0.53$, $p < 0.001$); education ($r = 0.54$, $p < 0.001$); and relationship with the opposite sex ($r = 0.43$, $p < 0.001$). Correlations for the chronic patients and their distant informants are far less impressive as shown in Table 2. Of the 21 functioning variables studied, only Welfare dependence ($r = 0.70, p < 0.001$) use of psychedelic drugs ($r = 0.97, p < 0.001$), alcohol

Table 2

Correlation Coefficients for Chronic Patients and Their Close and
Distant Informants for 21 Functioning Variables

Variables	Close	p	Distant	p
1. Education	0.53	<0.001	0.30	NS
2. Job	0.38	<0.001	0.14	NS
3. Housekeeping	0.06	NS	0.01	NS
4. Welfare dependence	0.59	<0.001	0.70	<0.001
5. Finances	0.21	<0.05	−0.02	NS
6. Living circumstances	0.25	NS*	−0.23	NS
7. Parents	0.07	NS	−0.01	NS
8. Relatives	0.20	<0.05	0.11	NS
9. Marriage	0.27	<0.05	0.12	NS
10. Children	0.62	<0.001	0.16	NS
11. Dating	0.43	<0.001	0.27	NS
12. Sex	0.38	<0.001	0.28	NS
13. Close friends	0.26	<0.01	0.07	NS
14. Neighbors	0.34	<0.001	0.32	NS
15. Relationship to others	0.17	<0.05	0.10	NS
16. Spare time interest	0.33	<0.001	0.19	NS
17. Religion	0.30	<0.001	0.44	<0.05
18. Drinking	0.55	<0.001	0.58	<0.001
19. Addictive drugs	0.74	<0.001	0.18	NS
20. Psychedelic drugs	0.65	<0.001	0.97	<0.001
21. Antisocial acts	0.53	<0.001	0.27	NS

*NS, Not significant because of small number of observations due to missing data.

Table 3
Correlation Coefficients for Acute Patients and Their Close and
Distant Informants for 21 Functioning Variables

Variables	Close	p	Distant	p
1. Education	0.59	<0.001	0.66	<0.05
2. Job	0.40	<0.05	0.48	NS
3. Housekeeping	0.26	NS	0.31	NS
4. Welfare dependence	0.70	<0.001	0.38	NS
5. Finances	0.30	NS	0.29	NS
6. Living circumstances	−0.40	NS	0.82	NS*
7. Parents	0.45	<0.05	0.21	NS
8. Relatives	0.54	<0.01	0.85	<0.01
9. Marriage	−0.04	NS	−0.19	NS
10. Children	0.41	NS*	0.52	NS
11. Dating	0.45	<0.05	0.30	NS
12. Sex	0.50	<0.05	0.24	NS
13. Close friends	−0.30	NS	0.09	NS
14. Neighbors	0.37	<0.05	0.38	NS
15. Relationship to others	−0.03	NS	0.13	NS
16. Spare time interest	0.15	NS	0.40	NS
17. Religion	0.41	<0.05	0.44	NS
18. Drinking	0.64	<0.001	0.66	<0.05
19. Addictive drugs	0.58	<0.001	−0.13	NS
20. Psychedelic drugs	0.77	<0.001	0.77	<0.01
21. Antisocial acts	0.38	<0.05	0.99	<0.001

*Not significant because of small number of observations due to missing data.

abuse ($r = 0.58, p < 0.001$), and religion ($r = 0.44, p < 0.05$) areas produced significant correlations indicative of a degree of concordance.

The correlation coefficients for the acute patients and their close and distant informants on the 21 functioning variables are presented in Table 3.

As can be seen there, the highest relationship between the patients and close informants was obtained for use of psychedelic drugs ($r = 0.77$, $p < 0.001$), Welfare dependence ($r = 0.70$, $p < 0.001$), alcohol abuse ($r = 0.64$, $p < 0.001$), education ($r = 0.59$, $p < 0.001$), use of addictive drugs ($r = 0.58, p < 0.001$), and relationship with relatives ($r = 0.54, p < 0.001$).

As was the case with the chronic patients, the correlations for acute patients and their distant informants on the 21 psychosocial functioning dimensions are mostly insignificant (see Table 3). Significant agreement was obtained for antisocial acts ($r = 0.99$, $p < 0.001$), relationship with relatives ($= 0.85$, $p < 0.01$), use of psychedelic drugs ($r = 0.77$, $p < 0.01$), education ($r = 0.66, p < 0.05$), and alcohol abuse ($r = 0.66, p > 0.05$).

Results for the 21 stress variables for chronic and acute schizophrenics and their close informants are presented in Table 4. Examination of Table 4 reveals that most of the obtained correlations for the chronic group, although statistically significant, are of low magnitude accounting for only 4 to 12% of the variance. The areas of stress where agreement between the chronic patients and their close informants may be considered to be present are: education ($r = 0.19, p < 0.05$), management of finances ($r\ 0.19, p < 0.05$), living circumstances ($r = 0.22, p < 0.01$), relationship with parents ($r = 0.35, p < 0.05$), close friends ($r = 0.22, p < 0.05$), and others in the community ($r = 0.28, p < 0.001$). None of the correlations for chronic patients and their distant informants on the 21 stress variables reached statistically significant levels.

For the acute group and their close informants, statistically significant correlations of moderate magnitude were found for the following dimensions: education ($r = 0.45, p < 0.01$); work history ($r = 0.42, p < 0.05$); relationship with parents ($r = 0.49, p < 0.01$); relatives ($r = 0.41, p < 0.05$); and opposite sex peers ($r = 0.58, p < 0.01$). None of the correlations for the acute patients and their distant informants for the same stress variables were found to be significant.

Table 4

Correlation Coefficients for Acute and Chronic Patients and
Their Close Informants for 21 Stress Variables

Variables	Acute	p	Chronic	p
1. Education	0.45	<0.01	0.19	<0.05
2. Job	0.42	<0.05	0.16	NS
3. Housekeeping	0.25	NS	0.16	NS
4. Welfare dependence	0.57	NS*	0.23	NS*
5. Finances	0.32	NS	0.19	<0.05
6. Living circumstances	0.09	NS	0.22	<0.01
7. Parents	0.49	<0.01	0.35	<0.001
8. Relatives	0.41	<0.05	0.16	NS
9. Marriage	−0.29	NS	0.18	NS
10. Children	−0.08	NS	−0.05	NS
11. Dating	0.58	<0.01	0.21	<0.05
12. Sex	−0.11	NS	0.20	<0.05
13. Close friends	−0.07	NS	0.22	<0.05
14. Neighbors	0.06	NS	0.15	NS
15. Relationship to others	−0.19	NS	0.28	<0.001
16. Spare time interest	0.05	NS	0.13	NS
17. Religion	0.08	NS	0.08	NS
18. Drinking	0.34	NS	0.24	NS*
19. Addictive drugs	0.00	NS	0.12	NS
20. Psychedelic drugs	0.71	NS*	0.05	NS*
21. Antisocial acts	0.00	NS	0.33	NS*

*Not significant because of small number of observations due to missing data.

Attitude Toward Posthospitalization Adjustment

The last series of data analyses dealt with degree of concordance between patients and their informants regarding attitudes toward posthospitalization adjustment. Chi-square tests of independence were used to test agreement in attitudes toward medication use, outpatient care, change in living circumstances, relationship with spouse and friends, procurement of job, and continued reliance on public assistance. The results indicate that significantly more informants (79.7%, N = 169) than patients (65.0%, N = 146) believe that medication use could be helpful in the maintenance of the patient in the community (X^2 = 13.24, df 1, $p < 0.001$) as would outpatient aftercare (X^2 = 20.13, df 1, $p < 0.001$; informants 88.2%, N = 194; patients 71%, N = 162). A greater proportion of informants (50.2%, N = 111) than of patients (38.2%, N = 87) indicated that change in living circumstances may also be advantageous for the patients' posthospital adjustment (X^2 = 6.59, df 1, $p < 0.001$), as well as the procurement of a new job (informants 60.3%, N = 126; patients 49.1%, N = 112, X^2 = 5.25, df 1, $p < 0.05$). Although more informants than patients (53.7%, N = 108 vs. 42.9%, N = 73) stated that obtaining a new boy–girl friend would ameliorate the patients' condition (X^2 = 4.26, df 1, $p < 0.05$), fewer informants than patients (66.8%, N = 133 vs. 79.2%, N = 175) felt that getting along with spouse or friends would help the patients' mental health in the posthospitalization period (X^2 = 8.13, df 1, $p < 0.05$).

FAMILY CONFLICT OF EXPECTATIONS AND PATIENT READMISSIONS

The obvious discrepancies in expectations and attitudes regarding the posthospitalization period raised the issue of whether this condition might lead to rehospitalization of the patient. In order to test this hypothesis a second study was undertaken in which the lack of congruence in attitude and expectations between patients and their close informants were analyzed as predictors of patient readmission.

In this second study about the informant–patient agreement or conflict, only close relatives (spouses, parents, and siblings) were used as informants since it has been shown that they give the most reliable estimates of the premorbid functioning. The subjects of the second study were 112 of the chronic patients used in the first study. Each patient in this study was discharged from Bellevue Hospital when considered improved by the ward psychiatrist. The subjects were followed up for a period of 18 months after discharge. Of the original 112 patients, 74 were readmitted to Bellevue or some other psychiatric facility in New York City. Thirty-eight of the former patients did not require rehospitalization during the 18-month observation period.

Twelve areas of the patient's posthospitalization behavior in the community were selected for study. These were: attendance at a clinic or visiting a private psychiatrist, regular use of prescribed medication, housekeeping, seeking work (and what type), receiving and continuing on welfare, associating with friends, type of living arrangements preferred, self-reliance of patient, drinking behavior, drug use, doing housework (if appropriate for patient), and change in personality and abilities. The information obtained from both patients and the informants was based on a structured interview conducted by the project psychiatrist and a clinical psychologist during the patient's hospitalization period.

In order to achieve maximum objectivity with informants, they were approached tactfully, allowed to ventilate guilt feelings, and assured that the information provided would not be used to establish blame for either the present illness or its recurrance. As in the first study, the informants were asked to refrain from providing any information of which they were not sure.

During the interview the patients were asked to respond to 12 dichotomous items which revealed their attitudes and expectation in the 12 areas of posthospital functioning. Each family member responded to the same items, with the patient as the referrent.

The first step in data analysis involved establishing the degree of congruence between the patient and his close relative on each of the 12 dichotomous items. There were 24 possible matches for each patient–informant pair. Because of varying amounts of missing data, the percentage of matches was used as the indicator of patient–family member agreement.

In the next step, designed to determine the relationship between the patient–informant agreement and the patient readmission status, the percentage of matches for the patients who were rehospitalized were compared with those of the patients who were not readmitted. The mean percentage of matches for the readmitted group was 48.1%, while the mean for the nonreadmitted subjects was 56.9%. Because of the nature of the scoring system used, a nonparametric statistical test, a median test was used to compare percentages of agreement with the informant for the readmitted and nonreadmitted subjects. Results indicated that the nonreadmitted group demonstrated a significantly higher degree of agreement with family members than did subjects requiring hospitalization ($X^2 = 6.17, p < 0.02$).

In the third step, the rate of congruence between patients and their informants regarding beliefs about the efficacy of posthospital intervention and change in psychosocial patterns for community adjustment was determined. Nine areas were studied which could be divided into three major aspects of community functioning: (1) psychiatric intervention (aftercare) and medication; (2) adjustment in interpersonal relationships; and (3) instrumental functioning.

The rate of congruence between patients and their informants was then evaluated in relation to readmission status by means of two by two chi-square tests of independence. The results indicated that of the nine comparisons made, only one reached an acceptable level of statistical significance. The variable which significantly differentiated readmitted from nonreadmitted was job seeking in the posthospitalization period. Whereas 73.68% (N = 28) of the nonreadmitted patients agreed with their informants that seeking new employment would be beneficial to their community tenure, only 47.22% (N = 34) of the readmitted subjects similarly agreed. Of those pairs that disagreed, 52.78% (N = 38) were readmitted and 26.32% (N = 10) were not. These differences produced a chi-square of 7.08 ($p < 0.01$), suggesting that lack of agreement between patients and informants on the seeking of employment by the patient after hospitalization appears to be significantly associated with short-term readmission.

PATIENTS' USE OF COMMUNITY AFTERCARE PROGRAMS

The stabilization of the patient in the community appears to depend greatly on the use of aftercare programs, such as drug treatment and psychosocial therapy combined with a positive attitude towards employment. Recent research suggests that rehospitalization of chronic schizophrenic patients can be significantly reduced by psychoactive drugs. Phenothiazine was particularly effective early in the treatment with diminished effectiveness over time (12). Further studies confirmed the effectiveness of phenothiazine treatment in prevention of hospitalization in ambulatory schizophrenic patients (13, 30).

Supporting evidence for the importance of phenothiazine treatment in maintaining community tenure of schizophrenics comes from several drug withdrawal studies. Caffey et al. (7) reported that gradual reduction of active medication produced a high incidence of deteriorated behavior. In a more recent study Prien and Cole reported that withdrawal of tranquilizers has less deleterious effects for patients on low dosages than for patients receiving moderate to high dosages. The latter group, upon withdrawal, shows relatively high relapse rates. In a study of 71 chronic schizophrenic inpatients over 6 months, other authors found support for the Prien and Cole (28) findings that best results with chlorpromazine are obtained with higher doses in younger patients who are hospitalized for less than 10 years. Moderate dosages of 300 mg appear to achieve as much as higher dosages in patients who are hospitalized longer than 10 years (8).

There are widely disparate results concerning the value of aftercare when outpatient treatment combines psychotropic medication and psychotherapy. May and Tuma (24), for instance, suggested that whereas medication appeared to affect the outcome with schizophrenics, psychotherapy, whether or not combined with medication, was generally ineffective. By contrast, Karon and Vandebos

(20), found that medication was particularly effective in the treatment of schizophrenics by an experienced psychotherapist; patients seen by supervisors showed more balanced and longer lasting changes. In a more recent article, May *(23)* presented overwhelming evidence in favor of the efficacy of antipsychotic drug therapy. He warns, however, that there is also reasonably good evidence that milieu care and rehabilitation produced beneficial results, particularly in the outpatient settings. It should be also pointed out, says May, that drugs, particularly in large doses, are not beneficial to all patients just as psychotherapeutic efforts do not succeed in all cases.

Lowered rehospitalization rates due to the combined effect of neuroleptics and brief psychotherapy (21.6%) were reported by Mendel and Rapport *(25)*. Orlinsky and D'Elia *(27)*, in studying schizophrenic patients discharged from Illinois state hospitals, found that the effectiveness of clinic attendance was moderately associated with time between hospital discharge and first clinic visit and the number of clinic visits. Treatment offered in the clinic consisted of medication, followup interviews, and, in some cases, weekly individual or group psychotherapy and milieu therapy. A higher proportion of attenders than of nonattenders maintained community tenure at each point of follow-up from 90 to 730 days after discharge. However, no crucial cut-off point in time was found for initial clinic contact, and the number of clinic visits did not seem to differentially affect outcome to a significant degree, although some trends were found suggesting that the lower interview group had a higher rehospitalization rate after 1 year of observation.

More recently, Hogarty *et al. (18)* studied the effectiveness of maintenance phenothiazine therapy in combination with major role therapy designed to reintegrate the patients into their expected occupational roles. The results indicated that, while only 48% of the drug takers relapsed after 17 months of community tenure, 80% of the placebo patients were rehospitalized. Major role therapy, by contrast, was relatively ineffective in delaying relapse. It should be pointed out, however, that the combined chlorpromazine and major role therapies had a beneficial effect on the community adjustment of schizophrenics during the 2 year period following discharge *(19)*.

Despite the generally favorable reports on the beneficial effects of aftercare programs and their increasing availability, the national rate for rehospitalization of schizophrenics has remained at a fairly constant rate of 34% *(36)*.

There appears to be a contradiction between the usefulness of therapeutic interventions as a means of increasing community tenure of schizophrenics and relatively high and stable readmission rates, in spite of the availability of therapeutic interactions. We therefore undertook a study to test the hypothesis that schizophrenics underuse available facilities because of their underestimation of the value of continuing treatment after discharge. The aims of the study were twofold. First, an attempt was made to examine the attitudes of schizophrenic patients regarding the value of medication, regular aftercare, and the seeking of gainful employment as factors in posthospital adjustment. Second, the study sought to explore the extent of the actual utilization of programs allegedly beneficial in posthospital adjustment.

The study was conducted with the original sample of 641 schizophrenics seen at Bellevue Psychiatric Hospital. Twenty-eight questions regarding the patients' attitudes toward medication, aftercare, employment, welfare dependence, and hospitalization, comprising the index of the SSFIPD, served as measures. The 28 questions were first submitted to a correlational analysis to identify the significant and nonoverlapping dimensions measured by the individual items. Four variables, thus obtained, formed the basis for the analysis of the attitudinal components of the therapeutic interventions studied. These were: medication use, clinic attendance, employment (unemployed, employed part-time, employed, full-time), and welfare dependence. Information obtained from reliable informants was used to check the accuracy of the patients' statements.

The results are presented in two sections. The first section explores the significance of the behavioral vs. attitudinal dimensions on medication, aftercare, employment, and welfare variables for chronic and acute patients, based on the data obtained upon their first admission to the project. The second section presents quantitative analysis of the relationship of these variables to readmission.

COMPARISON OF ATTITUDES AND BEHAVIOR OF CHRONIC AND ACUTE SCHIZOPHRENICS IN REGARD TO MEDICATION, AFTERCARE SERVICES, AND EMPLOYMENT

Results regarding the implementation of instruction by the chronic schizophrenic group to continue medication following discharge, in the period between their last hospitalization and admission to the project, revealed that of the 516 chronics examined 58.8% (N = 216) reported either total nonuse of the prescribed medication or, at best, irregular use of it. In fact, only 151 patients of the entire sample of 516 or 29.3% reported strict compliance with the recommended drug regimen between their hospitalizations. Yet, an additional check with their informants revealed that only 19.8% of these cases (rather than 29.3%) had faithfully followed directions in regard to use of medication between admissions.

This extreme noncompliance with instructions for continuation of medication is perhaps more striking when viewed vis a vis this group's expressed attitudes about the value of medication in their posthospitalization adjustment. Of the 216 chronic patients who were remiss in the use of drugs between their hospitalizations, 67.8% indicated that they believed regular use of medication would be helpful to them following their current hospital stay. The attitudinal data regarding the value of medication obtained from the 125 acute schizophrenics, whose admission to Bellevue represented their first psychiatric hospitalization, reveals a similar trend: 60% (N = 75) of acute cases expressed a positive attitude toward medication as an aid in posthospitalization adjustment. This noticeable discrepancy between the generally positive attitude toward medication, and the marked failure in its actual use among these patients may be due to their lack of understanding of the importance of these remedial recommendations. Further questioning revealed that both acute and chronic patients would discontinue medication if (1) they felt they no longer needed it (chronics 52.3%, acutes 47.2%); (2) taking of the medication interfered with their activities (chronics 52.5%, acutes 48%); (3) made them feel different from others (chronics 39.1%, acutes 39.2%); and (4) they felt no difference in their condition after forgetting to take medication (chronics 45.2%, acutes 45.6%). Of the 516 chronics 83 (16.1%) felt that they would take medication if someone reminded them to or gave it to them on a regular basis, 310 (60.1%) felt they needed no reminders, 24 (4.7%) reported that reminders would help but such a program cannot be carried out, and 97 (18.8%) indicated that they would not take medication in any case. The corresponding data for 125 acutes regarding supervision of medication revealed that 24 (19.2%) would find it helpful, 2 (1.6%) could not have such supervision, 71 (56.8%) indicated that they needed no reminders, and 57 (45.6%) stated that they would not take medication in any case.

Furthermore, results pertaining to the utilization of and attitude toward professional aftercare indicate a trend similar to that already found for medication. Of the 516 chronic patients, 227 or 44% admitted that they did not seek outpatient treatment, be it in a clinic or with a private psychiatrist, and 143 of the 516 (27%) reported irregular attendance of outpatient services. Only 146 (28%) of these 516 chronic patients claimed to have followed through with a consistent aftercare program between hospitalizations. These findings, again, are in marked contrast with the expressed attitudes of both chronic and acute patients regarding the value of this posthospitalization assistance. Thus, 72.1% of the chronic patients questioned stated that attending a mental health clinic subsequent to discharge is beneficial to their mental health. Of special interest in this connection is the additional finding that the favorable responses toward enrolling in an outpatient program increased to 87.2% among the chronic group when the factor of doctors' recommendation was added. Among the acutes, 56% expressed the belief that aftercare is a valuable adjunct to posthospitalization adjustment, and 80% indicated that they would use outpatient services if instructed to do so.

The third therapeutic variable in posthospitalization adjustment, that of employment vs. welfare, revealed less of a discrepancy between behavioral manifestation and attitudes for both chronic and acute patients as compared with that obtained for medication and outpatient care variables. On the basis of the first interview at key admission, it was found that 71.9% (N = 371) of the 516 chronic patients were reported to be unemployed, only 13.4% (N = 69) were employed full-time, and 39.7% (N = 205) received welfare prior to the current hospitalization. Inquiry as to the patients' attitudes toward employment as a valuable aid to adjustment indicated that 50.8% (N = 262) of the patients in the chronic group expressed a belief in the value of gainful employment as an aid in posthospitalization adjustment, whereas 49.2% (N = 254) felt that it would be of no significant value. Among the 125 acutes 37.6% (N = 47) were found to be unemployed, 36.8% (N = 46) were working full-time, and 20% (N = 25) were receiving welfare at the time of their hospitalization. At the same time 49% (N = 64) of these patients disclosed that getting a new job would be of value. In addition, both groups agreed that living on welfare is not beneficial to their mental health (chronics, 67.2%; acutes 79.2%). The reliability of the patients statements was explored further at readmission.

Significance of Medication, Aftercare, and Employment Variables for Readmission

The follow-up data provided the check for the attitudinal statements made by both chronic (N = 349) and acute (N = 70) groups regarding the studied variables, and furnished information as to the relationship between the utilization of these therapeutic interventions and the need for rehospitalization.

Table 5 presents the results pertaining to compliance with instructions on medication and aftercare and findings regarding the employment variable, for readmitted and nonreadmitted groups of chronic and acute schizophrenics comprising the follow-up sample. Of the 258 chronics who were rehospitalized during the observation period of 2 years, 86.8% (N = 224) were readmitted to Bellevue, 13.2% (N = 34) were rehospitalized at other facilities, and 26.1% (N = 91) of the total group of 349 did not need hospitalization during the same period. Of the 70 acutes available to the follow-up observation, 11.4% (N = 28) were readmitted to Bellevue, 4.3% (N = 3), to other hospitals, and 55.7% (N = 39) were not readmitted during the same interval.

Examination of Table 5 reveals that only 127 out of 349 or 36.4% of all chronic patients, and 19 out of 70 or 25.7% of the acute counterparts comprising the follow-up sample, complied with their recommended drug regimen, and 144 out of 349 or 41.3% of the chronic and 27 out of 70 or 38.6% of the acute group sought outpatient services on a regular basis.

In order to determine whether regular medication use is associated with lessened likelihood of readmission, a 2×2 contingency table was set up to test the relationship between medication use and readmission for both chronic and acute follow-up samples as shown in Table 6. Examination of Table 6 reveals that in the chronic sample, nonuse of prescribed medication appears to be highly related to readmission, and by the same token, regular use of medication appears to be highly associated with nonrehospitalization during the observation period ($X^2 = 18.33$, df 1, $p < 0.001$). For the acute sample, however, regular

Table 5

Follow-Up Study to Determine Correlation of Medication Use, Aftercare, and Employment with Readmission of Chronic (N = 349) and Acute (N = 70) Patients

Variable	Readmitted to Bellevue with SSFIPD		Short interval readmission and readmission to other hospitals		Total readmitted		Total nonreadmitted	
	Number	Percent	Number	Percent	Number	Percent	Number	Percent
Chronic patients								
Regular medication use	114		144*		258		91	
Regular clinic attendance	26	22.8	51	35.4	77	29.8	50	55.0
Employment status	26	22.8	55	38.2	81	31.4	53	69.2
Total employed	114		138†		252†		80	
Working part-time	20	17.5	40	29.0	60	23.8	34	42.5
Working full-time	3	2.6	11	7.8	14	5.6	6	7.5
Housewife-student	12	10.5	21	15.2	33	13.1	19	23.8
Unemployed	5	4.4	8	5.8	13	5.2.	9	11.3
Welfare assistance	23	20.2	39	28.3	62	24.6	16	20.0
	71	62.3	59	42.8	130	51.6	30	37.5
Acute patients	11		20**		31		39	
Regular medication use	5	45.5	5	25.0	10	32.3	9	23.1
Regular clinic attendance	5	45.5	5	25.0	10	32.3	17	43.6
Employment status	11		19†		30†		38†	
Total employed	7	63.6	9	47.4	16	53.3	9	23.7
Working part-time	1	9.1	4	21.1	5	16.7	6	15.9
Working full-time	4	36.4	5	26.3	9	30.0	13	34.2
Housewife-student	2	18.2	0	0	2	7.7	1	2.6
Unemployed	0	0	5	26.3	5	16.7	20	52.6
Welfare assistance	4	36.4	5	26.3	9	30.0	9	23.7

*Of the 144 patients not readmitted with the SSFIPD, 43 were tested with a short form of the SSFIPD, 67 were tested with a short infrmant follow-up form, and 34 admitted to other hospitals were tested with the informant follow-up form.

†These numbers represent a smaller number of cases than the total sample due to missing data on the employment variable.

**Of the 20 patients not readmitted with the SSFIPD, 3 were tested with a short form of the SSFIPD, 8 were tested with a short informt follow-up form, and 9 admitted to other hospitals were tested with the informant follow-up form.

Table 6

Medication Use by Readmission Status for Chronic and
Acute Schizophrenic Samples

Chronic sample					
Readmission status	N	Regular medication use		None-use of medication	
		N	%	N	%
Readmitted	258	77	29.8	181	70.2
Nonreadmitted	91	50	54.9	41	45.1

$$X^2 = 18.33, df\,1, p < 0.001$$

Acute Sample					
Readmitted	31	10	32.2	21	67.7
Nonreadmitted	38	9	23.7	29	76.3

$$X^2 = 0.6263, df\,1, p > 0.05$$

medication use appears to be independent of readmission status, as indicated in the lower part of Table 2 ($X^2 = 0.6263, df\,1, p > 0.05$).

The comparisons of readmitted and non-readmitted chronic and acute samples on the variable of clinic attendance are presented in Table 7. As can be seen from Table 7, readmission in the chronic groups appears to be significantly associated with nonuse of outpatient services following hospitalization, whereas regular attendance appears to prevent and/or delay rehospitalization within the observation period ($X^2 = 39.72, df\,1, p < 0.001$). No significant differentiation was obtained for the acute sample, however, in terms of readmission and clinic attendance variables ($X^2 = 1.15, df\,1, p > 0.05$).

As regards employment, of the 258 chronic patients requiring rehospitalization, at either Bellevue or other facilities, 24.6% (N = 62) were unemployed between hospitalizations, 5.6% (N = 14) worked only part-time, 13.1% (N = 33) were fully employed, 5.2% (N = 13) had the status of student or housewife, and 51.6% (N = 130) were on welfare during the observation period. Of the 91 chronic patients not requiring rehospitalization during the same interval, 20.0% (N = 16) were unemployed, 7.5% (N = 6) were part-time employees, 23.8% (N = 19) worked full-time, 11.3% (N = 9) were students or housewives, and 37.5% (N = 30) received welfare benefits.

Of the acute patients available to the follow-up and readmitted during the observation period to either Bellevue or other facilities, 9 out of 30 or 30% received welfare assistance between hospitalizations, 16.7% (N = 6) were unemployed during that time, 16.7% (N = 5) worked part-time, and 30.0% (N = 9) were fully employed or enjoyed the housewife-student status (N = 2;

Table 7

Clinic Attendance by Readmission Status for Chronic and
Acute Schizophrenic Samples

Readmission status	N	Regular attendance		Nonattendance	
		N	%	N	%
Chronic sample					
Readmitted	258	81	31.4	177	68.6
Nonreadmitted	91	63	69.2	28	30.8

$X^2 = 39.72, df\ 1, p < 0.001$

Acute sample					
Readmitted	31	10	32.3	21	67.7
Nonreadmitted	38	17	44.7	21	55.3

$X^2 = 1.15, df\ 1, p > 0.05$

7.7%). Of the 39 acutes who were not rehospitalized during the follow-up interval, 23.7% (N = 9) were on welfare, 52.6% (N = 20) were unemployed, 15.9% (N = 6) worked on a part-time basis, and 36.8% (N = 14) were employed full-time (including students and housewives) (see Table 5).

The effect of employment status on readmission was tested by means of a 2 × 3 contingency table as shown in Table 8. The categorization of the employment variable for the purposes of this analysis involved combining the part-time employed with the fully employed and the student housewife category on the assumption that all of these subdivisions reflect a form of employment and can be treated as one category of this variable. Examination of Table 8 reveals that reliance on welfare assistance appears to be highly associated with readmission in the chronic group ($X^2 = 10.55$, df 2, $p < 0.01$). For acute patients the data were insignificant ($X^2 = 1.21\ df\ 2, p > 0.05$).

Table 8

Employment History by Readmission Status for Chronic Schizophrenics*

Readmission status	N	Welfare recipients		Unemployed		Employed	
		N	%	N	%	N	%
Readmitted	252	130	51.6	62	24.6	60	23.8
Nonreadmitted	80	30	37.5	16	20.0	34	42.5

$X^2 = 10.55, df\ 2, p < 0.01$

*Note: this analysis is based on a smaller number of cases due to missing data on this variable.

The results clearly imply that nonuse of medication, noncontinuance of aftercare subsequent to discharge, and dependence on welfare appear to be significantly associated with the need for rehospitalization for the chronic schizophrenic sample in this study. By contrast, these variables do not appear to account significantly for readmission of the acute schizophrenic patients.

To determine whether or not welfare recipients differ from nonrecipients regarding the use of medication and outpatient care, and to examine its effect on readmission, two additional 2 × 2 contingency tables were set up comparing readmitted versus nonreadmitted chronic schizophrenics with welfare and non-welfare subjects on the variables of clinic attendance and medication use as shown in Table 9. The results indicate that 57.8% of welfare recipients attending clinics were readmitted within the 2 year observation period as compared with 10.6% of their nonwelfare counterparts. By the same token, 89.4% of nonwel-fare chronic sample attending clinics was not rehospitalized during the same period as compared with 42.2% of the welfare cases. As regards medication, 57.8% of welfare recipients as compared with 26.3% of nonrecipients taking medication were readmitted during the follow-up period, and 73.7% of medica-tion users, not on welfare, as compared with 42.2% of welfare medication takers, did not require rehospitalization during the two-year interval. These results suggest that, whereas ambulatory treatment contributes significantly to non-

Table 9
Clinic Attendance and Medication Use by Readmission
and Welfare Status for Chronic Schizophrenics

| | | Clinic attendance | | | |
| | | Readmitted | | Nonreadmitted | |
Welfare status	N	N	%	N	%
Welfare	23 (19)†	19 (11)†	82.0 (57.8)†	4 (8)†	18.0 (42.2)
Nonwelfare	66	7	10.6	59	89.4

$$*X^2 = 39.34, df\ 1, p < 0.001$$
$$**X^2 = 17.03, df\ 1, p < 0.001$$

| | | Medication use | | | |
| | | Readmitted | | Nonreadmitted | |
Welfare status	N	N	%	N	%
Welfare	19	11	57.8	8	42.2
Nonwelfare	57	15	26.3	42	73.7

$$X^2 = 6.31, df\ 1, p < 0.02$$

*Yates correction applied.
†Represents claimed attendance. In reality only 11 subjects attended the clinic regularly.
**Chi-square based on adjusted frequencies.

rehospitalization of chronic nonwelfare schizophrenics, welfare dependence appears to play a decisive role in readmission independent of the type of the intervention used.

In order to determine more precisely the extent to which the variables of medication use, aftercare attendance, and employment history predict the need for readmission, a discriminate function analysis (2) was performed utilizing the following six variables: medication use and clinic attendance; full-time employment; part-time employment; unemployment; housewife–student status; and dependence on welfare assistance. Because the acute sample was too small to obtain reliable classification by discriminant function analysis, this method was applied to the chronic sample only.

Results (presented in Table 10) indicate that for the chronic schizophrenic sample, the analysis correctly identified 78.5% of the cases as to their actual readmission status, based on the six variables employed. Unemployment and dependence on welfare assistance ranked as the two most discriminating of the variables, nonuse of medication and clinic nonattendance ranked last, with housewife–student status, part-time and full-time employment, as intermediate in value.

It appears that although nonuse of medication and clinic unattendance are associated with readmission, unemployment in general, and dependence on welfare in particular, may be thought of as especially contributing to need for rehospitalization in this sample of chronic schizophrenic patients.

The Main Factor Responsible For Patient Misuse of After Care

The last factor contributing to the tenure of the schizophrenic patients in the community is related to his conception of "right to nontreatment" as a function of the level of awareness of degree of his illness. This factor points to the accumulating evidence about the underuse of available community resources designed to help the schizophrenic in his extramural adjustment, and raises important issues regarding the prevalent practice in discharge of this type of patient. In the current version of the New York State Mental Health Law conditional discharge, assuming some control over the discharged patients' compliance with ambulatory remedial procedures to assure greater success in the readjustment of the exhospitalized schizophrenic patient, is conspicuous by its absence. Based on the physical model of illness, the law presupposes that the psychotic expatient, particularly the schizophrenic, is healthy enough at time of discharge to assume responsibility for his acts, and to participate in the aftercare program voluntarily in order to assure his continued psychological well being. Furthermore, in case of exacerbation of his illness, he is seen as aware of his disruptive and maladaptive behavior, and is expected to seek treatment to ameliorate his condition. Contrary to expectation, however, this appears to be

Table 10

Discriminant Function Analysis: Values for Medication, Clinic Attendance,
and Employment History Variables Differentiating 78% of
Readmitted Chronic Schizophrenics

Variable	Relative ranking values
Never employed	1.00
Welfare assistance	0.80
Nonstudent–housewife	0.71
Part-time employed	0.70
Full-time employed	0.53
No medication and nonclinic attendance	0.47

rarely the case. As Rothman (31) and others have pointed out, schizophrenic patients, coming primarily from the lowest socioeconomic strata, show generalized resistance toward the use of remedial programs and have a drop-out rate of about 75% for aftercare (15, 20). The lack of awareness of the schizophrenic patient in need of treatment can be further inferred from the fact that, on the average, only 3.9% of the patients requiring hospitalization are self-admitting, the rest are referred by the family, police and other social agencies (29).

In addition, in the eyes of the Mental Health Law and some proponents of noncontrolled community treatment, the schizophrenic expatient, without active and florid symptoms, is expected to understand his relationship to the community, and be competent in judging his behavior in line with social expectations upon hospital discharge. Yet, it has been shown that 1 year after hospital release 89% of schizophrenics function below the level of an average person, failing to perform socially expected roles, particularly in terms of self-support, according to both his family and himself (32).

The aim of the study reported below was to examine the contribution of the schizophrenics' lack of insight into the nature of his illness which leads to the underuse of posthospitalization treatment, within the existing systems of aftercare. As a result of investigating such variables as level of functioning, reaction to stress between hospitalizations, attitudes toward posthospitalization treatment, all previously discussed, it was hypothesized that the schizophrenics' lack of awareness of the extent of his residual psychological impairment prevents him from using posthospitalization care even in the face of his progressive social dysfunction, resulting, all too often, in his readmission.

The study was conducted on 641 schizophrenic patients of both sexes who served as subjects for the entire project.

Psychiatric history, given by the patients themselves, and pertaining to reasons for admission, type of admission (voluntary vs. induced), and length of illness prior to current hospitalization was obtained from the first part of the SSFIPD. A global measure of premorbid psychosocial functioning based on the SSFIPD, and already discussed in detail in previous chapters, was also employed. In addition to the SSFIPD, mental status evaluation of the patient upon admission was obtained by means of the Problem Appraisal Scale described in Chapter 2.

The results are presented in three parts. First to be examined is the extent of the patients' awareness of their mental condition on admission. The second part of the results pertains to the patients' degree of insight into their illness between hospitalizations. Finally, the follow-up data on the patients' insights are studied in relation to readmission.

Reasons for admission, as given by the patients themselves, were used to determine the pattern of presenting problems upon hospitalization by both the acute and chronic schizophrenics. Eight reasons for hospitalization were considered: antisocial acts, confusion, inappropriate behavior, bodily problems, drug and alcohol abuse, depression, and vagrancy. Each patient was permitted to list multiple reasons for admission. The most frequent presenting problem was confusion; 76.4% of the chronic schizophrenics ($N = 394$) and 72% of the acute patients ($N = 90$) reported disorientation as a primary reason for hospitalization. Inappropriate behavior ranked second in importance, with 51.7% of the chronics ($N = 267$) and 46.4% of the acutes ($N = 58$) listing objectionable behavior as responsible for their admission. Depressive symptoms ranked third as presenting problems with 30.6% of the chronic patients ($N = 158$), and 37.6% of the acute patients ($N = 47$) reporting behavior manifesting depression. Bodily problems, antisocial acts, drug and alcohol abuse, and vagrancy problems were approximately equally distributed among the two types of schizophrenics and accounted for substantially smaller proportions of presenting problems on admission (16.1% was the average percent for chronic patients, 11.2% for the acute counterparts).

Point biserial correlations were used to determine the differences, if any, between the degree of insight into illness, as seen by the patients, and that determined by the psychiatric evaluation of the schizophrenics. Reasons for admission were used for this purpose. Results of the analyses are shown in Table 11.

Examination of table 11 reveals that psychiatric evaluation and self-report data yielded significant, although low level correlations for confusion ($r = 0.198$, $p < 0.05$), and low to moderate correlations for depressive symptomatology ($r = 0.377$, $p < 0.001$), and alcohol abuse ($r = 0.452$, $p < 0.001$). The correlations between patient self-reports and psychiatric assessments for bodily problems, antisocial acts, inappropriate behavior, and level of patient's insight into his mental condition failed to reach acceptable levels of significance for both groups of patients (chronics and acutes).

The degree of the patients' insight into their illness and the severity of the illness, as judged by the psychiatrist on the basis of a mental status examination, was also investigated. The obtained correlations between the patients' lack of

Table 11

Correlations of Patients' Self-Appraisal and Mental Status on Reasons
for Admission: Chronic and Acute Schizophreniacs

Self-report variables	Mental Status Evaluation	
	Acute	Chronics
Bodily problems	0.01	0.10
Antisocial acts	0.01	0.01
Confusion	0.20*	0.07
Inappropriate behavior	0.06	0.02
Depression	0.38†	0.37†
Drug or alcohol abuse	0.31	0.45†
Awareness of illness	0.02	0.03

*$p < 0.05$.
†$p < 0.001$.

awareness of their mental condition, and severity of illness, as judged by the psychiatrist on admission, failed to reach acceptable levels of significance for the acute sample ($r = 0.089$, $p > 0.05$); for the chronic patients the relationship between these two variables reached moderate magnitude ($r = 0.313$, $p < 0.001$), suggesting that the more the patient tends to deny his illness, the more likely is the psychiatrist to judge him as severely ill.

To investigate whether or not the specific reasons for admission are associated with type of admission (self or voluntary hospitalization versus induced admission), chi-square tests were performed separately for the acute and chronic patients, using presenting symptoms and type of admission as the test variables. None of the 2 by 3 contingency tables comparisons yielded significant results, suggesting that type of admission (self vs. induced) tends to be independent of the specific reasons for admission to a psychiatric facility.

The degree of the patients' insight into their illness and its effect on their functioning in the community was further investigated by ascertaining the relationship between insight on admission, comprehensive mental status, the amount of hospitalization during the 5 years preceding the current admission, and subtype of schizophrenia. The correlation matrix computed for the combined acute and chronic patient samples using the four variables mentioned above produced only a few statistically significant correlations. For the schizoaffective type of schizophrenics, a correlation of 0.24 was obtained ($p < 0.05$) between confusion (defined as inability to understand bizarre behavior or actions) as a presenting symptom and the amount of previous hospitalization, suggesting that the greater is the amount of previous hospitalization, the more likely is the patient to be readmitted because of symptoms of confusion. For the paranoid schizophrenics, a statistically significant but low level correlation ($r = 0.20, p < 0.05$) was obtained between total mental score on admission, and confusion as the reason for admission. Since the correlation accounted for only 4½ of the variance, it suggests rather weak agreement between the psychiatric evaluation of the patient and the latters' own appraisal of his mental condition.

Follow-up observation of the patients permitted the evaluation of the relationship between the patients' recognition of his own mental condition (based on self-report), the psychiatrist's assessment of the patients' mental state, and the need for rehospitalization within the 2 year observation period. The point biserial correlations computed for the 114 readmitted and 91 nonreadmitted chronic patients, and for 11 readmitted and 37 nonreadmitted acute schizophrenics failed to reveal any significant relationship between mental status scores and patients' self-reported awareness of confusion and inappropriate behavior. These results suggest that the level of the patients' insight into their illness bears little relationship to the mental status evaluation of admitting psychiatrists, either on admission or on readmission.

To determine more precisely whether or not lack of insight on the part of the patient, or the severity of his illness as judged by the psychiatrist is differentially related to readmission, point-biserial correlations were computed for lack of insight, serverity of illness, and readmission status for acute and chronic schizophrenics. Results indicated that lack of insight appeared to be unrelated to readmission status in either group (chronic $r = 0.003$, $p > 0.05$: acute $r = 0.005$, $p > 0.05$). The point-biserial correlations testing the association between severity of illness as determined by the psychiatrist and readmission status, failed to disclose a significant relationship between these variables for the acute schizophrenic patients, and a weak, though statistically significant relationship for the chronic counterparts ($r = 0.12$, $p < 0.05$). It would appear that in this sample, at least, severity of illness may be independent of readmission status for the acute schizophrenics, whereas for the chronic patients, severity of the illness may be associated with the need for rehospitalization.

DISCUSSION

We have presented a set of data attesting to a multidimensional level of factor such as interaction between the patient and informant, the attitude of the patient toward community treatment, the influence of his residual mental defect on his acceptance of any formulation of treatment for him influencing the schizophrenics' tenure in the community. What is important at this time is to evaluate separately these factors and to discuss their importance within the framework of the patients' adjustment to the community.

To start with, the significance of the involvement of family members and of the use of after care deserves reevaluation in the light of the studies reported above. One of the most striking findings has to do with the role of the relatives as potential therapeutic agents helping the patient maintain community tenure. The extent to which close family members are aware of the patient's condition, and are able to interact with him, despite the numerous differences in expectations and attitudes, may well determine, in the long run, the course of the schizophrenic's posthospital life.

The observed deficiency of close family members in evaluating the stresses in the life of the schizophrenic is particularly important. It minimizes their therapeutic value because they are unable to connect the schizophrenic's maladaptive behavior with the stress he experiences.

The lack of concordance between the attitudes and expectations of patients and their close relatives regarding post-hospitalization life becomes crucial in many cases when the patient is returned to the community in the care of his relatives. Of particular importance in this connection, are the attitudes toward psychiatric aftercare (including continued medication) and toward reorganization of social and personal life, especially employment plans and living arrangements, since they have an important effect on the patients' ability to remain free of hospitalization. It is, therefore, of special interest that the basically positive attitude of the close informants toward the available therapeutic forces and resources is met with a basically negative attitude on the part of the discharged schizophrenics. The findings strongly suggest that the very factors which may assure the patient's successful social reintegration into the community are perceived by them as either unimportant or irrelevant. For instance, patients appear to be unmotivated to seek consistent outpatient care and unaware of the beneficial effects of continued medication regimen. Even in the area of family interaction, schizophrenics appear to be unmotivated to improve relationships with spouses, friends, and boy friends or girl friends. The drastic contrast in expectations between the family and the patient predictably leads to continuous friction, resulting in further impairment of the latter's post-hospital adjustment. It is interesting that in the recent enthusiasm to provide community based treatment so little attention has been given to the former patients' attitudes. As has been shown here, the discrepancy between the ex-patients's expectations and attitudes and those of his close relatives can have only detrimental results. By contrast, acceptance of the former patient by his family, with harmonious interaction, generated by the willingness of both parties to deal with the adjustment problems openly and constructively would facilitate his social reintegration. Such therapeutic patient–family relationships, however, presuppose relatively congruent expectations. Brown, Birley, and Wing (5) provide independent evidence that negatively expressed emotion directed toward the patient by relatives is frequently associated with a relapse. Our own study has shown the importance of similar expectations in minimizing the need for rehospitalization. After all, conflict in expectations can only lead to increased stress for the patient and ill feeling for the family. The resultant loss of family support in the context of mounting tension results almost invariably in renewed breakdown. Therefore, more effort should be directed toward involvement of family members in the rehabilitation of schizophrenic patients. If it is adjustment that one seeks for the posthospitalized patient, then an active effort must be made to bridge the gap between his attitudes and expectations and those of his family. Our study reveals a marked discrepancy between the expressed positive attitude of both types of schizophrenics toward medication, outpatient therapy, and the need for gainful employment, and their behavioral noncompliance with these procedures. The study has corroborated the often observed clinical phenomenon of incongruences between intention and act on the part of schizophrenic patients which, apparently, continues even following discharge. This finding has far reaching implications. The first of these is the need for awareness, on the part of community treatment planners, of the schizophrenics' basic inability to follow through on a plan of action. This inability is well reflected in the reasons for noncompliance given by the patients themselves. Some patients felt that consistent medication use and participation in outpatient therapy made them different from others (39.1% of the chronic and 39.2% of the acute patients reported this as a reason for noncompliance). Some felt that these procedures interfered with their activities (52.5% of the chronics and 48.0% of the acute schizophrenics reported this). These findings are consistent with the conclusions reported by Klein and Davis that the drug resistance of psychiatric patients is associated with their refusal to accept the reality of their illness (21). It is of interest to note that although 67.2% of the chronic and 79.2% of the acute patients disapproved of welfare dependence as detrimental to their mental health, there was scant evidence that either group of patients had made any effort toward gaining financial independence. The new, liberal concept of treatment assumes that the postpsychotic patient is able and willing to carry out psychiatric recommendations. The present results suggest that the psychiatrist's well-intentioned instructions have a good chance of meeting with verbal acceptance, but not behavioral compliance. Consequently, it is advisable to institute a more structured control at the time of discharge. This would probably make aftercare of schizophrenics more productive for the patient and less frustrating for the psychiatrist.

Of special interest, and ironically in opposition to the liberal treatment concept, is the apparently detrimental effect of prolonged Welfare dependence, originally conceived as a humanitarian act of aiding the sick and disabled. The present evidence unequivocally shows that dependence on public assistance impairs readjustment efforts of schizophrenics in general, and the chronic ones in particular. Welfare recipients have significantly higher readmission rates than their nonwelfare counterparts. The readmissions of Welfare recipients appear to be independent of other factors affecting readmission rates such as continued medication and clinic attendance.

The clearly demonstrated relationship for chronic patients between medication use, outpatient treatment, and nondependence on Welfare, on the one hand, and delayed hospitalization, on the other hand, does not hold up for acute patients. This may be because many acutes suffer a transient psychotic episode which does not affect their general way of life. In addition, as a group, the acute schizophrenics have more integrated personalities than the chronics. Therefore, they are more likely to find sufficient social support on their return to the community; this minimizes medication use, outpatient treatment, and the effect of dependence on welfare. By contrast, continued use of medication and the support provided by aftercare offer chronic patients a chance for marginal adjustment. Dependance on welfare, however, decreases their self-esteem, discourages productive participation in community living, and encourages overdependence.

The Mental Hygiene Law presupposes that the schizophrenic is able to seek help voluntarily and makes compulsory institutionalized treatment a thing of the past. The question remains, however: what does this new attitude mean to the patient in terms of his "right to treatment?" Greenblatt *(16)*, discussing the legislative and judicial decisions responsible in part for the closing down of state mental hospitals, argues that some of the new laws have been used as an excuse for not treating psychotic patients.

The results of the third study support the clinical observation that schizophrenics are insufficiently aware of the severity of their mental condition to seek voluntary hospitalization. This point has been particularly attested to by the discrepancy seen in the psychiatric evaluation of the schizophrenics and the patients' own evaluation of their mental condition. Although a large proportion of schizophrenics attribute hospitalization to symptoms of confusion, they fail to acknowledge inappropriate behavior as presenting problems. Yet, the latter provides more exact evidence of the patients' mental condition than does the former, since inappropriate behavior is an indication of severe illness. Even accepting confusion as a predominant reason for admission, only 33.5% (173) of the 516 chronic patients, and 22.4% (28) of the 125 acute schizophrenics, were admitted voluntarily. The remaining 67.5 of the chronic schizophrenics and 78.6% of their acute counterparts were hospitalized for antisocial behavior including criminal acts, drug and alcohol abuse, and/or vagrancy.

The length of onset of illness also does not seem to act as an incentive for seeking psychiatric help between the onset and psychiatric hospitalization. Apparently schizophrenics do little to seek help voluntarily but wait until their uncontrollable condition precipitates forced hospitalization. Similarly, at discharge, most of the schizophrenic patients have not recuperated despite the abatement of their florid symptoms. Residual psychological deficits lead to short-term readmissions as the stresses of living in the community exacerbate the illness. The factors that play a decisive role in the maintainance of community tenure reflect the schizophrenic's underlying fragility.

An important question must be asked: to what extent is a discharged patient doomed to be rehospitalized? To answer this question, prognostic factors must be reevaluated in order to design proper therapeutic interventions to attain the goal of successful community adjustment. Any realistic treatment effort must take into account the patient's many difficulties in coping with daily living.

REFERENCES

1. Alivisatos, G., and Lyketsos, G.: A preliminary report of research concerning the attitude of the families of hospitalized mental patients. *Int. J. Soc. Psychiat.* **10**, 37–44, 1964.
2. Anderson, R.L., and Bancroft, T.A.: "Statistical theory in research." McGraw-Hill, New York, 1952.
3. Arbogast, R.C.: The effect of family involvement on the day care center treatment of schizophrenia. *J. Neur. Ment. Dis.* **149**, 277–280, 1969.
4. Brown, G.W., Carstairs, G.M., and Topping, E.: Post hospital adjustment of chronic mental patients. *Lancet* **2**, 685, 1958.
5. Brown, G.W., Monck, E.M., Carstairs, G.M. and Wing, J.K. Influence of family life on the course of schizophrenic illness. *Brit. J. Prev. Soc. Med.* 16, 55–68, 1962.
6. Brown, G.W., Birley, J.L.T., and Wing, J.K.: Influence of family life on the course of schizophrenic disorders: a replication. *Brit. J. Psych.* **121**, 241–258, 1972.
7. Caffey, E.M., Diamond, L.S., Frank, T.V., Gresberger, J.C., Herman, L., Klett, C.J., and Rothstein, C.: Discontinuation or reduction of chemotherapy in chronic schizophrenics. *J. Chronic Dis.* **17**, 347–358, 1964.
8. Clark, M.L., Ramsey, H.R., Rahhal, D.K., Serafetinides, E.A., Wood, F.D., and Costiloe, J.P.: Chlorpromazine in chronic schizophrenics. *Arch. Gen. Psychiat.* **27**, 479–483, 1972.
9. Deykin, E.: The reintegration of the chronic schizophrenic patient discharged to his family and community as perceived by the family. *Mental Hygiene* **45**, 235–246, 1961.
10. Ellsworth, R.B. *Nonprofessionals in psychiatric rehabilitation.* New York: Appleton-Century Croft, 1968, pp. 143–147.
11. Ellsworth, R.B., Childers, L.F.B., Arthur, G. and Kroeker, D. Hospital and community adjustment as perceived by psychiatric patients, their families and staff. *J. of Cons. Psych. Mon. Suppl.,* 1968, 32, No. 5, Part 2, pp. 1–41.
12. Englehardt, D.M. Rosen, B., Freedman, N., Mann, D., and Margolis, R.: Phenothiazines in prevention of psychiatric hospitalization II. Duration of treatment exposure. *JAMA* **186**, 981–983, 1963.
13. Englehardt, D.M., Rosen, B., Freedman, N., and Margolis, R.: Phenothiazines in prevention of psychiatric hospitalization *Arch. Gen. Psychiat.* **16**, 98–101, 1967.
14. Folkard, S.: Comparative study of attitudes to rehabilitation of psychiatric patients. *Brit. J. Prev. Soc. Med.* **14**, 23–27, 1960.
15. Greenblatt, M.: "Drugs and Social Therapy in Chronic Schizophrenics." Charles C. Thomas, Springfield, Ill., 1965.
16. Greenblatt, M.: Historical forces affecting the closing of mental hospitals. In "Proceedings of a Conference on the Closing of State Mental Hospitals." pp. 3–17. Stanford Research Institute, Menlo Park, Calif., 1974.
17. Hammer, M.: Influences of small social networks as factors on mental hospital administers. *Human Organization* **22**, 243–251, 1964.
18. Hogarty, G.E., Goldberg, S.C., Schooler, N.R., and Ulrich, R.F.: Drug and sociotherapy in the aftercare of schizophrenic patients. II. 2 year relapse rates. *Arch. Gen. Psychiat.* **131**, 603–608, 1974a.

19. Hogarty, G.E., Goldberg, S.C., Schooler, N.R., and Ulrich, R.F.: Drug and sociotherapy in the aftercare of schizophrenic patients. III. Adjustment of nonrelapsed patients. *Arch. Gen. Psychiat.* **131**, 609–618, 1974b.

20. Karon, B.P., and Vendenbos, G.R.: Experience, medication, and the effectiveness of psychotherapy with schizophrenics. *Brit. J. Psychiat.* **116**, 427–428, 1970.

21. Klein, D.F., and Davis, J.M.: "Diagnosis and Drug Treatment of Psychiatric Disorders." pp. 17–32. Williams & Williams, Baltimore, 1969.

22. Kreisman, D.E., and Joy, V.D.: Effects of attitudes of patient families on outcome. *Schiz. Bull.* (No. 10), 34–35, 1974; **Fall.**

23. May, P.R.A.: Rational treatment for an irrational disorder: what does the schizophrenic patient need? *Am. J. Psychiat.* **133** (a), 1008–1012, 1976.

24. May, P.R.A., and Tuma, A.H.: Treatment of schizophrenics: an experimental study of five treatment methods. *Brit. J. Psychiat.* **11**, 503–510, 1965.

25. Mendel, W.M., and Rapport, S.: Outpatient treatment for chronic schizophrenic patients. *Arch. Gen. Psychiat.* **8**, 190–196, 1963.

26. Niskaven, P. & Pihkaner, T.A. Attitudes of the relatives of schizophrenic patients. *Acta Psychiatrica Scandinavica*, 48, 178–185, 1972.

27. Orlinsky, N., and D'Elia, E.: Rehospitalization of the schizophrenic patient. *Arch. Gen. Psychiat.* **10**, 47–53, 1964.

28. Prien, R.F., Cole, J.O., and Belkin, N.F.: Relapse in chronic schizophrenics following abrupt withdrawal of tranquilizing medication. *Br. J. Psychiat.* **115**, 679–686, 1968.

29. Rock, R.S.: "Hospitalization and Discharge of the Mentally Ill," p. 83. University of Chicago Press, Chicago, 1968.

30. Rosen, B., Engelhardt, D.M., Freedman, N., and Margolis, R.: Hospitalization proneness scale as a predictor of response to phenothiazine treatment. *J. Nerv. Ment. Dis.* **146**: 476–480, 1968.

31. Rothman, T. (ed.): Comparing therapeutic results of community care in early schizophrenics. In "Perspectives in the Treatment of Schizophrenia." pp. 124–148. Crown Publishing Co., New York, 1970.

32. Schooler, N.R., Goldberg, S.C., Boothe, H., and Cole, J.O.: One year after discharge: community adjustment of schizophrenic patients. *Am. J. Psychiat.* **123**, 986–995, 1967.

33. Simmons, O.G., and Freeman, H.E.: Familial expectations and posthospital performance of mental patients. *Human Relations* **12**, 233–242, 1959.

34. Small, J.G., Small, I.F., and Gonzales, R.: The contribution of the informant in psychiatric evaluation. *Int. J. Neuropsychiat.* **1**, 446–451, 1965.

35. Stevenson, I.: *"Medical History Taking."* P.B. Hoeber. New York, 1969.

36. Taube, C.A., and Redick, R.: Utilization of mental health resources by persons diagnosed with schizophrenia. NIMH Statistical Report, NIMH, Rockville, Md., May, 1972.

CHAPTER 11

Prognosis in Schizophrenia as Related to Treatment

In the preceding chapters, we have described and evaluated the predicting power of prognostic factors associated with the rehospitalization or absence of rehospitalization of schizophrenics. As you have seen, our research raises serious questions as to the validity of some of the existing prognostic indicators, particularly in the light of the new approach to the treatment of schizophrenics in the community.

Let us now review the findings pertaining to factors that appear to have value in predicting the schizophrenics' community tenure in order to help ascertain to what extent these prognostic variables should influence the course of therapy.

PREDICTION OF ILLNESS OUTCOME

As we have discussed in the previous chapters, for each particular area related to the development of schizophrenia, researchers made attempts to identify the predictive factors for good or bad outcome. The old classification, which distinguished recoverable schizophrenics from those that would not recover (going into chronicity), developed by Langfeldt (25), Leonhardt (27), Schneider (34), and Zigler and Phillips (49), was based on clinical observations of some weak criteria appearing to differentiate the favorable from the unfavorable courses of the illness. Yet, the alleged prognostic factors, treated either as isolated variables or in combination, should have had enough power to decide the outcome of the disease. However, in making these assumptions, the interaction of the schizophrenic with his total psychosocial environment was minimized; and this very factor which generates the internal over external stress experienced by the patient may lead to his hospitalization.

The problem has been even further complicated by the introduction of drug therapy that has considerably changed the picture of the former chronic institutionalized schizophrenic. The institutionalized chronic has now become primarily a pseudoambulatory schizophrenic characterized by repeated hospitalizations.

In this context, because of the changing course of schizophrenia, it seems that any attempt to deal with long-term prognostic indicators in this illness necessitates the study of schizophrenics starting at their initial acute psychotic episode, precipitating the first hospitalization. The advantage of this approach becomes apparent when we consider that the group of acute schizophrenics (first hospitalization cases) represents either true schizophrenics or persons with schizophrenic-like psychoses, the differentiation of whom can only be made at some later date when the course of the illness becomes clear. Ideally, the acute group should be followed up for a considerable period of time, using all the presently available scientific evaluation instruments to determine the basis for the separation of true schizophrenics who become chronics from those who do not but who develop episodic schizophrenia-like psychosis (3, 4). At the same time, the acute group should be compared with the chronic one (already on the course of progressive deterioration) to help identify the common elements which may hold an answer to the variables which identify the prognosis of schizophrenia (39).

At the present time our knowledge of predictive factors in schizophrenia appears to be limited despite extensive attempts to implicate various domains of behavior in the search for reliable prognostic signs (42). Perhaps the most serious error made in this search has been the emphasis on finding a single predictor or a set of a few specific variables to account for the outcome of such a complex disease as schizophrenia. This approach may have often provided researchers with an illusion of the extent of the influence of one decisive factor in the patients' mental decompensation.

It has been generally believed that sociodemographic data may yield the key to the outcome of schizophrenic illness. Yet, as we have shown in Chapter 3, dealing specifically with these indicators, no significant prediction of outcome (rehospitalization) was possible for the acute schizophrenic group on the basis of the commonly employed sociodemographic variables of education, employment history, occupation, or marital status. For the chronic group, the differentiation of readmitted and nonreadmitted patients, obtained from the variables of employment history, occupation, and marital status, can best be ascribed to the varying degrees of instrumental social functioning present at the time when illness became self-evident (41). It appears that social competence may be an after-effect or at best a built-in-effect rather than a predictive variable as claimed by some theoretically inclined researchers (48). If a complexity of psychosocial factors affects the life of the schizophrenic in the community, then only a comprehensive evaluation of their social functioning in their "natural habitat," where the interaction among all the important dimensions constituting their lives takes place, can demonstrate the true important aspects precipitating rehospitalization of some patients but not others. Needless to say, this approach is even more important in the observation of the chronic patients who, because of a more fragile personality structure have a more impaired ability to reintegrate into the community and are subject to faster decompensation under social stress.

Interestingly enough, in the careful study of psychosocial functioning, evaluated by the SSFIPD, it was found that schizophrenics have full cognizance, in retrospect, of the factors which might have precipitated their hospitalization, compounded with the general impairments in their social performance.

After the delineation of specific problems in functioning, for acute and chronic schizophrenics, as mentioned in Chapter 4, it would seem that the problem of identifying readmission factors has been solved. Naively, we could rest complaisant that the disturbed interactions with parents, friends, and loved ones lead the acute schizophrenics to rehospitalization, while for the chronic patients the inability to integrate even marginally within their community settings would bring them back to the hospital. Obviously, this is an oversimplification of the complex problem.

Superimposed on it and interacting with it, there is another dimension widely investigated in relation to prognosis, that of the influence of after care, which has been assumed to be of importance in helping schizophrenics maintain community tenure. It basically consists of crisis intervention and drug therapy. All the data point in the direction that drug therapy plays a major role in arresting or holding back the rehospitalization of schizophrenics, providing a chance for these individuals to readjust to the extramural living at a higher level. With this in mind, the course of disease seems to be altered from the classical view. It might be said that if all the schizophrenic patients had continued on medication while in the community and had received after care supervision perhaps all the other predicting factors (instrumental functioning and interpersonal relationships) would not have the same significance for outcome.

Without any intention to complicate the already complex problem of prediction, a third set of elements may also enter the prediction equation: the patient's life upon return to the community—as determined by his reacceptance into the family and his subsequent interactions with them during community tenure. Assuming that the extent of the divergence in expectation toward reorganization of life after hospitalization was not as great or as extensive as suggested by the data presented in Chapter 10, some of the rehospitalizations could have been avoided. It is well known that the stronger the family support for the posthospitalized patient, the greater the chance of his reintegration into the family life and the community at large (6).

Finally, the level of acceptance of the patient in the community must be considered. This study has shown that patients who are able to work, and find even a relatively acceptable job, have lessened their chances for readmission as compared with those who are rejected by the work forces of the community. It is really ironic that the schizophrenics released into the community and left pretty much to their own devices, subsisting on public assistance, have been readmitted time and again, continuing the cycle as rejects of the community (40).

But even if all the above factors contributing to the outcome could be successfully implemented, we still do not always know why some schizophrenics end up in the hospital. We know, for instance, that about 15 to 20% of the chronic schizophrenics, in back wards of psychiatric facilities, do not respond to medication at all (47). It may well be that constitutional factors, whether specifically genetic or not, hold the final key to the enigma of schizophrenia, which we are as yet unable to control through either chemical or psychosocial therapeutic means.

Within this framework of reference, understanding the limitations in our current ability to help hard core schizophrenics, we still must use all available research data to attempt to create the optimal environmental conditions for helping these patients maintain their community tenure. The approach to this problem became even more complicated, despite the use of more sophisticated techniques, when the treatment of schizophrenics was shifted from institutional care to voluntary therapeutic intervention in community settings.

GENERAL PROBLEMS OF COMMUNITY TREATMENT

Evaluation of treatment results in noninstitutional settings are far from optimistic (11, 22, 23, 32, 43, 45). Even if chronic schizophrenics appear to maintain community tenure, they are functioning at a generally marginal level (13, 41) regardless of the type of therapeutic intervention used (2). Part of the problem appears to stem from the inclination of Community Mental Health Centers to treat less seriously disturbed patients rather than the chronic schizophrenics and other deteriorated psychotics (33, 35). This problem is all the more serious when one considers that the schizophrenics' lack of insight into their illness and negativistic response to supportive intervention adds substantially to the underuse of available therapeutic facilities in the community, compounding the problem of treatment attitudes of the health providers. As has been shown, on the average only 40% of the chronic and 30% of the first-time admitted schizophrenic patients follow through with the recommended posthospitalization instructions (40).

The reported successes with some groups of patients who respond to the follow-up treatment (7, 8, 20, 45) tend to blur the issue of the efficacy of current community mental health programs. However, a closer scrutiny of their data indicates a rather loose definition of adjustment to the community, mainly reduced to absence of violent behavior on the part of the patient. Frequently, the present solutions for reintegration of schizophrenics into the community are merely substitutions for institutionalization with boarding home or half-way house existence, which do not appear to have any lasting therapeutic effects. These types of milieu not only seem to fail in providing the schizophrenic with an opportunity for meaningful integration into community living but also do not appear to diminish rehospitalization rates, perhaps because these solutions represent nothing more than small community-based wards *(19, 22, 31)* where patients retreat from the world to a greater extent than they did in state hospitals *(23)*. Reich and Siegal's *(32)* more graphic description attests to the less publicized effects of rooming houses, foster homes, and hotel environments on chronic psychiatric patients: ". . . here the discharged patients are frequently clustered—unsupervised, unmedicated, uncared for, frequently the prey of unscrupulous and criminal elements . . . The state hospital back wards may be no worse, and in some respects better, than a coffin-like room at a deteriorated inner-city hotel or Bowery flop house.''

But even the customary therapeutic aftercare programs appear to lack specific goals aimed at helping the patient's readjustment to his community. All too often, mental health centers appear to be satisfied with patients' readjustment if these individuals produce evidence of some level of activity in community settings no matter how irrelevant. Even the most stringent criteria of adjustment tend to be restricted in scope and operationally defined in broad categories of employment versus unemployment status, or degree of passive participation in social activities as discussed in Chapter 3 *(43)*.

The problem faced by the community psychiatrist is whether deinstitutionalization works as some of the literature or verbal pronouncement of its administrators attempt to convey. The approach has to have a more scientific basis than just that of a social action directed at ameliorating the dehumanizing conditions in mental hospitals. Research on the community treatment is inconclusive if not controversial. For instance, even against the overwhelming data on the efficacy of drugs in the treatment of schizophrenia, some clinicians presently attempt to minimize if not to discount their role, emphasizing only the socialization program *(29)*. The same debate supported by scanty data affects also the use of various modalities of psychosocial treatment.

In fact, a recent study done at Bellevue, with 100 chronic schizophrenics, evaluating the effectiveness of various aftercare programs available to these patients discharged into the community, supported the previous contention about the limitedness of the help offered to them. The subjects of this study were drawn from Bellevue MHC and Fountain House. They had an average number of 3.94 hospitalizations and were assigned to the most commonly used forms of aftercare treatments such as: medication follow-up and crisis intervention when necessary, regular psychotherapy, and socialization and comprehensive rehabilitation. In addition, all subjects were receiving regular psychotropic drugs in combination with the above forms of treatment. Their community adjustment was assessed in terms of social functioning and stress, degree of mental illness, and type of diagnostic subclassification. The results suggested that the group of patients who

Table 1

Means, Standard Deviations, and Analyses of Variance of Functioning,
Stress, and Total Adjustment Scores of SSIAM and SSFIPD
for Treatment Groups*

Variable	Medication N = 40		Socialization N = 25		Psychotherapy N = 20		Rehabilitation N = 15		
	X̄	S.D.	X̄	S.D.	X̄	S.D.	X̄	S.D.	F
Deviant									
behavior (SSIAM)††	6.87	1.56	7.50	1.19	5.82	1.44	7.03	1.89	4.38**
Distress (SSIAM)	4.46	1.17	4.73	1.05	3.91	1.05	3.96	0.86	2.77*
Total Adjustment									
(SSIAM)	6.08	0.21	6.60	0.92	5.20	1.13	6.04	1.35	2.70†
Functioning									
(SSFIPD)	2.05	0.21	1.96	0.22	2.23	0.24	2.12	0.23	5.53**
Stress (SSFIPD)	2.43	0.25	2.30	0.28	2.41	0.28	2.47	0.22	1.58
Total Adjustment									
(SSFIPD)	2.24	0.19	2.13	0.20	2.32	0.25	2.30	0.17	3.69†

*High SSIAM scores indicate maladjustment; High SSFIPD functioning and adjustment scores indicate high functioning. The SSFIPD stress scores are scored in the opposite direction.

†$p > 0.05$.

**$p > 0.01$.

††Gurland BY, Yorston NJ, Stone AR et al. The structured and scaled interview to assess maladjustment (SSIAM) description rationale and development. *Arch. Gen. Psychiatry* 27: 259–264, 1972.

benefited most from the program were those on medication as well as in psychotherapy, while the medicated group of patients in socialization showed the poorest adjustment. The psychotherapy group manifested higher level of adjustment with lower level of stress as compared to the socialization group which showed opposite trends. The medication group with only crisis intervention came second in their social integration into the community, followed by the rehabilitation patients of Fountain House who were somewhat similar to the poorest performers—the socialization group (see Table I).

A few conclusions can be drawn from these findings. The first one supports the data presented in Chapters 4 and 5 which shows the negative correlation between stress and functioning previous to hospitalization of schizophrenics. The data indicate that even after the minimum of 1 year of community follow-up, stress continues to interfere with the activities of the chronic patients in the community, affecting their total functioning as clearly demonstrated in the socialization group. In fact, any therapeutic process applied to schizophrenics attempts to cope at least with this problem of control of stress. Although there appear to be differences between the levels of stress experienced by patients in various types of therapy, the overall stress is high, regardless of the therapeutic intervention. Psychotherapy, individual and group, seems to be more stress-controlling than socialization where the stress is highest. Although in a particular form of socialization with a highly structured environment such as Fountain House, the patients who otherwise function at very low levels appear to have a lower level of stress, this is mainly true because they feel comfortable enough in the protective environment offered them under the supervision of a continuous mental health staff. Yet, for the patients in Fountain House who have a better level of functioning, it is not different than for those from Bellevue who reported the same amount of stress. Both of these groups of patients were in psychotherapy.

The subjective stress experienced by patients in all modalities of treatment found further support in the amount of anxiety and depression found during their mental evaluation. There appears to be an extremely close parallelism between the stress presented by the patients in each treatment group and their level of anxiety and depression found in mental status. The exception was present only in the rehabilitation group from Fountain House where the patients did not experience subjective stress, anxiety or depression due to their obliviousness to their surroundings, and nonparticipation in any active program which would further their social involvement regardless of the attempts of the staff. This particular group from Fountain House presented the second highest rate of rehospitalization to the socialization group from Bellevue (see Table II).

The second interesting finding regarding the relationship between community adjustment and diagnostic subclassification gave us some clue as to the basic difficulties encountered in the rehabilitation of some patients as compared to others. It has been shown that schizoaffectives, regardless of the form of treatment, are adjusting better to the community than do chronic undifferentiated schizophrenics who apparently have the worst community integration. The paranoids appear to have a intermediate level of adjustment. This supports, to some extent, the findings of Zigler and Levine who suggested that paranoids have better coping mechanisms on the cognitive level than do the undifferentiated patients *(50)*. If the diagnosis subclassification is correctly identified by the First Rank Schneiderian criteria, then the relationship between any form of therapeutic treatment and the type of schizophrenia includes a genetic-biological

Table 2

Correlations of PAI Total Mental Status, Anxiety, and Depression Scores
With the SSFIPD Total Stress and Functioning Scores*

	Anxiety	Depression	Total MS	Total stress	Total functioning
Anxiety		0.56	0.70	0.60	−0.38
Depression			0.67	0.38	−0.42
Total MS				0.48	−0.43
Total stress					0.41

*All correlations are significant at the 0.001 level.

factor which complicates the prediction of outcome. However, the whole debate about adjustment of hard-core chronic schizophrenics in the community becomes a highly rhetorical issue if we consider that 68.68% of these studied schizophrenics are on welfare, 4.4% have never been employed, 12.13% receive disability or are on supplemental programs, and only 3.03% work full time. This excludes 4.04% of patients who are students and 4.04% who are housewives. The situation doesn't look any brighter when we consider the patients' marital status with 58.5% single, 24.2% separated, and only 8.1% married. It seems that it is not enough to discharge the patient into the community, only to exchange his institutionalization for an illusion of community integration where the services provided are meaningful only for a restricted category of patients and inadequate for the hard-core schizophrenics of long-standing illness.

If the current extramural therapeutic programs do not do their intended job, this might be remedied by reconceptualizing community adjustment to include all the facets of schizophrenic psychosocial functioning within noninstitutionalized settings. One important aspect in such a revision in thinking about adjustment necessitates cognizance of the factors contributing to the patient's progressive decline in social functioning in the course of his episodic hospitalizations. By the same token, it is equally important to give full recognition to the importance of stress experienced by the patient at his given level of adjustment and the amount of stress that he is able to absorb at his particular level of functioning.

As presented in the above data, stress experienced by the schizophrenics in the context of their marginal level of functioning suggests that their inability to deal with events and situations is responsible for the impaired functioning, even when the demands encountered in extramural living are minimal (17).

At present, the most fruitful therapeutic approach toward alleviating the patient's stress incurred in social interactions appears to be maximization of the patients' learning ability to control stressful environmental influences. Such a treatment program would require the development of new coping skills specific for the patient in dealing with his daily interaction which produces stress in him.

In the final analysis, it appears that the treatment of schizophrenics should be a highly individualized one since only this type of approach can provide a chance of success in balancing off the two sets of divergent forces controlling the outcome of an act. One force is represented by the attitude and motivation of the patient which are influenced by his thinking defect and shape his appraisal of reality. The other force reflects the tasks and demands which must be met if community integration is to be achieved. This balance is indeed a very precarious one; in order to function, the schizophrenic has to be able to learn to control and to process the information input overload which he receives from the environment. According to Broadbent (5), his difficulty consists of making errors continuously in appraising environmental pressures. As a result his adjustment is inadequate and inappropriate. His distorted evaluation of a task is unlikely to automatically increase the level of his anxiety and stress, thus negatively influencing his ability to function in a particular situation. At the same time, any unrealistic expectation, unmet by the reality of his living, increases his phychological disintegration. In view of these considerations the schizophrenics' adjustment to community living has to be evaluated in terms of several variables: (1) the patient's response to medication; (2) his interaction with his family; (3) tolerance level to sudden environmental changes; (4) capacity and opportunity for gainful employment; (5) treatment based on social reconditioning which permits creating new patterns of functioning through reinforcement of successful activities that can be realized in daily life; and, finally, (6) an acceptance by the schizophrenic of his deficits. Apparently, the most important tool of keeping the schizophrenics in the community is related to the proper administration of drugs.

As regards the patients' tolerance of drugs, there is a widely held misconception that more or less all tranquilizing medication has the same effect, and the choice of a specific drug is dictated solely on the basis of minimal side effects. In reality, the psychopharmacology of tranquilizers represents at least 4 major groups of interrelating acting medications all bringing somewhat different response from the patient. Awareness of this fact makes it necessary to carefully evaluate and observe the response which each of these groups of drugs may produce in each individual patient.

In this context, a discussion of the psychopharmacological mechanisms of action of drugs might be warranted.

Due to the work of the Swedish pharmacologist Arvid Carlsson and others, we have gained some general indications of how neuroleptics, such as phenothiazine,work in the brain *(9)*.

The activity of neuroleptics in the brain attempts to elucidate indirectly the biological mechanisms of schizophrenia. All neuroleptics have a basic common property; that of inhibitory action on dopaminergic neurotransmissions. Dopamine is mainly produced in three brain regions: nigrostriatal, mesolimbic, and tuberoinfundibular from the arcuate nucleus to the median eminence. These three regions are affected in specific ways by the neuroleptics (tranquilizers) by their extrapyramidal symptoms, antipsychotic actions, and endocrine reactions. Since each tranquilizer has a different degree of response in its antipsychotic and extrapyramidal actions, it is only natural to suspect that antipsychotic activity takes place in the limbic system while their extrapyramidal one takes place in the striatum. Some of them, like thioridazine, affect sexual endocrine functions. This assumption is supported by the fact that tranquilizers that have a low effect on the extrapyramidal side—like thioridazine or clozapine sulpiride—have a stronger effect on the limbic structure.

In general, the neuroleptic–tranquilizer compete with dopamine receptor bindings by blocking the dopamine receptors at the level of postsynaptic neurons. The first proof that this may be so came from the observation that after the administration of phenothiazine there is an increase of dopamine metabolites in the brain. Research has indicated that there is direct relationship between the amount of phenothiazine (chlorpromazine) administered and the increase in dopamine metabolites *(15)*. The dopamine metabolites are increased parallel with the release of dopamine by the neuroleptics. In other words, dopamine neurons fire more rapidly due to the phenothiazine intake. Furthermore, we now know that a particular enzyme, neurotransmitter adenylate cyclase (AMP) responds to dopamine accumulation, serving as an indicator for the level of dopamine receptor activity. Neuroleptics have the property of inhibiting the effect of dopamine in the adenylate cyclase proportionally to its clinical activity *(1)*. In this sense, fluphenozine is approximately six times as potent as chlorpromazine, while haloperidol appears to be half as potent in vitro as chlorpromazine in competing for the dopamine receptor bindings. Yet this creates controversy since butyrophenone (haloperidol) is much more potent clinically per milligram than chlorpromazine. Bearing these facts in mind, the only clinical indication for the potency of a particular drug is based on the observation of the effect of the drug on symptom reduction. Thus far, it appears that phenothiazine with a triflumethyl substitute in the ring A of dopamine is more potent than that with alkylamine side chains, and most potent of all is hydroxy-ethyl-piperazine side chains such as fluphenazine. All phenothiazine and butyrophenones have antipsychotic effects, but they do not cure schizophrenia. This explains why schizophrenic patients should be maintained on drugs on long-term basis *(16, 18)*.

The findings regarding the therapeutic values of these antipsychotics do not answer the question as to which drug is most beneficial for a particular patient. It appears that differences in metabolism, rate of absorption, and accumulation at receptor site vary from individual to individual influencing the therapeutic response. The widely held notion that hyperexcitable patients respond best to chlorpromazines while the withdrawn patients respond best to fluphenazine does not appear to hold ground when verified by research. According to an NIMH study *(10)* apathetic and retarded patients did respond well to chlorpromazine therapy. However, for unknown reasons some patients are refractory to some antipsychotics while responding very well to others.

It is important at this point to mention some of the misleading concepts about the use of mega dosage of antipsychotics. Studies addressed to this problem indicate that the use of high dosage—does not accelerate or improve the condition of the patient. For instance, the study of Wijsenbeck *et al.* compared trifluoperazine (Stelazine) in an average dosage and a high dosage (up to 700 mg./day), and found that the results were basically the same. Recently, two new antipsychotics were introduced to the market, which have different chemical structure from the more known ones, such as phenothiazine, thioxanthenes, or butyrophenones. They are molindone and dibenzoxazepine compound (Loxapine). These drugs have basically the same effects as phenothiazine, and more or less the same side effects *(36)*.

Antipsychotic treatment raises three major problems. One of these is the interaction with other drugs which might make them less potent. An example is

Gelusil, which interferes with the absorption of chlorpromazine, or phenobarbitol or other barbiturates, which result in faster metabolism of chlorpromazine.

The second aspect is related to the long-term side effects described as tardive dyskinesia and due to long-term processes in the extrapyramidal function. Unfortunately, all the existent antipsychotics could produce toxicity affecting the extrapyramidal system. Although not yet fully tested, the new class of antipsychotics, such as clozapine and pimozide, appear not to affect the extrapyramidal system; however, their clinical validity and efficacy has yet to be proven.

The third related problem is the length of maintenance therapy and its value against relapses. It is important to note that a study done in this direction indicates that patients maintained on antipsychotics have a lower rate of relapse than those on placebo. In a study sponsored by NIMH (30), seventy-two percent of patients on placebo relapsed as compared with 16% of those who were drug treated.

The role of neuraleptic drugs in the maintenance of schizophrenics in the community does not require further discussions since at least a dozen studies have documented this point fully. Yet the relapse of patients taking drugs has remained quite high varying from study to study: 48%, Goldberg (14); 5%, Caffey (8); and 20%, Prien et al. (30); 33%, Leff and Wing; 15% (26), Engelhard et al. (12). This means that the drugs have a limited effect in controlling the stress undergone by the patient in his interaction with the environment, or it is quite possible that the patient does not take his medication regularly. These two variables are more likely to be controlled with reeducational, rehabilitative programs which should be instituted immediately after the patient's discharge.

The maintenance of this type of therapy requires a reeducative effort, particularly with schizophrenic patients. The central part of this effort is getting the patient to accept the value of medication and its role in ameliorating his condition. At the point when the schizophrenic patient understands that the tranquilizer represents for him what insulin does for the diabetic, true cooperation of the patient is obtained and the relationship between the schizophrenic and his therapist becomes highly productive in helping the patient deal with the pressures encountered in community living.

Obviously the patient does not live in a vacuum. He has a family and friends who represent a potential first line of support in his readjustment efforts (44). Utilization of this important resource should not be minimized in the treatment plan. It seems imperative that the close relatives be made aware of the change in mental state which the patient undergoes as he moves from one situation to another, or faces a variety of events, and the importance of tolerance of these manifestations be pointed out to the family members. Through these manipulations the patients' lives can be made more bearable within the social environment since family support and their understanding of the patients' behavior tends to reduce the level of stress within family settings. As is discussed in the previous chapter, it was found that although close relatives are well aware of the difficulties affecting the functioning of the patient, they are unable to understand the amount of stress which the patient experiences in internalizing his own inability to respond appropriately to the environment.

Within this context a harmonious plan of action between the therapist, the patient and a member of the family should be devised to help eliminate both unrealistic motivations and aspirations of the patient and the unreachable expectation of the family, which can become another source of conflict, unnecessarily increasing the patient's level of stress leading to rehospitalization. The goals derived from such a cooperative effort should be based squarely on true and realistically perceived limitations of each individual patient. Persuasion should be used to make the outlined goals acceptable to the family and to the patient. Once such goals are delineated, their implementation should proceed in a step-wise fashion, thus initiating a process of helping the patient obtain a realistic level of integration into the community. The often heard complaint of the family that the patient is lazy should be interpreted as inertia in functioning and part of the patient's intolerance to changes which requires not only psychiatric attention by also family support to help the patient overcome the fear of facing the whole gamut of social responsibilities upon discharge. It is imperative that the family understands that the discharged schizophrenic patient is only partly recovered psychologically, and actually very poorly adjusted from the social point of view. Cognizance of repeated attempts and failures in the long rehabilitative process before the patient reaches a relatively acceptable level of social integration will go a long way to make the treatment successful.

The therapeutic value of gainful employment in the process of schizophrenic patients' rehabilitation should be given special attention (44), irrespective of the quality this work may represent or its social status equivalent. Convincing the patient of the value of work is particularly important. Rehabilitation in terms of gainful employment should again be approached in a step-by-step fashion. Beginning at a realistically low job level, which might start with vocational placement with a few specific agencies that accept these former patients in simple jobs such as messenger, stock room boys, or mail room, or maintenance workers, etc., he should be progressively encouraged to reach his current potential which will permit him to perform his work role comfortably and without self-induced stress. In this connection it is important to emphasize to the patient that though it might appear that the work now offered to him is below his previous level of employment, no work is humiliating since the process of working itself is therapeutic. It is also important to point out to the schizophrenic that by accepting his limited possibilities, he is likely to be able to function in the community, thereby regaining a sense of self-esteem as a productive member of his social group.

It is obvious that the patient's functioning at work will be affected not only by the pressures of the job itself but also by the social interactions with co-workers and supervisors. In widening the social contacts of the patient one must assume that the schizophrenic will be affected by many interpersonal situations which may produce crises. In general, interactions with the opposite sex, friends and neighbors are difficult for schizophrenics, not only because of their exaggerated sensitivity but also because of their tendency to all too easily misinterpret the meaning of interpersonal interactions. For this reason, the therapeutic effort must concentrate on correcting the interpretations of the patients' goals, choices, and interactions to help them obtain new perspectives that will serve as alternatives to the conditions which have led to a crisis or relapses in the past.

Throughout the rehabilitative procedure the life style which the patient develops in the community, particularly the positive aspects of it, should be reinforced according to the conditioning model. This procedure provides the patient with a sense of direction which guides his various activities. It is assumed that by the repetitiveness of the reinforcements the newly acquired behaviors will be incorporated into the patients' behavioral repertoires.

It is of particular therapeutic significance to point out to the patients that the new instrumental functioning level, whatever its intrinsic social value within the large social context, is still a means of providing them with a sense of satisfaction and the knowledge that they are able to function in life.

It must be clearly understood that none of the therapeutic recommendations for the rehabilitation of schizophrenic patients in community settings guarantees the elimination of hospitalization in the course of illness, on the one hand, or complete recovery on the other. These procedures, however, are based on our present knowledge of schizophrenia and are likely to provide a more realistic treatment program than those used currently in outpatient settings. The therapeutic approach outlined above makes no extravagant claims by either denying the existence of schizophrenic illness or by treating schizophrenics as the pariahs of our society. The therapeutic approach advocated here is merely offered in the hope that the procedures which are realistic in application and scientifically correct in conceptualization may help improve the lot of the schizophrenics discharged into the community, and to diminish their daily suffering in an environment which either rejects them or denies their existence.

The basic difficulty with the present therapeutic modalities offered to the patient are due to the tendency to place him in the form of therapy which fits the professional training of the therapist. On one hand, if the therapist is adhering to the etiological concept of schizophrenia as a disease due to the schizophrenogenic mother, to a family double-binding communication, to the parental, marital skewness, or to an amorphous style of communication, then obviously he will approach the therapy from the point of view of family reorganization of interaction and communication process. On the other hand, if the therapist is a behaviorist, then his model of therapy is that of attempting to modify behavior, cognitive and affective as well. His goal is to correct learning and to improve performance in order to reduce the subjective stress experienced by the patient. Since the behaviorist is mainly interested in the behavior which results in problems, he is not truly interested in their etiology. For instance, the anxiety of the schizophrenic is treated in the same manner as the anxiety of neurotics, disregarding the difference in the mental condition between these two categories of patients. No wonder that the results were, at best, mixed and attributed to the difference in the level of concentration of schizophrenic patients *(50)*. Yet, the value of behavioral therapy in changing the undesirable behavior of the patient has its merit. For instance, procedures of the token economy used with institutionalized patients could be applied successfully to socialization group-therapy in the outside setting for promoting the social interaction.

In contrast, individual therapy could draw heavily from the general psychodynamic and existential theories of human behavior in order to help the integration of the external experience of the patient within his ego level of organization and responsive capacities.

The therapeutic approach to schizophrenic patients has to be a multiphasic, holistic, and eclectic one, according to their needs at that time. The therapist has to use all available knowledge accumulated by the various schools of thought, based on their clinical and experiential research, in his effort to evaluate and control the symptoms and redirect and retrain the patient toward his new social reassignment and family interaction.

REFERENCES

1. Ayd, F.: Law and high dosage fluphenozine. *Intern. Drug Therapy Newsl.* **7**, 25–27, 1972.
2. Bellak, L. (ed.): "A Concise Handbook of Community Mental Health." Grune and Stratton, New York, 1974.
3. Bleuler, E. "Dementia Praecox or the Group of Schizophrenias." International Universities Press, New York, 1950.
4. Bleuler, M.: A 23-year Longitudinal Study of 208 schizophrenics and Impressions in Regard to the Nature of Schizophrenia. In *The Transmission of Schizophrenia.* (D. Rosenthal and S.S. Kety, eds.) pp. 3–12. Pergamon, Oxford, 1968.
5. Broadbent, D.E.: "Decision and Stress." Academic Press, London and New York, 1971.
6. Brown, G.W., Birley, J.L.T., and Wing, J.K.: Influence of Family Life on the Course of Schizophrenic Disorders: A replication. *Br. J. Psychiat.* **121**, 241–258, 1972.
7. Byrne, L., O'Connor, T., and Fahy, T.J.: Home behavior of schizophrenic patients living in community and attending day center. *Br. J. Psychiat.* **125**, 20–24, 1974.
8. Caffey, E.M., Diamond, L.S., Frank, T.V., Gresberger, J.C., Herman, L., Klett, C.J., and Rothstein, C.: Discontinuation or reduction of chemotherapy in chronic schizophrenics. *J. Chronic Dis.* **17**, 347–358, 1964.
9. Carlsson, H., and Luidquist, M.: Effect of chlorpromazine or holopendol on formation of three metoxy tyramine and normetanephrine in mouse brain. *Acta Pharmecol.* **20**, 140–144, 1963.
10. Cole, J.O., Goldberg, S.C., and Davis, J.M.: Drugs in the treatment of psychosis. Controlled studies. In "Psychiatric Drugs" (P. Solomon, ed.), pp. 153–180. Grune and Stratton, New York, 1966.
11. Donlon, P.T., Rada, R.T., and Knight, S.W.: The therapeutic aftercare setting for "refractory" chronic schizophrenic patients. *Am. J. Psychiat.* **130**, 682–284, 1973.

12. Engelhardt, D.M., Koren B., Freedman, D. and Margolis, R.: Phensthesque in the Prevention of Psychiatric Hospitalization. *Arch. Gen. Psychiat.* **16**, 98–101, 1967.
13. Fairweather, G.W., Sanders, D.H., and Maynard, H.: "Community Life for the Mentally Ill: An alternative to Institutional Care" Aldine, Chicago, 1969.
14. Goldberg, S.C., Mattsson, N., Cole, J.O. and Klerman, G.: Prediction of improvement in schizophrenia under four phenothiazines. *Archives of General Psychiatry,* 1967, 16, 107–117.
15. Goldberg, S.C., Frosch, W.A., Drossman, A.K., Schooler, N.R., and Johnson, G.F.S.: Prediction of response to phenothiazine in schizophrenia; A cross validation study. *Arch. Gener. Psychiat.* **26**, 367–373, 1972.
16. Goldberg, S.C. Schooler, R.N., Hogarty, G.E. and Roper, M.: Treatment of relapse in schizophrenic outpatients treated by Drugs and Socio-therapy. *Arch. Gen. Psy.* **34**, 171–184, 1977.
17. Harrow, M., Harkavy, K., Bromet, E., and Tucker, G.J.: A longitudinal study of schizophrenic thinking. *Arch. Gener. Psychiat.* **28**, 179–182, 1973.
18. Hogarty, G. and Ulrich, R.F.: Temporal effect of drug and placebo in delaying relapse in schizophrenic outpatients. *Arch. Gen. Psy.* **34**, 279–301, 1977.
19. Keskiner, A., Zalcman, M.J., Ruppert, E.H., and Ulett, G.: The foster community; a partnership in psychiatric rehabilitation. *Am. J. Psychiat.* **129**, 283–287, 1972.
20. Klein, J.E., Person, T.M., Itil, T.M., and Marchbank, G.: Significant social variables in favorable community adjustment of schizophrenics. *Public Health Briefs* **64**, 813–814, 1974.
21. Kraeplin, E.: "Dementia Praecox and Paraphrenia," Livingstone, Edinburg, 1919.
22. Lamb, R.H., and Goertzel, V.: Discharged mental patients. Are they really in the community? *Arch. Gen. Psychiat.* **24**, 29–34, 1971.
23. Lamb, R.H., and Goertzel, V.: High expectation of long-term state hospital patients. *Am. J. Psychiat.* **129**, 471–475, 1972.
24. Langfeldt, G.: The prognosis in schizophrenia and the factors influencing the course of the disease. *Acta Psychiat. Scand.* Supplement **13**, 1937.
25. Langfeldt, G.: Prognosis in schizophrenia. *Acta Psychiat. Neurol. Scand.* (Suppl 110), 1956.
26. Leff, J.T., and Wing, J.K.: Trial of Maintenance Therapy in Schizophrenics *Br. Med. Journal* **2**, 599–604, 1971.
27. Leonhardt, K.: The question of prognosis in schizophrenia. *Inter. J. Psychiat.* **2**, 633–635, 1966.
28. Morrison, J.: The Iowa 500. *Arch. Gen. Psychiat.* **29**, 678–682, 1973.
29. Mosher, L.R., Reifman, A., and Menn, A.: Characteristics of nonprofessionals serving as primary therapists for acute schizophrenia. *Hosp. Comm. Psychiat.* **24**, 391–396, 1973.
30. Prien, R.F., Levine, J., and Switalski, R.W.: Discontinuation of chemotherapy in classic schizophrenia. Results from two collaborative studies. *Hosp. Comm. Psychiat.* **22**, 20–23, 1971.
31. Rachlin, S.: The Case Against Closing of State Hospitals. In *State Mental Hospitals* (P. Ahmed and S.C. Plog, eds.), pp. 31–44, Plenum, New York, 1976.
32. Reich, R., and Siegel, L.: The chronically mentally ill: Shuffle to oblivion. *Psychiat. Ann.* **3**, 35–55, 1974.
33. Rieder, R.O.: Hospitals, patients and politics. *Schizophrenia Bulletin* **10** (Winter) issue No. 11, 9–15, 1974.
34. Schneider, K. "Clinical Psychopathology." Grune and Stratton, New York, 1959.
35. Scully, D., and Windle, C.: An empirical study of the impact of federally funded CMHC on state mental hospital utilization. Unpublished report, National Institute of Mental Health, Rockville, Md., 1974.
36. Serban, G.: Loxapine in Acute Schizophrenic Disorder. Therapeutic Research Press, **25**, **1**, 139–143, 1979.

37. Serban, G., and Gidynski, C.B.: Relationship Between Cognitive Deficit, Affect Response, and Community Adjustment in Chronic Schizophrenics. *Br. J. Psychiat.* **134**, 601–604, 1979.
38. Serban, G.: Mental Status, Functioning and Stress in Chronic Schizophrenic Patients in Community Care. *Am. J. Psychiat.,* **136, 7,** 948–950, 1979.
39. Serban, G., and Gidynsky, C.B.: Differentiating Criteria for Acute-Chronic Distinction in Schizophrenia. *Arch. Gen. Psychiat.* **32,** 705–711, 1975.
40. Serban, G., and Thomas, A.: Attitudes and behaviors of acute and chronic schizophrenic patients regarding ambulatory treatment. *Am. J. Psychiat.* **131,** 991–995, 1974.
41. Serban, G., Functioning and stress of schizophrenics in community adjustment, in Serban, G. (ed.) *New Trends of Psychiatry in the Community.* Ballinger Publishing Co., Cambridge, Mass., 1977.
42. Strrauss, J.S., and Carpenter, W.T. J.: The Prediction of Outcome in Schizophrenia. *Arch. Gen. Psychiat.* **31,** 37–42, 1974.
43. Smith, W.G., Kaplan, J., and Siker, D.: Community mental health and the seriously disturbed patient. *Arch. Gen. Psychiat.* **30,** 693–696, 1974.
44. Stein, L.I., and Test, M.A.: Training in community living: One-year evaluation. A symposium. Follow-up studies of community care. *Am. J. Psychiat.* **133,** 917–918, 1976.
45. Stevens, B.: Evaluation of rehabilitation for psychotic patients living in the community. *Acta Psychiat. Scand.* **49,** 169–180, 1973.
46. Wijsenbeek, J., Steiner, M., and Goldberg, S.C.: Trifluoperazine: A comparison between regular and high doses. *Psychopharmcologia,* **36,** 147–150, 1974.
47. Yolles, S.F.: Community psychiatry: 1963–1974. *J. Operational Psychiat.* **6,** 142–151, 1975.
48. Zigler, E., and Phillips, L.: Social competence and outcome in psychiatric disorder. *J. Abnorm. Soc. Psychol.* **63,** 264–271, 1962.
49. Zigler, E., and Phillips, L.: Social competence and the process-reactive distinction in psychopathology. *J. Abnorm. Soc. Psychol.* **65,** 215–222, Oct. 1962.
50. Zigler, E. and Levine, J.: Premorbid adjustment and paranoid-non paranoid status in schizophrenia: A further investigation. *Journal of Abnormal Psychol.* **82:** 189–199, 1973.
51. Zeisset, R.M.: Desensitization and relaxation in the modification of psychiatric patients' interview behavior. *J. Abnorm. Psychol.* **73**(1), 18–24, 1968.

Appendix A
M.A.A.I.S.*
(Motivation Bellevue Scale)

Date ....

....
Name   (last)   (first)

Project # ....

Occupation	(X₁)

(X_1)

```
Occupation

 1 ............................
 2 ............................
 3 ............................
 4 ............................
 5 ............................
 6 ............................
 7 ............................
 8 ............................
 9 ............................
10 ............................
```

Raw Score Factors

(Self Appraisal and Improvement)
General Goals:
$Y_1 = 0.4\,D2 + D3 + D4 + G2 + G3 + G4$

Vocational Aspirations:
$Y_2 = J4 + P4 + S4$

Vocational Self-Concept:
$Y_3 = J2 + J3 + P2 + P3 + S2 + S3$

Achievement:
$Y_4 = 0.6\,D1 + G1 + J1 + P1 + S1$

School-Grade (X_2)

1	2	3	4	5
7	8	9	10	11
6	7	8	9	10
12	13	14	15	16

Intelligence Factor (X_3)

Standardized Score Factors

(Self-Appraisal and Improvement)
General Goals:
$Y_1^S = Y_1 + .056\,X_1 - .721\,X_3 - 42.971$

Vocational Aspirations:
$Y_1^S = Y_1 - 13.013$

Vocational Self-Concept:
$Y_3^S = Y_3 - .949\,X_2 - 35.947$

Achievment:
$Y_4^S = Y_4 + .04\quad X_1 - .891\quad X_2 - .744$
$X_3 - 173\quad X_4 - 22.560$

	AGE	F	(X_4)
1	16–17	11	
2	18–19	12	
3	20–21	13	
4	22–24	14	
5	25–27	15	
6	28–31	16	
7	32–35	17	
8	36–40	18	
9	41–45	19	
10	46–52	20	

AGE
18–24
25–40
41–52

Total

$Z = .24\,Y_1^S - .72\,Y_2^S - .17\,Y_3^S - .01\,Y_4$

DID YOU EVER

Please indicate by writing 'no' or 'yes' whether you have (or have not) *ever engaged* in the following:

_____	graduate from a school	_____	earn respect
_____	have a job	_____	reach a goal
_____	sell things	_____	enjoy house-cleaning
_____	control temper	_____	accept responsibility
_____	draw sketches	_____	take photos
_____	do office work	_____	work with wood
_____	make good money	_____	help elect someone
_____	accept demanding tasks	_____	try to impress someone
_____	instruct or tutor someone	_____	play music
_____	drive a vehicle	_____	get bored/tire easily
_____	feel mentally well	_____	try not to daydream
_____	perform on stage	_____	work with people
_____	read much	_____	satisfy sexual needs
_____	dress properly	_____	work for government
_____	set or cut hair	_____	fix clothes
_____	investigate something	_____	help sick people
_____	fix things	_____	run errands
_____	lead a group	_____	own a home
_____	shop efficiently	_____	learn a skill
_____	maintain high standards	_____	understand yourself
_____	have a hobby	_____	worry about tomorrow
_____	fall in love	_____	go on a diet
_____	enjoy studying minds	_____	handle finances
_____	cook a meal	_____	serve food
_____	direct an activity	_____	have admirers

COULD YOU LEARN

Please indicate by writing 'no' or 'yes' whether you think you *could learn* (or not learn) any of the following:

_____	in school (now)	_____	to achieve respect
_____	a (new) job	_____	to be ambitious
_____	sales work	_____	to clean house/offices
_____	self-control	_____	to be responsible
_____	drawing	_____	photographic work
_____	clerical work	_____	wood work/finishing
_____	to earn more	_____	about politics
_____	to cope with challenges	_____	to impress people
_____	how to teach	_____	a musical instrument
_____	how to drive (better)	_____	to persevere/sustain effort
_____	to be mentally better	_____	to daydream less
_____	to act/perform	_____	to counsel people
_____	to read faster	_____	to function well sexually
_____	to dress better	_____	a civil service job
_____	hair styling/cutting	_____	to tailor clothes
_____	problem-solving	_____	to treat sick people
_____	mechanical work	_____	message delivery
_____	to direct organizations	_____	to keep up a home
_____	to shop on a budget	_____	a (new) skill
_____	better standards	_____	more about yourself
_____	a (new) hobby	_____	to plan ahead
_____	to love somebody	_____	weight control
_____	about human behavior	_____	bookkeeping/accounting
_____	to cook better	_____	food service
_____	to supervise work	_____	to be more popular

WOULD YOU LIKE

Please indicate by writing 'no' or 'yes' whether you *would like* (or not like) any of the following:

_____	being in school	_____	being respected
_____	working in a job	_____	to achieve your goal
_____	commercial selling	_____	cleaning work
_____	having self-control	_____	having responsibility
_____	sketching	_____	photographing
_____	typing, filing	_____	wood-working
_____	to increase your income	_____	political office
_____	challenging situations	_____	to impress people
_____	teaching	_____	to play an instrument
_____	to drive vehicles	_____	to pursue a task/goal
_____	to be mentally well	_____	to not live in fantasy
_____	stage acting	_____	to help people adjust
_____	to read better	_____	to improve sexually
_____	to dress well/better	_____	to serve in government
_____	to cut and set hair	_____	tailoring
_____	to solve mysteries	_____	giving medical treatment
_____	mechanics	_____	delivering things
_____	organizing people	_____	owning a home
_____	to shop thriftily	_____	to have a (new) skill
_____	higher standards	_____	to know yourself better
_____	to have a hobby	_____	planning the future
_____	falling in love	_____	to look physically well
_____	studying minds	_____	to work with records of money
_____	cooking	_____	serving meals
_____	to supervise work	_____	to be well known

WILL YOU BECOME

Please indicate by writing 'no' or 'yes' whether you *intend to be* (or not be) any of the following:

_____ a student or trainee	_____ a respected person
_____ a job-holder	_____ a "go-getter"
_____ a salesman/saleslady	_____ a house/office cleaner
_____ self-disciplined	_____ a responsible worker
_____ an illustrator	_____ a photographer
_____ an office worker	_____ a wood worker/finisher
_____ a high earner	_____ a politician
_____ resourceful/expedient	_____ impressive to/admired by others
_____ a teacher/instructor	_____ a musician
_____ a (good) driver	_____ highly efficient
_____ mentally healthier	_____ more realistic
_____ a performer	_____ a social worker
_____ a good reader	_____ sexually masterful/expert
_____ well-dressed	_____ a civil service employee
_____ a hair setter/cutter	_____ a tailor/seamstress
_____ an investigator/researcher	_____ a medic/nurse
_____ a mechanic	_____ a messenger
_____ a leader/manager	_____ a home owner
_____ a thrifty shopper	_____ a skilled worker
_____ follower of high standards	_____ more self-understanding
_____ a hobbyist	_____ future-minded
_____ in love	_____ physically fit
_____ a mental health worker	_____ a bookkeeper/accountant
_____ a cook/chef	_____ a waiter/waitress
_____ a foreman/supervisor	_____ a famous person

Appendix B

SAMPLE OF THE FUNCTIONING AND STRESS

QUESTIONS FROM SSFIPD

Instrumental Performance

Education 1

16. How far (did you go) (have you gone) in school? (Circle highest)

    00. Eighth grade not completed
    11. Eighth grade completed   27,28 __/__
    12. Tenth grade completed
    23. High school degree or equivalency certificate
    24. Two years' college completed
    25. College degree
    26. Entered graduate school
    27. Graduate degree

17. How much are you bothered (upset) by the level of education that you have achieved?

    0. Greatly bothered
    1. Somewhat bothered   29 _____
    2. Not bothered (Go to Q. 19)

19. How much education do you have compared to your family as a whole?

    01. Much less   33,34 __/__
    12. Less
    23. Same   ⎫
    24. More (higher)   ⎬
    97. INAP, No family   ⎭   (Go to Q. 21)
    98. Don't know

(If 19 Is 01 or 12, ASK 20)

20. Do you feel bothered (upset) by this?

    0. Greatly bothered   35 ____

    1. Somewhat bothered

    2. Not bothered

    9. INAP (No family or not less educated)

(If the person has left school or a training program without completing the degree or diploma he was working for)

24. Why did you leave school or training? (Circle more than one if necessary)

Yes	No	INAP or Never dropped out		Reason	
0	2	9	a.	Mental illness or nervousness in school	43 ____
0	2	9	b.	Unable to learn (schoolwork was above your head)	44 ____
0	2	9	c.	Asked to leave because of behavior	45 ____
1	2	9	d.	Couldn't afford to stay in school; felt school made no difference to future; or other "functional" reason (specify) _____	46 ____

If columns 43– 46 are 9, go to Q. 26

(If 24 not 9)

25. How do you feel about dropping out?

    0. Bad   47 ____

    1. Indifferent

    2. Good

    9. INAP (Never dropped out)   48 ____

34. In what ways has your education affected you in life?

    01. Made you feel inferior to other people

    02. Held you back in life   72,73 _/_

    03. Both 1 and 2

    14. Didn't affect you one way or another or don't know

    28. Helped you through life

35. Is there any problem that you had with education that upset you so much that it directly contributed to your hospitalization? (If yes) What was the problem?

    1. No problem (Go to Q. 37)

    2. Mentioned above in question ____   74,75,76 _/_/_

    3. Other (specify) _____

Job 1

37. What was (your) (his/her) work situation right before coming to Bellevue? (If previously hospitalized) What was (your) (his/her) work situation before going to that hospital?

    01. Never employed (Go to Q. 39).
    02. Unemployed or dropout   8,9 __/__
    11. Employed part-time—temporary work
    12. Retired
    21. Student (currently enrolled)
    22. Housewife
    23. Employed—on sick leave
    24. Employed full-time and working
    25. Student and employed
    26. Student and housewife
    27. Employed and housewife
    98. Don't know

40. Patient: What is the major reason for your present unemployment? Informant: As far as you know, what is the major reason for his/her present unemployment? (Circle all that apply)

    Code Instructions
    If 01–06 code '0' in col. 13, otherwise 9.
    If 11 or 12, code 1 in col. 14, otherwise 9.
    If 21–25, code 2 in col. 15, otherwise 9.

    01. Left because of nervous breakdown   13 ____
    02. Was laid off or fired because couldn't do job
    03. Was fired because of friction with supervisor   14 ____
    04. Was fired because of friction with co-workers
    05. Was fired because of irresponsibility (late, absent, goof off, drunk on job)   15 ____
    11. Left because of physical illness
    21. Left because of household or family responsibilities (woman)
    22. Left to retire
    23. Left to go to school
    24. Was laid off (for non-invidious reasons) or quit Other (specify)

    97. INAP., working or never worked
    98. Don't know

(If 40 is 01–05, go to Q. 42)

41. Was there any problem with the job before hospitalization?

    01. Was unable to concentrate or to function   16,17 __/__

    02. Was getting mentally ill

    03. Too depressed to work or go to work

    15. The job made (you) (him/her) too anxious—upset. Other (specify)

    _____

    29. No problem

    97. INAP. (Q. 40 is 01–05)

    98. Don't know

(If patient is student or housewife who is not expected and/or doesn't expect himself/herself to work, circle the Y below and go to Q. 48).

    Y.

42. How long have you been out of work?

    01. Over five years   18,19 __/__

    02. Over two, up to five years

    03. Over one, up to two years

    04. Over six months, up to one year

    15. Over three, up to six months

    16. Over one, up to three months

    27. Up to one month

    28. Employment terminated by present hospitalization

    97. INAP.

(If Q. 42 is 28 or 97, skip to Q. 47)

43. How troubled are you about being out of work (not working)?

    0. Very much troubled

    1. Troubled   20 ____

    2. Not at all or indifferent

    9. INAP.   21 __9__

(If 43 is yes)

46. What kind of difficulty (have you) (has he/she) had getting work? (Circle more than one if necessary)

    _____
    Code Instruction
    If 01–03, code 0 in col. 25; otherwise 9.
    If 14 or 15, code 1 in col. 26, otherwise 9.   25 ____
    If 26–27, code 2 in col. 27, otherwise 9.   26 ____
    If only 98, Don't know, is circled, code 8 in cols. 25–27. 27 ____
    _____

01. They constantly refuse to hire (me) (him/her) (unable to pass the interview)
02. Not hired because of (alleged) physical or mental problem
14. Not trying hard enough or other psychological reasons
26. Can't find work that (I am) (he/she is) qualified for Other (specify)

_____

98. Don't know

51. Would you like to change from your main line of work to a different kind of work? (If student or housewife with a job, ask about the job.)

    0. Don't want to work
    1. Very much
    2. Somewhat   42 _____
    3. No
    9. INAP. (45 is 02)

(If 45 is not 02 ''Not interested in work'')
52. Could you be satisfied if you did not get the type of work you want?

    01. Extremely dissatisfied   44,45 _/_
    12. Somewhat dissatisfied
    23. Doesn't matter
    24. Already have the kind of work I want
    97. INAP (45 is 02)

57. Has your ability to do your job over the last five years . . .

    01. Declined markedly
    12. Declined somewhat   56,57 _/_
    13. Fluctuated
    24. Remained the same }
    25. Improved   } (Go to Q. 59)
    97. INAP

(If declined)
58. Are you upset about this?

    01. Very upset   58,59 _/_
    12. Somewhat upset
    23. Indifferent
    24. Not at all
    97. INAP. (57 is 24 or 25)   60,61 _9/7_

59. Is there any problem you have with work or unemployment that upset you so much that it directly contributed to your hospitalization? (If yes) What was the problem?

    1. No problem (Go to Q. 61)   62 ____
    2. Mentioned above in question ____   63 ____
    3. Other (Specify) _____   64 ____

Housekeeping and Shopping 1

61. Do you have any difficulty getting things done at home?

    01. Unable to do the work altogether
    12. Often   66,67 __/__
    23. Sometimes
    24. None or rarely
    97. Not responsible for housework (Go to Q. 66)

63. What is the major factor interfering with your housework? (Circle more than one if necessary)

    No   Yes
    2   0   a. Uninterested or unable to start   69 ____
    2   0   b. Feeling confused—forgetful   70 ____
    2   0   c. Get bogged down by details   71 ____
    2   0   d. Never able to finish on time   72 ____
    2   0   e. Other (specify) _____   73 ____
                                                          74 _9_

64. How upset do you get about housework (or the complaints of other people, if any)?

    0. Very upset
    1. Somewhat upset   75 ____
    2. Not at all upset
    9. INAP.

68. Is there any problem you have with housekeeping and shopping that upsets you so much that it directly contributed to your hospitalization? (If yes) What was the problem?

    1. No problem (Go to Q. 70)   13,14,15 _/_/_
    2. Mentioned above in question _____
    3. Other (specify) _____
    9. INAP.

Welfare or Assistance Program (Workmen's Compensation, Veterans or Other Agency) 1

70. How much experience (have you) (has he/she) had in the past with Welfare?

    00. Almost entire life, childhood to present
    01. In and out of Welfare   17,18 _/_
    02. Most of adult life
    13. Grew up on Welfare
    14. Parents on Welfare for a while when growing up
    26. None or very little (emergency Welfare) (Go to Q. 72)
    98. Don't know

73. Did you work to supplement your Welfare or Assistance income with odd jobs (babysitting, neighborhood jobs, etc.)?

    0. No
    1. Yes   22 _____
    8. Don't know   9. INAP.
    9. INAP.

74. Do you feel that being on Welfare or Assistance is having a bad effect on yourself and your family?

    01. Upset by the change in social standards
    02. Upset by the bad effect of Welfare or Assistance (losing self-esteem)   23,24 _/_
    13. Somewhat
    24. Not at all
    97. INAP., Not on Welfare   25,26 _/_

77. Do you get upset by dealing with the personnel of the Welfare Department or other social agencies?

    0. Very much
    1. Somewhat   32 _____
    2. Little or not at all
    9. INAP., Not on Welfare

Finances 1

78. What is (your) (his/her) main source of income? Another? What is it?

    0. No income

    1. Own job   33 ____

    2. Spouse's job

    3. Relatives   34 ____

    4. Welfare or Assistance program

    5. Unemployment insurance   35 ____

    6. Illegal activity

    7. Other source (pension, etc.) (specify) _____

    8. Don't know

    9. No second or third mention

80. (If Patient) How well do you get by on your income?
(If Informant Lives With Patient) How (do you and he/she) (does your family) get by on your (Family) income?
(If Informant Does Not Live With Patient) How well does he/she get by on his/her income?

    1. Severe strain   37 ____

    2. Some strain

    3. Can live modestly

    4. Get by very well

    8. Don't know

81. How does (your) (his/her) present income compare with that of (your) (his/her) parents while (you were) (he/she was) growing up?

    1. Much lower   38 ____

    2. Somewhat lower

    3. The same

    4. Somewhat higher   (Go to Q. 83)

    5. Much higher

    8. Don't know

(If lower, 2 or 1 in Q. 81)

82. As far as you can tell, how (upset are you) (upset is he/she) about the drop in living standard?

    01. Very upset
    12. A little
    23. Resigned to it   39,40 _/_
    24. Not at all or a little upset
    97. INAP. (81 is 3,4,5, or 8)
    98. Don't know

Living Circumstances 1

88. How comfortable did (you) (he/she) feel in the last place (you) (he/she) lived before coming to the hospital?

    0. Didn't like home at all
    1. Comfortable only for short periods of time   51 ____
    2. Found home comfortable
    8. Don't know
    9. INAP. (Never had a home)

(If 89 not 0)

90. How upset are you about your living circumstances?

    0. Very upset
    1. Upset   54 ____
    2. Indifferent
    9. INAP. (89 is 0)   55 _9_

(If 89 not 0)

91. Have you done anything to improve your living conditions?

    0. No
    1. Tried without success   56 ____
    2. Tried with some success
    9. INAP. (89 is 0)

92. Is there any problem you have with finances, Welfare or living circumstances that upset you so much that it directly contributed to your hospitalization? (If yes) What was the problem?

    1. No problem (Go to Q. 94)
    2. Mentioned above in question ____   57,58,59 _/_/
    3. Other (specify) _____

Family Interaction

Parents

96. Was your family broken before you reached the age of sixteen?

    (1) How was your family broken? (Give first one if more than one)

        1. Divorce/separation/illegitimate
        2. Long term prison (Three years)   69 ____
        3. Long term mental illness (Three years)
        4. Death
        5. No

    (2) If so, how old were you?

        ____ . Age of patient at marked event   70,71 __/__
                                                           72 __9__

98. How (do) (does) (did) (you) (he/she) get along with (your) (his/her) parents
    (mother, father)? With the people whom (you think) (he/she thinks) of as
    (your) (his/her) parents?

    (Got) (gets) along with mother (or mother figure)

        01. Terribly
        12. Poorly
        23. Fair   74,75 __/__
        24. Well
        97. INAP. (No mother or recollection of her)
        98. Don't know

101. How much (do you) (does he/she) depend on either or both of (your)
     (his/her) parents for emotional, social or material support?

        10. Very much
        11. Somewhat   9,10 __/__
        22. Not at all or little
        98. Don't know
        97. INAP.

103. (Are you) (Is he/she) upset about any problem (you) (he/she) may have in asking for or getting help from (your) (his/her) parents?

    0. Very upset
    1. Somewhat   19 ____
    2. Not upset or a little
    8. Don't know
    9. INAP.

104. How much pressure (do you) (does he/she) think (you have) (he/she has) to take in living or dealing with either or both of (your) (his/her) parents?

    01. Very much   20,21 _/_
    12. Some
    23. None or a little
    24. Doesn't have dealing with parents
    97. INAP.
    98. Don't know   22,23 _9/7_

105. Is there any problem you have or had with your parents that upset you so much that it directly contributed to your hospitalization? (If yes) What was the problem?

    1. No problem (Go to Q. 107)
    2. Mentioned above in question ____   24,25,26 _/ /_
    3. Other (specify) _____

108. Generally speaking, how do you get along with your brother(s) (and/or) sister(s)?

With how many do you get along . . .

    a. Well ____   30 ____
    b. So so or no contact (not due to argument) ____   31 ____
    c. Badly ____   32 ____

(Code: 0 = None; 9 = No siblings)   33 _9_

110. How much do you depend on your brother(s) (and/or) sister(s) for emotional, social or material support?

    0. Very much
    1. Somewhat   36 _____
    2. A little or not at all
    9. INAP.

111. Do you ever ask for help from your brother(s) (and/or) sister(s)?
(YES) How often (do) (does) (he) (she) (they) give you the help you want?
How do you feel if your brother(s) (and/or) sister(s) don't give you the help you want?

    01. Very upset   37,38 __/__
    12. Somewhat upset
    23. Makes no difference
    24. They always give me help
    25. Don't ask for help
    97. INAP., No siblings

113. How well do you get along with the relatives (other than brother(s) and sister(s) on whom you depend most? (If more than one, the one with whom you get along best)

    01. Terribly   40,41 __/__
    12. Poorly
    13. Fair
    24. Well
    97. None

115. (Patient) How do you feel if your close relatives don't give you the help you want?
(Informant) How does (he/she) feel if (his/her) close relatives don't give (him/her) the help (he/she) wants?

    01. Very upset   44,45 __/__
    12. Somewhat upset
    23. Makes no difference
    24. They always give me help
    25. Don't ask for help
    98. Don't know
    97. INAP.

116. Is there any problem (you have) (he/she has) with (your) (his/her) brothers, sisters or close relatives that upset (you) (him/her) so much that it directly contributed to (your) (his/her) hospitalization?
(If yes) What was the problem?

     1. No problem (Go to Q. 118)
     2. Mentioned above in question _____   46,47,48 _/_/_
     3. Other (Specify) _____
     8. Don't know
     9. INAP   } (Go to Q. 118)

Marriage 1

(If ever divorced, separated or terminated common-law)
121. How many divorces, separations or terminations of common-law were initiated by you (him/her) and how many by (your) (his/her) spouse?

     a. _____ patient   56 _____
     b. _____ spouse   57 _____
     c. _____ mutual agreement   58 _____
     8. Don't know - Record this 8 in the appropriate column(s) for Q. 121.
     9. INAP. (120a and c are 0 or 120 is 9)

122. How did the (most recent) divorce, separation, death or termination of common-law relationship affect (you) (him/her)?

     01. Very upset   59,60 _/_
     12. Somewhat upset
     23. Did not care or mixed feelings
     24. Happy
     97. INAP. (118 is not 40 or 50 and 119 is 0)
     98. Don't know

Marriage 3

(If ever divorced, separated or terminated common-law)
123. Why did (your) (his/her) marriage(s) or common-law relationship(s) break up? (Circle # of times each reason applies)

INAP	Don't know	2 or more	1	No	Reason		
9	8	0	0	2	a.	Patient couldn't function sexually (frigidity—impotence)	61 _____
9	8	0	0	2	b.	Spouse couldn't function sexually (frigidity—impotence)	62 _____
9	8	0	0	2	c.	Sexual incompatibility—different sex needs	63 _____
9	8	0	0	2	d.	Patient unable to support family (husband) or patient unable to take care of house and children (wife)	64 _____
9	8	0	0	2	e.	Spouse unable to support family (husband) or spouse unable to take care of the house and children (wife)	65 _____
9	8	0	0	2	f.	Unfaithfulness on the part of spouse or patient	66 _____
9	8	0	0	2	g.	Couldn't get along with each other	67 _____
9	8	0	0	2	h.	Interference from relatives or parents	68 _____
9	8	0	0	2	i.	Nonacceptance of (your) (his/her) mental illness by spouse	69 _____
9	8	0	0	2	j.	Differences on how to bring up children	70 _____
9	8	0	0	2	k.	Out of love—loss of interest—(either party)	71 _____
9	8	0	0	2	l.	Patient's antisocial behavior (drinking, drugs, physical violence, prison)	72 _____
9	8	0	0	2	m.	Spouse's antisocial behavior (drinking, drugs, physical violence, prison)	73 _____
9	8	0	0	2	n.	Differences on money matters	74 _____
9	8	0	0	2	o.	Other is S	75 _ __
9	8	0	0	2	p.	Other is NF	76 _____
					q.	Other (Specify):	

126. What problems leading to conflict in the present marriage/relationship upset you most? (Very much = 0; Somewhat = 1) (Circle more than one if necessary) (If INAP., code 9)

Very Much	Somewhat	No			
0	1	2	a.	Patient can't function sexually (frigidity, impotence)	10 _____
0	1	2	b.	Spouse can't function sexually (frigidity, impotence)	11 _____
0	1	2	c.	Sexual incompatibility—different sex needs	12 _____
0	1	2	d.	Patient unable to support family (husband) or patient unable to take care of house and children (wife)	13 _____
0	1	2	e.	Spouse unable to support family (husband) or spouse unable to take care of the house and children (wife)	14 _____
0	1	2	f.	Unfaithfulness on the part of spouse or patient	15 _____
0	1	2	g.	Can't get along with each other	16 _____
0	1	2	h.	Interference from relatives or parents	17 _____
0	1	2	i.	Nonacceptance of your mental illness by spouse	18 _____
0	1	2	j.	Differences on how to bring up children	19 _____
0	1	2	k.	Out of love—loss of interest (either party)	20 _____
0	1	2	l.	Patient's antisocial behavior (drinking, drugs, physical violence, prison)	21 _____
0	1	2	m.	Spouse's antisocial behavior (drinking, drugs, physical violence, prison)	22 _____
0	1	2	n.	Other (Specify)_____	
				(1) Other is S	23 _____
				(2) Other is NF	24 _____

128. Does the way in which the differences in your marriage are usually dealt with or solved upset you?

    0. Very upset   43 _____
    1. Somewhat or a little upset
    2. Not at all
    9. INAP.   44 _____

130. How do you feel when your spouse/partner is not concerned with your work and problems?

    0. Very upset   46 __9__
    1. Somewhat upset
    2. Indifferent
    2. Spouse/partner always shows concern
    9. INAP.

(If marital relationship or functional equivalent)

131. Is there any problem you have with your marriage/relationship that upset you so much that it directly contributed to your hospitalization? (If yes) What was the problem?

    1. No problem (Go to Q. 133)   47,48,49 _/_/_
    2. Mentioned above in question ____
    3. Other (Specify) _____
    9. INAP. (Go to Q. 133)

Children 1

137. If some of (your) (his/her) minor children are not living with (you) (him/her), (are you) (is he/she) upset about the arrangement?

    01. Upset regardless of place   57,58 _/_
    12. Upset because with agency
    13. Upset because in foster home
    14. Upset because with parents
    15. Upset because with relative
    26. Not upset
    97. INAP. (All living with patient)
    98. Don't know

(If child (children) is (are) living with patient)

139. How much time do you spend with your child (children) at home?

    01. None   61,62 _/_
    02. Rarely
    13. See them on weekends
    24. One hour a day
    25. A lot
    97. INAP. (136 is 0)

140. How upset do you feel about your relationship with or the doings of your children (or the one who causes you the most upset)?

    0. Very upset   63 ____
    1. Somewhat
    2. Not at all or a little upset
    9. INAP. (136 is 0)   64 _9_

(If there are children at home)

143. How much trouble do you have taking care of your children? Are you troubled or guilty about any difficulty you might have in caring for your children?
(Circle one stress and one functionability item)

    01. Unable to care for them   68,69 _/_
    02. A lot of trouble, but able to care for them
    13. Some trouble, but able to care for them
    24. No problem
    97. INAP., no children at home
    98. Don't know

    01. Troubled or guilty because someone else has to take care of them
                                            70,71 _/_
    12. Troubled or guilty about not being able to take good care of them
    24. No guilt or troubled feelings
    97. INAP., no children at home

145. Is there any problem you have with your children that upset you so much that it directly contributed to your hospitalization? (If yes) What was the problem?

    1. No problem (Go to Q. 147)   73,74,75 _/_/_
    2. Mentioned above in question ____
    3. Other (specify) _____

Social-Interpersonal Interaction

Dating

150. How interested (are you) (is he/she) in dating the preferred or opposite sex?

    01. Wants to have nothing to do with them   14,15 __/__
    02. Tries to avoid their company
    13. Indifferent
    14. Somewhat interested
    25. Very interested
    98. Don't know

153. (Do you) (does he/she) have difficulty getting or holding a girlfriend (boyfriend)? (Mark one for getting and one for holding)

Getting: 00. Not interested   18,19 __/__
            01. Very much
            13. Somewhat
            25. Never
            98. Don't know about getting

Holding: 00. Can't get one   20,21 _9/7_
            01. Very much
            13. Somewhat
            25. None
            98. Don't know about holding

(If 153 is 01 or 13 for either getting or holding)
154. How much do you worry, get upset about it (the area of greater difficulty)?

    0. Very upset   22 _____
    1. Somewhat upset
    2. Doesn't matter
    9. INAP. (153 is not 01 or 13 for getting or holding)

155. How do you usually feel when you are dating (your preferred sex)?

    0. Feel uneasy or guilty   23 _____
    1. Feel indifferent
    2. Feel good
    9. INAP.

Social-Interpersonal Interaction

Sex 1 (to be asked of everybody)

158. In general, do you have or have you had difficulty in developing a sexual relationship with a member of the preferred sex?

    01. Have not tried   32,33 _/_
    02. Unable to develop a sexual relationship (always have difficulty)
    03. Usually have difficulty
    14. Sometimes have difficulty
    25. Rarely or never have difficulty (Go to Q. 160)

(If 158 not 25)
159. Are you worried about your difficulty in developing a sexual relationship with a member of the preferred sex?

    0. Extremely worried   34 ____
    1. Moderately worried
    2. Indifferent
    9. INAP., (158 is 25)

(If any sexual difficulties cited in Q. 160)
161. How much are you worried by your sexual difficulty?

    01. A great deal   44,45 _/_
    12. Somewhat
    23. Not at all or a little
    97. INAP. (no sexual difficulty in Q. 160)

(If separated or not married, circle Y below and go to Q. 166)

    Y.   46 _9_

166. Is there any problem you have with dating and/or sex that upset you so much that it directly contributed to your hospitalization? (If yes) What was the problem?

    1. No problem (Go to Q. 168)   54,55,56 _//_
    2. Mentioned above in question ____
    3. Other (Specify) _____

Social Life—Close Friends 1

168. (Do you) does he/she) find it hard to make friends?

    0. Yes   58 ____
    1. Not interested
    2. No
    8. Don't know

170. Does it upset (you that you) (him/her that he/she) don't/doesn't have any, or that (you don't) (he/she doesn't) have more close friends?

    0. Very upset   61 ____
    1. A little or somewhat upset
    2. Not upset
    8. Don't know
    9. INAP.

174. How well do you get along with your friends?

    0. Poorly   68 ____
    1. Fair
    2. Well
    9. INAP., has no friends (Go to Q. 176)

(If 176 response not 9)
177. How (were you) (was he/she) affected by the loss of a close friend for one reason or another?

    0. Felt badly   15 ____
    1. Moderately upset
    2. Not upset
    8. Don't know
    9. INAP., (176 is 9)

Social Life—Neighbors 1

178. How friendly are you with your neighbors?

    01. Unfriendly   16,17 __/__
    02. Indifferent or little contact
    13. Somewhat friendly
    24. Friendly
    97. INAP.

181. Are you upset by any aspects of your relations with the people in your building or neighborhood? (e.g., Don't get along, not enough contact, etc.)

    0. Very upset   22 ____

    1. Somewhat upset

    2. Not upset or a little upset

Social Life—Relationship to Other People 1

182. How do you feel you are treated by people in general? (Circle more than one if necessary) (This is a geometric code. Sum the responses and put the total in col. 23–24)

    01. Feel they take advantage of me   23,24 _/_

    02. Feel they act insultingly

    04. Feel they avoid, dislike or ignore me

    20. Fairly   25,26 9/7

183. How do you feel about dealing with authorities (police, court, hospitals)?

    0. Very upset   27 ____

    1. Somewhat or a little upset

    2. Indifferent

186. Do you usually stay by yourself? (If yes) Is this because you are uneasy with other people? (If don't stay by self) Are you uneasy with other people?

    01. Yes, stay by self, due to uneasiness   30,31 _/_

    02. Stay by self, but not due to uneasiness

    23. Don't stay by self, but feel uneasy

    24. Don't stay by self, and don't feel uneasy

190. How active is (your) (his/her) social life?

    0. Inactive   37 ____

    1. Somewhat active

    2. Active

    8. Don't know

191. How (do you) (does he/she) feel about (your) (his/her) social life as a whole?

    01. Upset   38,39 _/_
    12. Displeased
    23. Indifferent
    24. Pleased
    98. Don't know

Social Life—Spare Time Interest

192. How often do you read a book for pleasure?

    0. Not at all   40 ___
    1. Rarely
    2. Often or usually

196. How often do you engage in some hobby?

    0. Not at all   44 ___
    1. Rarely
    2. Often or usually

    (If any hobby) What hobby?

(If 1 or 2 in any of Q's 189–196)
197. How much are you upset by an inability to pursue any of the following because of lack of funds? (Circle more than one if necessary) (Code instructions: 0 if very much checked; 1 if somewhat checked; 2 if not checked; 9 if enough funds)

Very much	Somewhat	Not			
0	1	2	a.	Movies—theaters _____	45 ___
0	1	2	b.	Sports events _____	
0	1	2	c.	TV watching _____	
0	1	2	d.	Making small trips ____Number	
		2	e.	None of events	46 ___

(If yes)
200. How upset are you because of your difficulty in traveling or taking a walk?

    0. Very upset
    1. Somewhat
    2. Not at all or a little upset
    9. INAP. (199 is no)

Social Life—Religion 1

202. How strong are your religious beliefs?

    1. None or slight   59 _____

    2. Moderate

    3. Strong

    4. Extremely preoccupied with religious thoughts

Social Maladaptive Activities

Drinking 1

208. If (you drink) (he/she drinks), to what level of inebriation (do you) (does he/she) go? (Circle highest level)

    00. Getting "the shakes"   10,11 _/_

    01. Losing consciousness

    02. Losing track of everything

    03. Getting drunk

    15. Getting high (feeling good)

    27. Doesn't drink or casual social drinking

         Other (Specify) _____

(If 207 is 14,15, or 26 and 208 is 27 or 28, circle Y below and go to Q. 214)

    Y.

210. What are (your) (his/her) main reasons for drinking? (Circle up to three if necessary)

    1. To be able to work   13,14,15 _/_/_

    2. To relieve mental distress (anxiety, depression)

    3. To take his/her mind off personal problems

    4. To relate to others socially or sexually

       Other (Specify) _____

    8. Don't know

    9. INAP., does not drink

    0. No second or third reason given

211. Does (your) (his/her) drinking upset you because it interferes with . . .

		Yes	Somewhat	No	INAP	
a.	Working	0	1	2	9	16 ____
b.	Family life	0	1	2	9	17 ____
c.	Social life	0	1	2	9	18 ____
d.	Sexual life	0	1	2	9	19 ____

Number of problems created by drinking   20 ____

213. Do you feel that drinking has something to do with making (you) (him/her) mentally ill or bringing (you) (him/her) to the hospital?

    0. Yes, does make me ill   22 ____
    1. Sometimes
    2. No
    8. Don't know
    9. INAP.

Drugs—Addictive 1

215. What (do you) (does he/she) take? (Circle more than one if necessary)

    Code Instructions:
    This is a geometric
    code. Sum the total of responses and
    put the total in cols. 24–25.

    01. Heroin   24,25 __/__
    02. Barbiturates
    04. Speed or other amphetamines
    08. Others (specify) _____
    97. None (2 in Q. 214)
    98. Don't know

217. What is (your) (his/her) main reason for taking drugs?

    1. To be able to work   28 ____
    2. Relieve mental distress (anxiety, depression)
    3. To take his/her mind off other things (family, sex, etc.)
    4. Other (specify) _____
    8. Don't know
    9. INAP., does not take drugs

218. Does (your) (his/her) taking drugs upset you because it interferes
     with. . . .

		Yes	Somewhat	No	INAP	
a.	Working	0	1	2	9	29 _____
b.	Family life	0	1	2	9	30 _____
c.	Social life	0	1	2	9	31 _____
d.	Sexual life	0	1	2	9	32 _____

Drugs—Psychedelics

222. How many "trips" did you have?

    20. None   37,38 __/__
    11. One
    02. Two
    03. Three
    04. Four
    05. Five
    06. Six
    97. INAP., never took drugs
    98. Don't know how many

223. How many "bad trips" did you have?

    0. More than one   39 _____
    1. One
    2. None
    9. INAP.

224. Do you think that drugs have something to do with making you mentally ill
      or bringing you to the hospital?

    0. Totally   40 _____
    1. Partly
    2. Not at all
    9. INAP.

Antisocial Acts 1

227. (Patient) Have you ever been arrested for . . .
     (Informant) As far as you know, has he/she ever been arrested for . . .

		Yes	No	Don't know	
a.	Disorderly conduct	0	2	8	44 ____
b.	Vagrancy	0	2	8	45 ____
c.	Traffic violations (red light, speeding)	0	2	8	46 ____
d.	Public alcoholic intoxication	0	2	8	47 ____
e.	Other misdemeanors	0	2	8	48 ____
f.	Possession of drugs	0	2	8	49 ____
g.	Pushing drugs	0	2	8	50 ____
h.	Robbery	0	2	8	51 ____
i.	Assault	0	2	8	52 ____
j.	Prostitution	0	2	8	53 ____
k.	Other sexual offense(s)	0	2	8	54 ____
l.	Setting fire	0	2	8	55 ____
m.	Others (Specify)				
	0. Other is F	2	2	8	56 ____
	2. Other is LF	1	2	8	57 ____
	8. Other is NF	0	2	8	58 ____

(Number of reasons for arrests: 00 = No arrests; 98 = Don't know on all)   59,60 __/__

(If 228 not 9, INAP., patient denies charges)
229. What condition (are you) (is he/she) in when (you break) (he/she breaks)
     the law?

          1. Alcoholic intoxication   67 ____
          2. Drug intoxication
          3. In need of money for drugs
          4. Feeling mentally ill
          5. Other (specify) _____
          8. Don't know
          9. INAP. (228 is 7)

232. How did you feel about being arrested or convicted?

      01. Very bad   71,72 __/__

      02. Bad

      13. Indifferent

      24. Good

      97. INAP.

Conclusions of Attitudes and Expectations

Plans After Leaving Hospital

262. Which of the following do you think will be very helpful for your mental health? (Every line should be answered), and for those that do not comply, code 9.

It will not help	Somewhat	Yes			
0	1	2	a.	Taking medication	51 ____
0	1	2	b.	Seeing a psychiatrist regularly	52 ____
0	1	2	c.	Going back to your job	53 ____
0	1	2	d.	Getting a new job	54 ____
0	1	2	e.	Getting along with your (spouse, friends, etc.)	55 ____
0	1	2	f.	Getting along with your children	56 ____
0	1	2	g.	Getting along with your parents	57 ____
0	1	2	h.	Living on Welfare	58 ____
0	1	2	i.	Taking a long rest	59 ____
0	1	2	j.	Living alone	60 ____
0	1	2	k.	Staying in a psychiatric hospital	61 ____
0	1	2	l.	Different social milieu	62 ____
0	1	2	m.	Hobby	63 ____
0	1	2	n.	A new boyfriend/girlfriend	64 ____
0	1	2	o.	Other (specify) _____	65 ____

                                                           67 __9__

                                                           68 __9__

Index

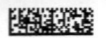